Community health

Community health

C. L. ANDERSON, B.S., M.S.P.H., Dr.P.H.

Former Professor and Head, Hygiene and
Environmental Sanitation, Oregon State University,
Corvallis, Oregon

RICHARD F. MORTON, M.B.B.S., M.P.H., F.A.C.P.M.

Department of Social and Preventive Medicine,
University of Maryland, School of Medicine,
Baltimore, Maryland

LAWRENCE W. GREEN, B.S., M.P.H., Dr.P.H.

Professor and Head, Division of Health Education,
Department of Health Services Administration, The Johns Hopkins
University, School of Hygiene and Public Health,
Baltimore, Maryland

THIRD EDITION

with 106 illustrations

The C. V. Mosby Company

Saint Louis   1978

The C. V. Mosby Company
11830 Westline Industrial Drive, St. Louis, Missouri 63141

Library of Congress Cataloging in Publication Data

Anderson, Carl Leonard, 1901-
   Community health.

   Bibliography: p.
   Includes index.
   1. Public health. 2. Public health—United
States. I. Morton, Richard F., 1924-
joint author. II. Green, Lawrence W., joint
author. III. Title. [DNLM: 1. Community
health services—United States. 2. Public health—
United States. WA900 AA1 A83c]
RA425.A68 1978   362.1   77-23864
ISBN 0-8016-0182-7

GW/CB/B 9 8 7 6 5 4 3 2 1

PREFACE

This is a book about community health rather than about personal hygiene. Personal health practices are critical to the success of community health programs, but it is the approach to such practices through the planning and promotion of programs for *populations* that distinguishes community health from medicine and self-care. Community health encompasses medical and self-care activities, but its concern is with the coordination and integration of these activities with the needs, goals, and resources of whole communities.

Community health is more concerned with the availability and accessibility of adequate resources for the care of a few. This book will dwell more, therefore, on questions of distribution, participation, and organization than on questions of biomedical processes and techniques; more on prevention than on cure; more on the dissemination and application of health knowledge than on its source or its control; and more on communities than on individual patients.

Just as the individual faces health problems, the community also faces health problems that must be solved. In the solutions to community health problems some unique promotional approaches are emerging. In the United States federal funding to state and county health departments and for medical and hospital facilities and services has had a catalytic effect, but other resources and efforts have also been important in community health advances in the past decade. Much of this edition is directed to a discussion of these recent advances.

Ironically, with all of mankind's collective health efforts, the United States and other Western nations appear to have reached a plateau in life expectancy and in the death rate. Perhaps man is approaching his biologic limits in both of these respects. Certainly, to break away from these plateaus will require ingenuity and concerted effort in dealing with human health on all levels and in all aspects. Yet minimization or correction of such adverse factors as smoking, alcoholism, other drug abuse, injuries, and malnutrition presents opportunities for extending life expectancy. This applies to the community as well as to the individual.

Population change and the possibility of a population exceeding the supply of energy arouse concern. Zero population growth is still some distance in the future, but great strides have been made in extending family planning to all segments of communities.

Federal legislation such as the Traffic and Motor Safety Act has given impetus to renewed efforts to reduce motor vehicle injuries, but thus far the nation has not truly come to grips with this destructive force in our midst. Congressional indifference and languid resignation of the public must be replaced with a vigorous, scientifically based program to deal effectively with this ubiquitous threat.

Recreational and fitness programs to promote mental, social, and physical health are given primary emphasis in American society, although proper recognition is given to the role of recreation in the correction of disabilities and in rehabilitation. With each passing year the role of the community becomes more important in providing a recreational program to meet the needs of most of the community's citizenry. Recreation and fitness as an investment in health is not a new concept, but the resurgence of interest in fitness is a societal change of major significance for health.

Alcoholism as an inborn defect of metabolism and treatment for alcohol and other drug addictions are of interest and concern to every community in America. Like many other health problems, drug abuse has long been with us, and, like other health problems, it has multiplied in gravity at a geometric rate. As with most such problems, virtually all citizens in a community can make a contribution to the solution of drug abuse.

Health maintenance organizations, health systems agencies, and proposed national health insurance programs are reviewed in this edition. Projection of present thinking to a future national medical care program demands that the nation define its problem in precise terms, obtain all possible facts, analyze these facts carefully, and then come to a definite conclusion. This is a monumental decision. In Chapter 18 some guidelines for analysis of proposals for national health care are offered.

The National Health Planning and Resources Development Act of 1974 has revamped comprehensive health planning on state and local levels. The nation, and likewise the community, can no longer afford to approach health problems so inefficiently as in the past.

The continuing reorganization of federal health services is presented in both discussion and diagrammatic form. Different roles of the various divisions of the health services are explained by means of a presentation of the organization and the administration of the services. Recent developments in international health are similarly reviewed.

The pace of developments and the growing breadth and complexity of community health have suggested the collaboration of three authors in this revision. A community health educator and a physician—both with experience at local, state, national, and international levels of health practice and research —have joined the original author, an environmental health specialist and public health generalist, to provide breadth and balance in all areas covered.

C. L. Anderson
Richard F. Morton
Lawrence W. Green

CONTENTS

PART III

Preventing disorders and disabilities

PART I

Overview

1 ▪ THROUGH THE CENTURIES

The history of public health might well be written
as a record of successive redefinings of the unacceptable.

Sir Godfrey Vickers

Understanding and appreciation of any field of social significance are based on a knowledge of its historical development. Community health promotion has had as much impact on a time and its people as any of the other great social forces or disciplines. Historically, health has been interwoven with the philosophy, religion, economic conditions, form of government, education, science, aspirations, and folklore of any given period. Because of the organic relationship that exists between health and human advancement, the history of community health reflects man's advances and declines.

Civilization depends on the quality and distribution of health in the general population. Health in turn is dependent on human advancement in various spheres. Accounts of public health at a given period should be cast in the total framework of the time. Community health is not something apart from the life of the time—it is a result of life-styles as well as a barometer of that period in history.

Community health promotion is constantly evolving; it has never fully arrived. Community health practice today is not isolated from the past; it is built on and retains the best of the past. A new discovery may lead to the abandonment of a well-accepted practice, or it may lead to a new method of applying what has been an accepted health principle. Vestiges of health advances of the past serve as a heritage from the intrepid scientists and other pioneers in man's continual quest for better health and periodic redefinition of unacceptable conditions.

The history of efforts to promote community health reflects on all the health and parahealth professions, including sociology, education, nursing, civil engineering, pharmacy, medicine, nutrition, food technology, entomology, biology, journalism, and a host of other professions whose services have related to community health activities. These fields constitute those professional segments whose services contribute tangibly to community health, and, in turn, are enhanced by community health promotion.

CONCEPT OF COMMUNITY HEALTH PRACTICE

C.-E. A. Winslow, one of the leading figures in the history of public health, characterized public health practice as the science and art of preventing disease, prolonging life, and promoting health and well-being through organized community effort for the sanitation of the environment, the control of communicable infections, the organization of medical and nursing services for the early diagnosis and prevention of disease, the education of the individual in personal health, and the development of the social machinery to assure everyone a standard of living adequate for the maintenance or improvement of health.

Organized community effort is the key to community health. There are some things the individual can do entirely alone, but many health benefits can be obtained only through united community effort. Communi-

3

ty health promotion is necessary to make the fruits of health science available to all citizens.

HISTORY OF COMMUNITY HEALTH
Egyptian and Babylonian health practices

One of the earliest sources of information on ancient health practices comes from the papyri. The papyrus discovered by Edwin Smith indicates the early use in Egypt of prescriptions, particularly of opium, minerals, and root drugs. The association of moon and lunatic arose from the relationship of religion and astrology. ℞ was the astrologic sign of Jupiter, under whose protection medicine was placed. Alcoholic intoxication was thought to be due to the spirits of the fruit that was used in making the beverage. Pharmaceutical preparations played an important role in attempts to treat disease, although most of the successes are attributed to placebo effects. Medication was not universally available or acceptable.

Hammurabi, a great king of Babylon who lived around 2000 B.C., formulated a set of laws called the Code of Hammurabi that governed the conduct of physicians and provided for health practices. The code also regulated and defined unacceptable conduct in general.

Excavations have revealed that the Egyptians had community systems for collecting rain water and for disposing sewage. Herodotus, in the fifth century B.C., described the hygienic customs of the Egyptians. Personal cleanliness, frequent baths, and simple dress were emphasized. Earth closets were in general use. Yet from the standpoint of community health practice, the Egyptians went backward as the centuries advanced. Greek health practices were destined to go far beyond those of the Egyptians and Babylonians.

Hebrew Mosaic Law

Early Hebrew society contributed greatly to the advancement of community health. It extended Egyptian concepts of disease and the promotion of health through the regulation of human conduct by the Mosaic Law or Code. Human conduct is fundamental in all health—community as well as personal. With the Hebrews, a weekly day of rest was a health as well as a religious measure. Family relations and sexual conduct were directed to the best interests of personal, family, and community health. While the Hebrews had rather crude concepts of the spread of disease, they did make concerted efforts to prevent disease spread. The first practice of preventive medicine was the segregation of lepers, as recorded in Leviticus. Recognition that eating pork at times resulted in illness led the Hebrews to regard pork as unclean and to forbid it in the diet.

The Mosaic Law or Code encompassed many subjects, including health. It provided for (1) personal and community responsibility for health, (2) maternal health, (3) communicable disease control, (4) segregation of lepers, (5) fumigation, (6) decontamination of buildings, (7) protection of water supplies, (8) disposal of wastes, (9) protection of food, and (10) sanitation of camp sites. Without the aid of fundamental knowledge of the nature of infectious disease, the health efforts of the Hebrews were not highly effective. Nevertheless, they defined unacceptable conditions and mobilized community forces against them.

The glory of Greece

The Greek era in history extends over many centuries, but the Classic Period was the years 460 to 136 B.C. The Greeks excelled in physical aspects of personal health. Games, gymnastics, and other exercises were directed toward their definition of physical strength, endurance, dexterity, and grace. Harmonious development of all faculties was the guiding philosophy. While athletic prowess may not have received the acclaim it does today in America, the Greeks did glory in the well-developed athlete. Exercise was supplemented by measures in personal cleanliness and dietetics. The Classic Period of Greece is characterized by its emphasis upon the individual. As a consequence, very little attention was given to environmental sanitation.

Perhaps because of their narrow concerns with health the Greeks did not borrow from other nations. The Hindus of ancient India had practiced surgery for at least a century, but there is no evidence that the Greeks utilized the Hindu methods of surgery, despite Alexander's conquests on the Indian subcontinent.

The Roman empire

With the destruction of Corinth in 146 B.C., the health knowledge and health practices of the Greeks migrated to Rome and were welcomed by the rising Roman empire. However, in the philosophy of the Romans, the state and not the individual was of primary importance. To the Romans, the individual existed merely to serve the state. With this extreme emphasis on the state, it is not surprising that the influence of Greek hygiene should soon fade through neglect.

The Romans had a special talent for military science, and their administrative and engineering attainments were reflected in their many community health projects. At all times the welfare of the state was primary and that of the individual was subservient. The registration of citizens and slaves and the taking of a periodic census were community health measures, though their primary purpose was doubtless mercenary. Regulation of building construction, the prevention of nuisances, and the destruction of decaying goods and buildings were measures that are still practiced in the modern state. Building regulations provided for ventilation and even for central heating. Town planning was directed toward sanitation measures as well as toward other needs. Public sanitation was promoted through the construction of paved streets with gutters. Street cleaning and repair were standard procedures in the interest of sanitation, though modern health officials regard these measures as being of esthetic rather than of direct health importance. Drainage networks carried off rain and other water, all of which was of some health significance. Removal of garbage and rubbish, though desirable in any society, was not of as great health significance as the Romans contended. Public baths were promoted as community health measures. Although street cleaning, garbage removal, and public baths were of minor health value, several other measures promoted by the Romans were of significant importance to health.

Roman officials had sufficient understanding of health to provide a protected water supply for their cities. Water was brought to Rome from great distances via aqueducts, some of which are still incorporated into the water system of Rome. City sewerage systems were built, and some of these drains are still part of the sewerage system of the city. This ability of the Romans to design and construct public water and sewerage systems enabled Rome to grow to a city of 800,000 population during the reign of Julius Caesar. This in contrast to the Greeks, who depended upon family wells and private refuse disposal, which limited the size to which their cities could grow. Corinth at the pinnacle of its greatness had a population of only 35,000.

The downfall of the Western empire was related to degeneration—"where wealth accumulates and men decay." The term Byzantine, which refers to the Eastern Roman empire, connotes luxury and sloth. Even in this atmosphere, Galen (A.D. 130-201) did some experimentation relating to health, but his extreme dogmatism limited the value of his work. Contrasted to the attempt of Galen to understand disease is the statement of Saint Augustine (A.D. 353-430): "All diseases are to be ascribed to demons."

Dark ages

The early years (A.D. 476-1000) of the medieval period of history are usually referred to as the Dark Ages. Western civilization was in a chaotic, almost formless state. The only existing science was fostered by the state and was but a trifle. Virtually the entire emphasis of the time was on the spiritual aspects of life because the clergy were the only educated class. Rejection of the body and glorification of the spirit became the accepted pattern of behavior. It was regarded as immoral to see one's body. People seldom bathed, and they used dirty garments. The use of perfumes appears to have stemmed from the attempt to conceal body and other unpleasant odors about the person. The more one could neglect and abuse one's body, the more esteemed one was. A legendary example of body neglect is of Saint Stylites, who sat on top of a pole for 16 years in order to expose his body to the abuse of the elements. It was as though health itself had been defined as unacceptable. The poor diets of the time resulted in the use of spices to overcome the bad odor and the foul taste of the food.

During the sixth and seventh centuries, Mohammedanism arose. After the death of Mohammed, a series of pilgrimages to Mecca began. Each pilgrimage was followed by a cholera epidemic. All through history migrations have been a vehicle of disease spread.

The spread of leprosy was from Egypt to Asia Minor and then to Europe. Most nations decreed lepers unacceptable and civilly dead. Lepers were required to wear identifying clothing and to warn of their presence by a bell or a horn. This isolation, however, together with the early death of lepers, virtually eliminated leprosy in Europe.

Medieval pandemics

The later medieval period, from A.D. 1000 to about 1453, is of special interest because of the severe pandemics of the time and the attempts to deal with the spread of disease. Disease was rampant and morals were low. Between the years 1096 and 1248, the six great crusades to the holy lands were of health significance. To provide crusaders who were fit for the long journey, attention was given to building up the best possible level of health. While the approach was somewhat that of the ancient Greeks in build-

ing up physical prowess, the general result was that of building up a better condition of well-being in that one segment of the population. However, in their journeys the crusaders picked up cholera, and the death rate among them was high.

In 1348, bubonic plague, or the Black Death, followed a devastating path from Asia to Africa, Crimea, Turkey, Greece, Italy, and up through Europe. Some idea of the devastation of the disease can be gathered by referring to the deaths in several of the large cities in Europe: Paris, 50,000; Seine, 70,000; Marseilles, 16,000 in one month; Vienna, 1,200 daily; Florence, 60,000; Venice, 100,000. Boccaccio reported that in the terrible outbreak of plague in Florence in this year, feelings, pity, and humanity were forgotten. Families deserted their sick. In Venice, the government appointed three guardians of public health, and in 1374 denied entry to the city of infected or suspected travelers, ships, or freight. In 1403 a quarantine of 40 days was imposed on anyone suspected of having the disease. In England two million died, representing approximately half the total population of the country. London had 100,000 deaths. Over a number of years London's deaths exceeded its births. If it were not for the influx of people from the rural areas, London's population would have declined steadily. Estimates that approximately 25 million people died of the Black Death in Europe attest to the virulence of the bubonic plague.

Control measures. Pandemics were attributed to storms, comets, famines, drought, crop failures, insects, and poisoning of wells by the Jews. However, discerning officials of various communities recognized the possible relationship of crowding, poor sanitation, and migrations to the outbreak and spread of disease, and some communities took steps to establish control measures. In 1377 at Rogusa it was ruled that travelers from plague areas should stop at designated places and remain there free of disease for 2 months before being allowed to enter the city. Technically, this is the first official quarantine method on record. In 1383, Marseilles passed the first quarantine law and erected the first official quarantine station.

Measures to control disease spread were not highly effective. The need was for a scientific understanding of the cause and nature of disease and its spread. Scholars of the time who turned toward the scientific approach to pestilence were open to surveillance and public persecution. As a consequence of such resistance, there could be little progress in man's understanding of disease.

Renaissance

The beginning of the Renaissance is associated with revival of learning that was germinating in Italy, stimulated by the fall of Constantinople in 1453. For many historians, the Renaissance as applied to western and northern Europe encompasses the period from A.D. 1453 to 1600.

From the standpoint of community health, the Renaissance was particularly important because of its movement away from scholasticism and toward realities. It was an age of individual scientific endeavor, and it ushered in a spirit of inquiry that would lead to the understanding of the cause and nature of infectious disease. The fifteenth and sixteenth centuries produced such distinguished figures as Copernicus, da Vinci, Vesalius, Galileo, and Gilbert. By the middle of the sixteenth century, scholars had differentiated influenza, smallpox, tuberculosis, bubonic plague, leprosy, impetigo, scabies, erysipelas, anthrax, and trachoma. Diphtheria and scarlet fever were not recognized as separate diseases but were recognized as being different from all other diseases. Fracastorius (1478-1553), a physician of Verona, recognized that syphilis was transmitted from person to person during sexual relations. Learning was advancing, but the resulting social concentration, expanding trade, and movement of populations tended to spread disease. Knowledge of communicable disease control lagged behind

disease spread, and great plagues still harassed Europe.

Colonial period

During the colonial period from 1600 to 1800, community health in America was dependent on developments in Europe. No account of this period would be complete without some mention of health problems in Europe and the contributions that European scholars made to health.

Community health in Europe. Between 1600 and 1665 Europe suffered three severe pandemics of bubonic plague. The plight of London indicates the severity of the outbreaks. In 1603, a sixth of London's population died of the plague. In 1625, another sixth was destroyed by the plague, and in 1665 one out of five of London's residents died from the same disease.

This same era produced Descartes (1598-1650), Voltaire (1694-1778), and Boyle (1627-1691). This last named scholar, a distinguished Englishman, made a prophetic pronouncement: "He that totally understands the nature of ferments and the fermentation shall probably be much better able than he who ignores them to give a fair account of certain diseases (fevers as well as others) which will perhaps be never properly understood without an insight into the doctrine of fermentation." William Harvey (1578-1657) fairly accurately described the circulation of human blood. In 1658, an English investigator, Sydenham (1624-1689), made a differential diagnosis of scarlet fever, malaria, dysentery, and cholera. Some historians contend that most of Sydenham's discoveries were accidental, but it should be acknowledged that chance favors the disciplined mind. Sydenham is generally regarded as the first distinguished epidemiologist.

Athanasius Kircher (1602-1680) examined the blood of victims of plague, using a microscope of 33 diameters, and thereby instituted a new method of study. In 1676 a Dutch draper and city hall janitor, Anton van Leeuwenhoek (1632-1723), using a microscope with magnification of 200 diameters, succeeded in seeing bacteria, protozoa, red corpuscles, and spermatozoa. Robert Hooke (1635-1703) also worked with the microscope, as did Marcello Malpighi (1628-1694), who studied the microscopic structure of tissues and laid some of the early foundations for histology.

In 1693 an astronomer, Edmund Halley (1656-1742), compiled the Breslau Table of births and funerals. This represented a contribution to the growth of vital statistics. In 1762 M. A. Plenciz, a physician of Vienna, studied scarlet fever and other infectious diseases and concluded that each infectious disease was caused by a specific kind of thing. While he did not identify "thing" factually, his theory predated the discoveries of Pasteur and Koch by a century.

Edward Jenner (1749-1823), a British physician and son of a Gloucestershire clergyman, scientifically demonstrated the effectiveness of smallpox vaccination. In 1796, using matter from pustules on the arm of a milkmaid who had contracted cowpox, Dr. Jenner vaccinated a young boy. Six weeks later he inoculated the boy with smallpox virus and demonstrated that the boy was immune to smallpox. Dr. Jenner demonstrated scientifically that inoculation with cowpox virus can produce immunity to the smallpox virus. He received his idea of inoculating with cowpox vaccine to prevent smallpox from the practice of English peasants of allowing themselves to contract cowpox in the knowledge that they would then be safe from smallpox. Reports indicate that some form of smallpox vaccination had been practiced in Turkey previous to Dr. Jenner's time, but he generally is credited with the first scientific vaccination against smallpox.

Health in the American colonies. There was little interest in community health in colonial America. Educated men of the time were mostly clergy, though some of them were professionally prepared in medicine. Community health action was taken only during epidemics and consisted essentially of isolation and quarantine. Sanitation consisted of community tidiness or general housecleaning.

Smallpox actually aided the white man in settling America. Introduced to the east coast by the Cabot and Gosnold expeditions, the disease eliminated so many of the Indians that the whites were able to colonize the area with little or no opposition. However, smallpox took its toll among the whites and obliterated some of the early settlements. Some notable pandemics were those of Massachusetts Bay colonies in 1633, New Netherlands (New York) in 1663, and Boston in 1752. Of Boston's 1752 population of 15,684, only 174 completely escaped the smallpox pandemic. During the life of George Washington, 90% of the people who attained the age of 21 had had smallpox, and 25% of those infected by smallpox died. The significance of public health in history is reflected by these statistics in the context of the 1977 announcement of the World Health Organization that the last few cases of smallpox in the world were isolated in Ethiopia, signaling the total eradication of this disease.

Yellow fever became a bigger scourge than smallpox in America during the eighteenth and nineteenth centuries. In 1793 Philadelphia had the greatest single epidemic in America. Of a population of about 37,000, more than 23,000 had the disease and over 4,000 of these died. A citizen's committee appointed to deal with the problem drew up the following set of regulations.

1. Avoid contact with a case.
2. Placard all infected houses.
3. Clean and air the sickroom.
4. Provide hospital accommodations for the poor.
5. Keep streets and wharves clean.
6. Encourage general hygienic measures such as quick private burials, avoidance of fatigue of mind and body, avoidance of intemperance, and adaptation of clothing to the weather.

Vinegar and camphor were used on handkerchiefs to prevent infection. Gunpowder was burned in the streets to combat the disease. Simple and perhaps as ineffective as these measures may have been, they represented a sincere attempt of communities to combat the disease based on the fragmentary knowledge people had of yellow fever. Frosty nights on October 17 and 18 ended the epidemic. Citizens of Philadelphia did not understand the "miracle," but from the vantage point of today we know that the frost killed the *Aedes aegypti* mosquito, the temporary host or vector for yellow fever. Modern health authorities are indebted to Dr. Benjamin Rush for a magnificent report of the Philadelphia epidemic published in 1815.

Health advances during the colonial period were made mostly during the eighteenth century. Occupational hygiene and the safety and well-being of the worker were given specific attention. Infant hygiene was not founded on any scientific basis but was represented in a humane attempt to give better care to the child. Mental hygiene was limited to a sympathetic understanding and care of the mentally disordered.

In 1639 the Massachusetts colony passed an act stating that each birth and death must be recorded, and the Plymouth colony did likewise. In 1647 Massachusetts Bay colonies passed regulations to prevent the pollution of Boston Harbor. Between the years 1692 and 1708, Boston, Salem, and Jamestown passed laws dealing with nuisances and offensive trades. In 1701 Massachusetts enacted legislation providing for isolation of smallpox cases and for ship quarantine.

Superstitions expressed in witchcraft and other practices of the time indicate that the colonial period in history was hardly one in which to expect any great advances in health science. In America during George Washington's time, the average duration of life was about 29 years. Measured by today's standards, the men who wrote the American Declaration of Independence and drew up the Federal Constitution were extremely young. Decidedly few of them were over the age of 40.

Boards of health were established in New York and Massachusetts in 1797 as a result of the yellow fever outbreaks. Local boards of health were established in Petersburg, Virginia (1780), in Baltimore (1793), in Philadelphia (1794), in New York (1796), and in Boston (1799). Paul Revere served as chairman of the Boston Board of Health. While all these were formally organized health boards, none of them functioned as boards of health function today.

Early national period

From 1800 to 1850 the United States experienced a rapid industrial expansion and an intense nationalism. As remarkable as the expansion was, public health activities were at a standstill, and many epidemics occurred. The rapid growth of cities outstripped other developments. Community health could hardly flourish under such conditions, and organized health measures were almost nonexistent.

Community health promotions in England. Developments in England in the first half of the nineteenth century were important for several reasons. Public health was officially recognized in England in 1837 when legislation relating to community sanitation was enacted. This indication of an awakening interest in community health led to the appointment of a factory commission to study the health conditions of the laboring population of the nation. Particular emphasis was placed on the study of child employment conditions. Edwin Chadwick, a civilian who had a special interest in social problems, was made secretary of the Factory Commission. In 1842 his "Report on the Inquiry Into the Sanitary Condition of the Laboring Population of Great Britain" appeared. Chadwick's colorful descriptions of the deplorable conditions of the time had more than just a popular appeal. They aroused the determination of well-meaning people to improve the conditions of the laboring class, particularly the child employment conditions. Chadwick's report pointed out that half the children of the working classes died before their fifth birthday. While the death rate and infant mortality rates do not indicate the complete picture of a nation or community, the length of life and the infant death rates

Table 1-1 ■ Mean age of death and infant death rates, England, 1842*

Class	Mean age of death		Infant deaths per 1,000 births (England)
	London	England	
Gentry, professional persons, and their families	44	35	100
Tradesmen, shopkeepers, and their families	23	22	167
Wage classes, artisans, laborers, and their families	22	15	250

*Based on Chadwick. See Richardson, B. W.: The health of nations. A review of the works of Edwin Chadwick, vol. 2, London, 1887, Longmans Green & Co.

reported by Chadwick indicate health conditions in which mere survival could be the sole health goal.

The impact of such appalling health conditions is reflected in the loss at an early age of some of England's outstanding literary figures of the time. Shelley died at the age of 30, Keats at 25, Byron at 36, Robert Burns at 37, Charlotte Brontë at 39, Emily Brontë at 30, and Ann Brontë at 29. On the continent, Chopin died at 40, Felix Mendelssohn at 38, and Franz Schubert at 31. One might speculate on what these master artists might have produced for mankind if today's knowledge of health could have been applied during their lives.

Chadwick's report led to the establishment of a board of health in 1848. John Simon was appointed first medical health officer of London. However, the general board of health lasted but 4 years. Perhaps England was not yet ready for the reforms that Chadwick's report pointed out. Perhaps his enthusiasm led to over-promotion. Nevertheless, his report stands as a landmark in the history of public health.

Health developments in the United States. Not until the close of the first half of the nineteenth century was there a significant American development in community health promotion. Lemuel Shattuck (1793-1859) drew up a health report that was to serve as a guide in the field of health for the next century. Shattuck successfully was a teacher, historian, sociologist, statistician, and state legislator. From the health standpoint he was a layman, but with an intense and intelligent interest in sanitation. He was appointed chairman of a legislative committee to study sanitation and health problems in the Commonwealth of Massachusetts. The report was written by Shattuck and published in 1850. This report revealed Shattuck's insight and foresight. It charted health pathways for generations to come, and many of its provisions have not yet been fully attained. The importance of this remarkable document can be appreciated by reviewing its various recommendations:

1. Establishment of state and local boards of health
2. Collection and analysis of vital statistics
3. Systematic exchange of health information
4. Sanitation programs for towns and buildings
5. System of sanitary inspections
6. Studies on the health of school children
7. Studies of tuberculosis
8. Study and supervision of health conditions of immigrants
9. Supervision of mental disease

10. Control of alcoholism
11. Control of food adulteration
12. Exposure of nostrums
13. Control of smoke nuisances
14. Construction of model tenements
15. Construction of standard public bathing and wash houses
16. Preaching of health from pulpits
17. Teaching the science of sanitation in medical schools
18. Prevention as a phase of all medical practice
19. Routine health examinations

Shattuck was considerably in advance of his time. In addition, he did not have the flair for writing that Chadwick possessed. He did not depend on vivid descriptions of appalling conditions. The report produced no results until 1869, when a Massachusetts state board of health was established. Its membership included both laymen and physicians. The Shattuck report served as the guide for the board in its early years of activity. The wisdom of Shattuck's report stands as a valued guidepost in the history of public health in America.

Modern era of health

The modern era of health is dated from 1850 to the present. It represents an organized, disciplined attack on problems of health and disease, growing out of a general recognition of the importance of a united public approach to health protection. In America, interest in community health became a necessity with the rapid expansion in the latter half of the nineteenth century and continuing on into the twentieth century. An indication of the inability to control disease is illustrated by the death rates in Massachusetts at that time. In 1880 the Massachusetts tuberculosis death rate was more than 300 per 100,000 population, and the infant mortality rate was 200 per 1,000 live births.

The modern era of health can be logically divided into four phases. The first phase (1850-1880) is properly called the *miasma* phase, the second phase (1880-1920) may be designated as the *disease control* phase, the third phase (1920-1960) is the *health promotion* phase, and the fourth phase (1960-present) is the *social engineering* phase.

Miasma phase (1850-1880). The term "miasma" literally means noxious air or vapor. During this period the approach to disease control was based on the misconception that disease was caused by noxious odors, dirt, and general lack of cleanliness. Diphtheria was thought to be caused by gases associated with putrefaction. The term "malaria" literally means "bad air." Because it was observed that people who ventured about at dusk were those who invariably contracted malaria, the common belief persisted that the disease was a result of the particular air existing at dusk. Here was an illustrious example of interpreting mere coincidence as a cause-and-effect relationship. Disease control efforts were directed entirely toward general cleanliness. Garbage and refuse collection became important to communities. Street cleaning was pursued relentlessly. These general cleanliness measures were not directed at the specific causes of disease and consequently were of little value in control.

Quarantine conventions were held in a number of cities. The first of these was a 3-day convention held in Philadelphia in 1857. The topics discussed indicate the interests of the fifty-four people who were in attendance: prevention of typhus, cholera, and yellow fever; port quarantine; stagnant and putrid bilge waters, droppings or drainage from putrescible matters; and filthy bedding, baggage, and clothing of immigrant passengers where they had been confined. The convention recommended the vaccination of all incoming immigrants. Other conventions were held in 1858, 1859, and 1860.

The first state health department was organized in Massachusetts in 1869, with Dr. Henry I. Bowdich as the first head. The Department's program was directed to the following six areas:

1. Professional and public education in hygiene
2. Housing

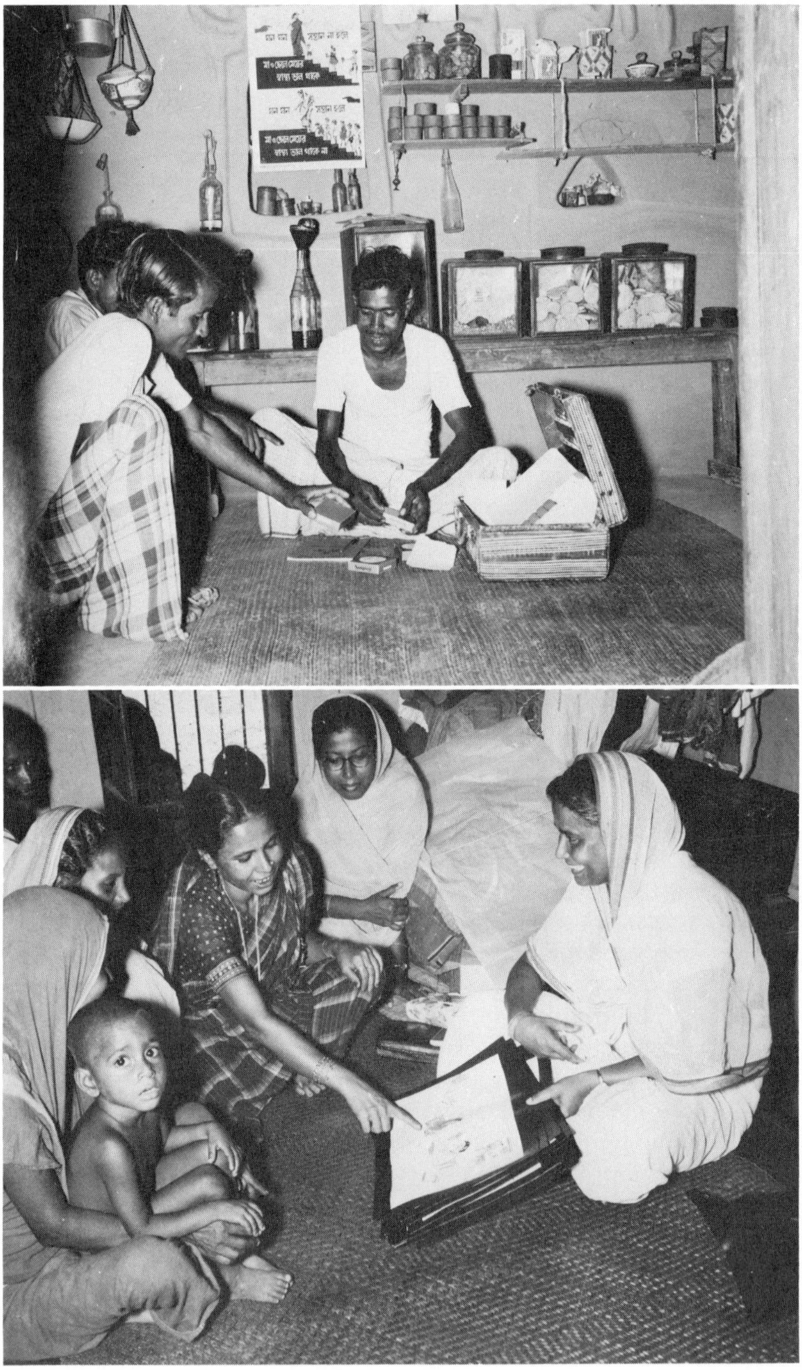

Fig. 1-1. Modern community health and contraceptive technology is delivered today in many developing countries through ancient channels of communication and distribution similar to those of the eighteenth and nineteenth centuries in Europe and America. (Courtesy Public Health Education Research Project, University of California, Berkeley)

3. Investigation of some diseases
4. Slaughtering
5. Sale of poisons
6. Conditions of the poor

Measured in terms of present standards in public health promotion, the program of the first state health department would rate rather poorly.

The American Public Health Association was founded in 1872 at Long Beach, New Jersey. Dr. Stephen Smith was the first president. The new association proposed to go considerably beyond the thinking of the quarantine conventions. Its program was to be much broader in scope and was to deal with sanitation, prevention and transmission of disease, and longevity, hospital hygiene, and all other health problems that arose that would be of interest and of concern to the public.

Public health teaching in America had its inception during this period. An English manual of hygiene by E. A. Parkes, professor of military hygiene in the army medical school of England, was published in 1859. The first as well as subsequent editions were in use in America. In 1879 A. H. Buck edited his pioneering text, *Hygiene and Public Health*. This volume deals with environmental sanitation, housing, personal hygiene, child hygiene, school hygiene, industrial hygiene, food sanitation, communicable disease control, disinfection, quarantine, infant mortality, and vital statistics. Several distinguished men contributed to the volume. Dr. J. S. Billings, who wrote the introduction, revealed magnificent foresight in writing on the jurisprudence of hygiene. His concepts, such as the following, are also enunciated by present leaders in public health.

1. County lines are not natural boundaries and have no relation to causes of disease.
2. Administrative health areas should be large enough and populous enough to require full-time sanitary and executive forces.
3. There should be nonpracticing full-time health officers with medical education.
4. The health officer should be especially trained for his job.
5. If a municipal board of health is properly constituted so that its relationship to the medical profession is harmonious, it should be charged with the supervision of all medical charities such as hospitals and dispensaries.

Schools of public health were not founded until a later time, but the seeds of professional public health preparation were being planted before the disease control phase of the modern health era was reached.

***Disease control phase** (1880-1920)*. This phase might be properly termed the bacteriology phase because it was initiated by the work of Louis Pasteur, Robert Koch, and other bacteriologists who demonstrated that a specific organism causes a specific disease. With the knowledge that an organism causes a certain disease, it was now possible to change from general measures in attempting to control diseases to specific measures in blocking the routes over which the causative agents would travel. As it became apparent that certain vehicles served as the means for the transmission of disease-producing organisms, attention was directed to such specific measures as the protection of water supplies, milk, and other foods, the elimination of insects, and the proper disposal of sewage. A natural further advance was the development of laboratory procedures.

The scientific productivity of the bacteriologists of this period is legendary. The French bacteriologist Louis Pasteur (1822-1895), in addition to demonstrating that a specific organism causes a specific disease, also made other outstanding contributions to the field of bacteriology. He disproved the theory of spontaneous generation, discovered the fowl cholera bacillus and the cause of silkworm disease, and, in addition, developed a method of inoculation against rabies. Robert Koch (1843-1910) discovered the tubercle bacillus and the streptococcus. He also discovered the cholera vibrio, which he demonstrated was transmitted by water, food, and clothing. In 1893 Theobald Smith of the United States Department of Agriculture showed that Texas fever in cattle was transmitted by ticks; thus the concept of an intermediate host, or vector, was established. In 1896 Dr. Bruce, a British army surgeon, demonstrated that African sleeping sickness was transmitted by the tsetse fly. In 1898 Sir Ronald Ross in India and Battista Grassi in Italy demonstrated that malaria was transmitted by the *Anopheles* mosquito. In 1900 Walter Reed, Jesse W. Lazier, James Carroll, and Aristides Agramonte demonstrated that yellow fever was transmitted by the *Aedes* mosquito.

Although Pasteur's work in the treatment of rabies was developed in 1883, it was not until 1894 that Emil von Behring (1854-1917) developed his procedure for use of diphtheria antitoxin for the successful treatment of diphtheria. In 1904 Sir Almroth Edward Wright developed the use of dead organisms for inoculation against typhoid fever. During this same period Lord Joseph Lister (1827-1912) developed the practical use of phenol (carbolic acid) as an effective antiseptic.

Official public health departments were staffed with bacteriologists, laboratory technicians, sanitarians, sanitation inspectors, sanitary engineers, quarantine officers, and others who specialized in disease control measures. With the extreme emphasis placed on isolation and quarantine during the first 2 decades of the twentieth century, one might with justification refer to these 20 years as the "tackhammer" period in public health history. To the public of that time, ubiquitous quarantine officers with their hideous placards were the identifying symbol of public health.

Limited as the health program of this period was, it did have a pronounced effect in reducing the death rate. A comparison of the death rate for 1930 with the average death rate for the years 1881 to 1885 indicated a pronounced reduction in deaths in western Europe and in the United States.

Health promotion phase *(1920-1960).* Medical examination of the men being inducted into the United States armed services during World War I was the first broad-scale barometer of the health status of the people of the United States. With health standards for induction lower than previously had prevailed, the armed services found it necessary to reject 34% of the men examined because of physical and mental disabilities. The nation was appalled to learn that 34% of its youth were unfit for military service. Professional health personnel analyzed the data obtained in the medical examination of draftees and arrived at a conclusion that was to change the course of public health in America.

Public health experts learned from the data that while communicable diseases had been controlled quite well, other health hazards and problems had been neglected. Many of the defects reported could have been prevented and most of the defects could have been corrected. It was clear that the public health program had neglected the citizen as an individual and that the future efforts of public health programs must be directed to individual citizens. It became apparent that it was necessary to build up and maintain the highest possible level of health for each individual citizen. The prevention of communicable disease was not enough.

State health departments began expanding their programs and directing their efforts toward health promotion as well as toward disease control. This required administrative reorganization within the state health departments and the inclusion of many new specialties in the health services.

In 1911, Guilford County, North Carolina, and Yakima County, Washington, organized the first full-time county health departments. The organization of official health departments on a county basis was slow in developing until the second decade of the positive phase of health promotion. Then, under the stimulus of financial support from such organizations as the Rockefeller Foundation, the Children's Fund of Michigan, the Kellogg Foundation, and the United States Public Health Service, county health departments became recognized as the desirable health unit in the age of modern transportation. County health departments with full-time professional personnel gradually displaced the city health departments with part-time health officers and non-professional personnel. Large metropolitan cities with full-time professionally prepared personnel still continue to function; but in 1969, of the 3,102 counties in the United States, more than 2,400 had full-time health services either on a district basis or on a single-county basis.

Voluntary health agencies had been established in the United States previous to 1920, but following this date these voluntary organizations played an increasingly important role in the promotion of health in the United States, particularly through health education. Voluntary health organizations are somewhat uniquely an American creation. Their contribution in bringing to public attention the importance of certain health problems and the necessary plan of action to solve these problems has been a force of infinite value in the promotion of health in America.

Social engineering phase (1960-present). By 1960 it had become apparent that technical health advances were not available to all people. Indeed, large segments of the community were completely isolated from developments in health. The husbanding of human resources required that the products of technologic developments be made available to every citizen. The social aspects of health were given a new priority.

To make the advances of health science available to all people posed a pyramid of problems because of the various individuals and groups incapable of utilizing health knowledge and health services. The poor —economically, educationally, socially, and otherwise—often missed the benefits of community health programs. Family and group health counseling were urgently needed. The approach had to be that of carrying health services to those who apparently were not availing themselves of the benefits of health programs. The "outreach" services of public health nurses thus became a mainstay of local health departments.

Migrant workers are an example of a group requiring health services adapted to their needs. There are other groups among the poor who also need special community health services. For all of these groups, more than health services is necessary. These groups need assistance in other aspects of wholesome living. Opportunities must be provided that enable these people to enrich their lives, limited though that enrichment may appear to be. This also calls for the enlistment of many community resources, voluntary and official agencies, in many different categories besides health.

Creating a favorable environment and favorable living conditions for these people means creating opportunities for self-improvement, calling for a form of social engineering not previously utilized for the betterment of the underprivileged. This approach has been criticized as paternalism and perhaps in some instances this is just criticism. Yet it need not be paternalism. To offer people more healthful channels of living and to help them develop the ability to guide their own mode of life is no more paternalistic than a college education.

The modern community health program covers all citizens of all ages but, of necessity, it must give a proportionately higher degree of attention to the "have-nots" among us, to the least knowledgeable, to the lower social, economic, and educational strata. The human ecology involved is apparent. The health of these people affects the health and economy of the entire community. Left to their own resources, many of the people in this category would decline in health and in their social condition.

Community health programs properly cannot overlook those least able to provide for their own health needs. These people are entitled to a better quality of health, an extended prime of life, and a greater life expectancy—the objectives of community health programs.

A recent trend in community health programs has been the funneling of federal funds through state and county health departments to provide for medical and hospital services for certain medically deprived groups in the community. Certain guidelines are laid down by the federal agencies, but within these stipulations health departments have considerable leeway in the use of these funds. Most of the funds go to practicing physicians for professional services rendered to citizens who otherwise would not have the medical care they need. This tendency to channel funds for medical services through the county health departments has cast an additional burden on the staffs of these local health departments because invariably no provision is made for additional personnel. If a national medical insurance program is instituted, county health departments would be relieved of the responsibility of administering funds for medical and hospital services.

SOME PUBLIC HEALTH MILESTONES OF THE PAST 2 CENTURIES

1777 General Washington inoculated entire Continental Army against smallpox
1780 Petersburg, Virginia, board of health created
1790 First United States census
1796 Scientific smallpox vaccination from cowpox
1798 Marine Hospital service established
First city health department, Baltimore Maryland
1831 New York City water supply provided
1832 England's Health and Morals Act passed
1842 Massachusetts registration of births and deaths
1844 Dorothea Dix crusade for humane treatment of mentally ill
1848 England's General Health Board created
1850 Shattuck's Massachusetts sanitary report
1851 European health conference
Paris sewer system installed

1860 Red Cross founded in Geneva, Switzerland
1869 Royal Sanitary Commission established in England
Massachusetts State Board of Health created
1872 American Public Health Association founded
1873 Germ theory of disease advanced
1879 Gonococcus identified
1880 Typhoid bacillus discovered
Pneumococcus identified
Malaria plasmodium discovered
1882 Tubercle bacillus discovered
1883 Rabies treatment successful
Cholera vibrio discovered
1884 Diphtheria bacillus identified
1889 Massachusetts Public Health laboratory and Johns Hopkins Hospital opened with new patterns of scientific health care
1893 Lawrence, Massachusetts, water treatment plant completed
1894 Diphtheria antitoxin successfully demonstrated
Pasteurella pestis, cause of plague, discovered
1895 Discovery of the x-ray
Cause of hookworm discovered
Relation of *Anopheles* mosquito to malaria established
1899 International Sanitary Bureau organized
1901 Infectious nature of yellow fever established
1902 United States Public Health Service established
Relation of *Aedes aegypti* mosquito to yellow fever demonstrated
1904 Typhoid fever immunization successful
1905 Spirochete of syphilis identified
1906 Pure Food and Drug Act passed
Standard methods of water analysis adopted
1908 Chlorination of Jersey City water supply
1909 Successful treatment of syphilis using arsphenamine
Hemophilus pertussis identified
1910 International Board of Health, Rockefeller Foundation, created
1911 Chemical nature of vitamin D (calciferol) discovered
Yakima County Health Department founded
Milk pasteurization proved effective
1913 Harvard School of Public Health established
Pellagra demonstrated to be a deficiency disease

1922 Insulin treatment of diabetes mellitus demonstrated
1923 Health Section of League of Nations founded
1925 Diphtheria toxoid used successfully
1930 National Institutes of Health established
1933 Influenza virus A identified
1935 Social Security Act passed
1941 Penicillin demonstrated
Papanicolaou developed cervical smear for cancer detection
1943 Streptomycin antibiotic effects demonstrated
1948 World Health Organization founded
1949 Cultivation of poliomyelitis virus
1952 Poliomyelitis vaccine successful field test
1954 Rubeola virus identified
1956 Poliomyelitis attenuated virus vaccine field test
1961 Peace Corps established
1963 Measles vaccine demonstrated successfully
1964 Mumps vaccine developed
Surgeon General's Report on Smoking and Health
1966 Rubella vaccine trial tested
1967 Medicare and Medicaid begin coverage
1969 Rubella vaccine introduced
1970 National High Blood Pressure education and screening programs begin
Occupational Health and Safety Act signed
1971 White House Conference on Aging
National health insurance plans introduced in Congress
1973 Health Maintenance Organization Assistance Act
1974 National Institute on Aging established
National Health Planning and Resources Development Act replaces Comprehensive Health Planning and Regional Medical Programs
1975 National Center for Health Education established
1976 Health Information and Health Promotion Act signed
1977 World Health Organization announced the eradication of smallpox in Asia

QUESTIONS AND EXERCISES

1. Why and how does a knowledge of the past in any field of human endeavor benefit those who now work in that field?
2. Illustrate how disease has altered the course of history.
3. Why should people in the parahealth professions have a broad knowledge of community health?
4. Why was the Mosaic Law or Code of special importance to the advancement of the community health movement?
5. Using examples, explain how the political philosophy of a nation affects its health program.
6. What specific lesson in health can the present generation gain from a study of health conditions during the Dark Ages?
7. To what extent did the Renaissance influence the direction of community health?
8. What, in your judgment, was the most important health discovery in Europe during the period of American colonization between 1600 and 1800?
9. Evaluate this statement. "Colorful reporting can get more public action than scientific fact."
10. Evaluate this assertion. "Lowering the death rate among laborers and their families does not improve their lot because it results in a surplus of laborers."
11. Appalling health conditions had an adverse effect on literary and musical productivity during the golden age of arts and letters in Europe. What factors in America today have a deterrent effect upon productivity in the field of arts and letters?
12. In 1850 Lemuel Shattuck listed a considerable number of health recommendations that were carried out in the next century. What health recommendations would you make for future America?
13. What questionable health practices in the miasma phase of health are still regarded by the general public as important to health?
14. What is the basis for the contention that scientific public health should be dated from 1880?
15. Why did the application of scientific methods have such a profound effect upon the death rate in Europe and the United States?
16. Why is the postponement of death not sufficient as the objective of a community health program?
17. Explain what is meant by the expression, "Public health is social engineering."
18. In what respects is the development of county health departments of more importance than the development of state health departments or the United States Public Health Service?
19. What single health discovery has been of greatest value to you?
20. What determines who benefits most from the present community health program?

REFERENCES

American Public Health Association: A half century of public health, New York, 1951, American Public Health Association.

Bartsocas, C. S.: Two fourteenth century descriptions of the "Black Plague," Journal of the History of Medicine 21:394, 1966.

Blake, J. B.: Public health in the town of Boston, 1630-

1823, Cambridge, Mass., 1959, Harvard University Press.

Buck, A. H.: Hygiene and public health, Philadelphia, 1879, William Wood and Co.

Calder, R.: The lamp is lit, the story of WHO, Geneva, Switzerland, 1951, WHO Division of Public Information.

Chapin, C. V.: A report on state public health work based on a survey of state boards of health, Chicago, 1916, American Medical Association.

Chapin, C. V.: The papers of C. V. Chapin, New York, 1934, The Commonwealth Fund.

Cowen, D. L.: Medicine and health in New Jersey, Princeton, 1964, Van Nostrand Co., Inc.

Duffy, J.: History of public health in New York City, 1625-1866, New York, 1968, Russell Sage Foundation.

Hanlon, J. J., Rogers, F. B., and Rosen, G.: A bookshelf on the history and philosophy of public health, American Journal of Public Health **50:**445, 1960.

Health in America: 1776-1976, Rockville, 1976, Health Resources Administration.

Henschen, F.: History and geography of disease, translated by Joan Tate, New York, 1966, The Delacorte Press.

History and American Public Health, American Journal of Public Health **55:**1, 1965.

Hobson, W.: World health and history, Baltimore, 1963, The Williams & Wilkins Co.

Koudelka, J. B.: Bibliography of the history of medicine in the United States and Canada, Bulletin of the History of Medicine **40:**547, 1966.

Leff, S., and Leff, V.: From witchcraft to world health, New York, 1957, The Macmillan Co.

Leff, S., and Leff, V.: Health and humanity, New York, 1962, International Publishers Co., Inc.

Lerner, M., and Anderson, O. W.: Health progress in the United States, 1900-1960, Chicago, 1963, University of Chicago Press.

Lewis, R. A.: Edwin Chadwick and the public health movement, 1823-1854, Clifton, N.J., 1970, Augustus M. Kelley, Publishers.

Means, R. K.: A history of health education in the United States, Philadelphia, 1963, Lea & Febiger.

Miller, G.: Bibliography of the history of medicine in the United States and Canada 1939-1960, Baltimore, 1964, The Johns Hopkins Press.

O'Brien, H. R.: Fifty years in public health, Camp Hill, Pa., 1967, Henry R. O'Brien.

Ravenel, M. P., editor: Half century of public health, New York, 1970, Arno Press, Inc.

Richardson, B. W.: The health of nations. A review of the works of Edwin Chadwick, vol. 2, London, 1887, Longmans Green & Co.

Rogers, F. B.: Man and his changing environment: historical perspective, American Journal of Public Health **51:**1637, 1961.

Rosen, G.: A history of public health, New York, 1958, MD Publications, Inc.

Rosen, G.: Preventive medicine in the United States, 1900-1975, New York, 1975, Science History Publication.

Rush, B.: Medical inquiries and observances, ed. 4, Philadelphia, 1815, University of Pennsylvania Press.

Shattuck, L., and associates: Report of the Sanitary Commission of Massachusetts, 1850, New York, 1948, Cambridge University Press.

Shryock, R. H.: Medicine and society in America, 1660-1860, New York, 1960, New York University Press.

Sigerist, H. E.: History of medicine, 2 vols., London, 1951, 1961, Oxford University Press.

Sigerist, H. E.: Landmarks in the history of hygiene, London, 1956, Oxford University Press.

Spiegelman, M.: Health progress in the United States, New York, 1951, American Enterprise Association.

Turner, C. E.: I remember, New York, 1973, Vantage Press.

Wain, H.: A history of preventive medicine, Springfield, Ill., 1970, Charles C Thomas, Publisher.

Wilcox, C.: Medical advance, public health and social evolution, New York, 1965, Pergamon Press, Inc.

Winslow, C.-E. A.: The untilled fields of public health, Science **51:**23, 1920.

2 ■ THE COMMUNITY AND ITS HEALTH

Social influences exert their power, either good or bad, upon all who come within their reach.

E. H. Janes, 1876

HEALTH FIELD CONCEPT

A working paper uses this new approach to formulate strategies for improving Canadian health (A New Perspective on the Health of Canadians, 1974). The health field concept (Laframboise, 1973) is a useful framework for categorizing the various factors that have an impact on the health of a community.

Four classifications are provided—human biology, environment, life-style, and health care organization. Human biology encompasses the health outcomes that directly derive from the biology of man. The genetics of the individual, growth, and aging are examples. Many diseases involve this component as a necessary substrate, and factors in the remaining three categories act on it.

Environment includes all those factors related to health that are external to the human body and over which the individual has little control yet over which the community may have a larger degree of control. Examples include safe, uncontaminated food, air, water, and drugs; control of air, water, and noise pollution; effective garbage and sewage disposal; and prevention of spread of communicable diseases. Providing a safe social environment by accident and fire prevention, gun control, and television programs that do not glorify and exploit violence are further examples. Urbanization, with resultant crowding and poor housing, is an environmental influence on community health.

Rapid social change with disintegration of established community values and their replacement by newer, untested mores may cause alienation and stress. Pursuit of private pleasure at the cost of common good may result in deterioration of community health, both physical and mental.

Life-style is the third category. This covers decisions by individuals that affect their health, including self-imposed risks such as cigarette smoking, overeating, drug addiction, alcoholism, promiscuity, careless driving, and failure to wear seat belts. Lack of exercise, recreation, or relief from pressure of work are further examples of self-imposed risks that are health hazards.

The fourth and last category is the one that has received the most attention and money and from which an unrealistic expectation of health improvement has developed. Health care organization is the category reserved for provision of health care. Elements are medical practice, nursing, hospitals, nursing homes, dental services, drugs, mental health, and other community health programs. An array of interventional methods, usually applied late in the natural history of disease, when little in the way of cure can be expected but much in the way of effort can be expended, are elements of this category. Society has developed a dependence on this category while overlooking the benefits to be derived from health-related changes in environment and life-style. This chapter will concentrate on community efforts in these latter two categories.

CONCEPT OF COMMUNITY

A community must be considered in terms of a social unit in which there is a transaction of a common life among the people composing the unit. It must be thought of in terms of a social group, functioning with reasonable harmony in promoting the many common interests inherent in society. It may exist in a fairly limited territory, but more and more the community is characterized by a constantly enlarging geographical expanse. Our concept of community has changed from the limited view that a city in its boundary constitutes a community to a consideration of the interaction in the common activities of life. A few decades ago a single large city was regarded as an independent community. Today we speak of a metropolitan area, implying that the entire area functions as a unified community. The Standard Metropolitan Statistical Area (SMSA) is a county or group of contiguous counties containing at least one city of 50,000 inhabitants or more. In the 1970 census there were 228 SMSA's in the United States. Sixty-nine percent of the population of the United States lived within a SMSA, 37.6% lived outside a central city, and 31.4% lived within one.

Certainly from the standpoint of health and particularly in the promotion of health it is necessary to think of the areas outside of the legal limits of a city as being an integral part of the total community. Erecting hospitals, establishing clinics, and providing other medical services today require planning based on the use of modern transportation and require an estimate of the health needs of the population served. Such planning is best accomplished by elected bodies including consumers as well as health providers. By so doing, it is possible to provide more complete facilities for all people living within the area and having a common interest in health facilities. It is interesting to observe that long-established industrial communities are adult-centered and suburbs are child-centered. To the suburbanites the needs of the children seem to command first priority. This is significant in health promotion.

Concisely stated, a community is a group of inhabitants living in a somewhat localized area under the same general regulations and having common interests and organizations. In terms of health promotion it would be unwise to limit the concepts of a community to a city, a village, or even a county. In its broadest sense a community may extend beyond the boundaries of one county and may even completely encompass another county. Not territorial boundaries, but common interests and common action should be the criteria for determining a community in terms of health and health promotion. A community consists basically of a relationship between people who live in an area by virtue of the things they have in common. Physical contours of a human settlement may be the most obvious characteristic of a particular community, but they do not fully define that community. Shared interest, perhaps membership in a large university, may define a community, or employment in a large plant may be the common bond.

COMMUNITY ENVIRONMENTAL FACTORS

In considering community factors that influence the health of the people, the general public tends to think largely in terms of population figures. The size of a city or the number of people living in a community is a significant factor in dealing with community health problems, yet from the community health standpoint a large city can be thought of as a group of villages, since varying economic factors and different influences can identify communities within the community. A number of community environmental factors must be recognized in dealing with community health problems. The physical environment, geography, climate, neighborhood, and industrial conditions all must be considered when appraising the health of a community. Some of these factors will have but a minor effect on health, while others may virtually identify the particular health problems peculiar to the community.

Physical environment and general conditions. The overall physical environment frequently identifies a community. Important to health, it often creates the particular background that accounts for the general health conditions existing within the community. Perhaps more important, the physical environment reflects the community's general health status. This applies to the mental, emotional, and social health of a community as well as to the physical health. The community that possesses a commendable orderliness usually reflects an awareness and a pride in the well-being of its citizens. In some instances it would be difficult to demonstrate a direct relationship between general objectionable physical conditions of a community and the low level of health possessed by its inhabitants. Scientifically it would be difficult to predict that merely changing the physical environment of a community would have a demonstrable effect on the health of the citizens. Yet the overall physical environment and general physical conditions of a community are significant, particularly as an index of health consciousness and community progress in health.

Geography, topography, and climate. Geography refers to the surface of the earth. Topography indicates the features of a region or locality. Together with climate, these two factors represent phenomena that give rise to special community health problems. Lowlands, marshy areas, and hot climates give rise to health problems not of particular concern to other areas. Dry, dusty areas may be confronted with certain health conditions differing from those of more humid areas. The minerals of an area, the types of soil, functions of rivers, canals, waterways, and harbors can be significant factors in determining the general health of the area. What people do with these natural resources is of health significance.

Neighborhoods. A neighborhood generally is thought of as being an area housing that population for which one elementary school is ordinarily required. Engelhart points out that each neighborhood should range in size from 1,000 to 3,000 families. This would mean a population (in the neighborhood) of about 5,000. However, areas deviating from this general pattern are common and can be designated as true neighborhood units.

The compactness and uniformity of neighborhoods vary. Some of the older, longer established neighborhoods have an amazing unity and rapport. Some of the newer neighborhoods, particularly in the suburban areas, frequently are neighborhoods in area only. Speculative building in the suburbs, combined with a mobile population, tends to produce communities of individuals who are almost transients, with scant allegiance to a common health standard. Time is needed before the influence of schools, churches, and community groups becomes established. In terms of social unity, neighborhood organization is extremely loose. The degree of neighborhood unity, past practices, leadership, and established standards all contribute to existing health conditions. More important, however, is the nature of the neighborhood unity that exists when a particular health problem arises that must be dealt with on a cooperative basis. Where a long-established neighborhood cohesiveness already exists, the necessary leadership and united support will be mobilized quickly and a program to solve the health problem will be initiated summarily. In a neighborhood where very little cohesiveness has been developed, valuable time will be consumed in the effort to mobilize the neighborhood's resources in dealing with the health problem requiring attention. Such a neighborhood may require several years to deal with a health problem that a more cohesive neighborhood will have well in hand in a matter of several weeks.

In many instances, a common health problem has been a highly important catalyst in unifying a neighborhood. A common concern about a situation that threatens health, or is important in the promotion of health, can bring people together, promote mutual respect, and provide a common purpose that will provide a sense of neighborhood unity that will be of value for years to come.

Solving neighborhood problems through wholesome neighborhood approaches is preferable to the exertion of legal means. Only when reasonably diligent effort on the part of the neighborhood has failed and the health problem jeopardizes the neighborhood should the extreme of resorting to legal means be employed.

In the modern community very few health problems arise that must be dealt with summarily. Sufficient time is usually available for working out a satisfactory solution. It is a fortunate neighborhood that has united to deal with problems in the past because of the unity such common purposes engender. It is a wise neighborhood that visualizes public health problems lying ahead and that has developed some form of organization and collective action to consider the health needs of the neighborhood and the action to be taken.

Industrial conditions. Health conditions and health problems can be identified with particular industrial conditions that prevail either within the community or that indirectly affect the community. A "garden city" or a residential community will not have some of the health problems that citizens in a highly industrialized community will encounter. An industry that causes a great deal of noise may create special problems of an emotional as well of a physical nature. The social health of the community can be affected by chemical plants creating obnoxious odors. A mining community or a logging community living in the shadow of extreme occupational hazards is a community different from one in which industrial accidents are not a significant factor.

In addition to the direct effect that a particular industry will have on the health of a community, there usually exists a secondary factor in the type of people an industry attracts to a city. Certain industries engage workers who have a high regard for health and who live under conditions conducive to the promotion of a high level of health. Other industries seem to attract the type of worker whose attitudes toward health tend to result in a community life in which health is not held in proper regard, and their general level of health tends to be at the lower end of the American health scale.

SOCIAL AND PSYCHOLOGICAL FACTORS

Communities are all different and the difference does not lie simply in the observable physical characteristics of the buildings, industries, and topography. Communities are identified by certain social and psychological factors that distinguish them. The traditions of the long-established community, social stratification in a community, the religious influences, the tenure of residence, and other sociological factors operate in giving a distinctive personality to a community. These same factors both directly and indirectly influence the health of the community. The recognition of health problems, the promotion of community health, and the ability to deal with health emergencies will be affected by the sociological and psychological influences that have evolved over the years.

Traditions and prejudices. Community health is not a static entity but is a process of continual change. New health problems, new aspects of old health problems, different health requirements, and new discoveries call for new approaches to health. In some communities long-established conventions, unwritten but generally understood, prove to be a barrier to attempts to deal with evolving health needs. In some instances these orally transmitted notions are not readily identifiable but appear as certain resistances in the form of "We have always done it this way." Perhaps an even greater obstacle to health advances in the community are certain preconceived judgments relating to certain health matters or health procedures. A health bias can be as deeply ingrained as a religious bias.

The inertia of habit and custom is a conservative force in the modern community.

Communities with broad social-mindedness and a concept of intercommunity and intra-community action provide the necessary tenable basis for dealing with health problems on the broad scale that modern living requires.

Socioeconomic status (SES). The population may be classified into subgroups on the basis of ranking, according to income, residence, occupation, or education. According to which of these four criteria are used, the resulting hierarchy is graduated and classified into upper, middle, and lower SES. SES determines life-style, which in turn governs environmental exposures, customs, and habits that affect health status. There is considerable overlap between income and residence as well as between occupation and education. The latter is the most powerful determinant of the four criteria with regard to influence on health-related behavior. Persons of high educational attainment often enjoy the best health status, and they respond to appeals from health professionals and modify their behavior in a positive, health-related manner, for example, smoking cessation, weight control, exercise programs, dental care, immunization status, etc. In contrast, persons of low educational level often suffer the worst health outcome and are difficult to persuade toward positive health behavior. There frequently exists a cultural barrier between the efforts of health professionals to educate and the perceptions of their clients with less education.

Regardless of the basis for social stratification, health problems affect all groups. Communicable diseases cut across all strata of society, though generally the lower strata are more affected than those higher up on the pyramid. However, prevention and control of communicable diseases among the less privileged groups indirectly protect and thus benefit the entire population. In general, public health activities are most needed by members of low-income groups and individuals of less educational attainment, but all people in a community will benefit from an overall community health program.

High-income families are more self-sufficient in health matters and are better able to avail themselves of the fruits of technological advancements. Their position enables them to obtain the best medical care, best hospitalization, and other services necessary to the protection of their health. Perhaps health cannot be purchased but, to a certain extent, health promotion and protection can be bought.

Social mores. Customs and habits imbued with ethical significance can have the force of laws. Usually the social mores of a community can serve as an asset in the promotion of community health. However, it may be necessary to change established customs in a community in order to obtain the necessary gains that modern health procedures can contribute. Modification of customs in a community usually represents a compromise. Attempts to eliminate or reverse a custom often generate hostile resistance to a health program.

Religious influences. Most American communities are composed of citizens of diverse religious faiths living in harmony, and no particular denomination or group of churches holds a dominating position in terms of community influence. The total effect is to elevate the general level of community life and provide a background in which community health promotion can flourish. This effect is achieved if those who provide the community's health leadership properly seek the support of the many church groups in the community. Health leadership must always be sensitive to possible conflicts, religious or otherwise, that may exist in a community.

Educational influences. A town with a majority of citizens who have a college education will provide an atmosphere more receptive to health program innovation than a community in which a small percentage of the people is graduated from high school. Communities in which a high proportion of the citizens have had a college education demand and support programs that provide the highest possible level of community health. While it is recognized that this type of community usually has the necessary means for providing the highest type of community health, this is not to imply that some communities of a lower educational level cannot and do not have community health of a high quality. Well-informed, public-spirited leadership can be the catalyst to provide the highest form of health in any community.

Political influences. Not all community health programs or factors are official or political in nature. Law enforcement is not a highly significant factor in modern community health promotion, yet the caliber of officials a community has and the extent of social-mindedness in its officialdom both directly and indirectly affect community health standards. The willingness of community officials to raise taxes for health promotion and their interest in giving a high priority to matters of health are significant in the final determination of the kind of health people of a community will have. However, even when official support of community health is inadequate, it is possible through other avenues, through other agencies, and through other means to promote a high level of community health.

Economic factors. The economic structure of a community has both a direct and an indirect relation to community health. The size of a trade area, the importance of farm people in a trade area, the diversity of industry, the fluctuations in the economy, and the extremes of rich and poor are of significance to health as a phase of the standard of living. Different economic conditions mean differences in the money available for food, clothing, housing, and other basic needs. It also means differences in money available for health facilities, health services, schools, sanitary facilities, leisure time activities, and general health promotion services.

The family income that an economy provides appears to be directly related to the level of health enjoyed by the people in a community. Surveys indicate that people in prosperous cities live longer than people who reside in low-income cities. It must be recognized that the factor of income may conceal several factors or variables. It may conceal the general educational and intellectual level of a people, and it may conceal groups that would tend to live longer under most circumstances. However, prosperous communities usually provide more and better health facilities than impoverished communities, a factor of no small importance in community health consideration.

Tenure of residence. Growth in population is a sign of a prosperous community and usually of a healthy community. Population growth may cause certain temporary displacements within a community that may be adverse to health promotion. Additional schools may be required and additional community services may be necessary. There may be some disorganization during the time between the occurrence of these new needs and their fulfillment. This is the experience of suburban communities adjacent to large metropolitan areas. In such communities the tenure of residence of a good many of the families is relatively short, but in this instance a high proportion of short-tenure residents can be an asset rather than a liability. Usually the newcomers are young couples with families of small children. In other communities where families are moving in and out constantly, an unfavorable health situation usually exists. A high number of transient families tends to lower the general health level of a community. It is recognized that modern America is a highly mobile nation, yet this mobility is a liability only in the case of those families that are constantly hedgehopping from one community to another. Health officials, state as well as local, have long recognized that these families create special health problems.

In many of the smaller villages of the nation there is a tendency for the younger people to move away, so that today most of the small rural and even nonrural villages are populated by older people. With a proportionately high percentage of their citizens over 65 years of age, these small communities find themselves faced with low birth rates, high death rates, and the special health problems of the elderly. Many of these communities are unable to provide the necessary health facilities and services for the health needs of their older citizens. Some communities are fortunate in being near to or part of a large community in which complete health services are available.

ORGANIZATIONAL FACTORS

In any community there will be a diversity of agencies and individuals providing services of direct and indirect health significance. Too frequently there is little coordination or integration of services, and considerable overlapping of functions frequently exists. Despite the lack of efficient teamwork, the fact that both tax-supported and nontax-supported health services are available is important to the health-conscious citizen who knows how to utilize health services to the best advantage for himself, his family, his neighborhood, and his community.

Tax-supported services. The official agencies that contribute to the health of a community usually touch the individual citizen directly. Some of the services given by these tax-supported agencies may be of an indirect nature, but the majority of their services directly affect individual citizens in their everyday living. Obviously, the most important of these tax-supported agencies is the county or the city health department. However, other official agencies also provide certain health services. These include the department of welfare, public hospitals, special boards and commissions, department of public works, public schools, local housing authority, county agricultural agent's office, and the police department. Each of these, individually and cooperatively, has an important role in community health promotion.

Nontax-supported services. Certain health services are available to citizens of most communities through voluntary agencies or organizations present in the typical community. Civic clubs, church groups, parent-teacher associations, Red Cross, visiting nurse associations, and the community hospital are classic examples. Special clinical services, as well as medical care and hospital service plans, may also be included.

Certain national voluntary health agencies may have an indirect effect on the health of any given community and in some instances may play a direct role in the health of individual citizens. These national voluntary health agencies serve several functions, such as education, demonstrations, supplementing official activities, supporting official health activities, and coordinating community health efforts. Some of these agencies are concerned with specific diseases. This group would include chapters of organizations such as American Cancer Society, American Heart Association, National Tuberculosis and Respiratory Disease Association, and National Foundation.

No discussion of nontax-supported services would be complete that omitted private practitioner services. Certainly the practicing physician, the dentist, the nurse, and other health specialists provide indispensable services to the community. The medical society, the dental society, and medical service plans must be included in any appraisal of nontax-supported health services in a community.

QUALITY OF HEALTH

Health is the ability to perform certain valued social roles.

Talcott Parsons

Many Americans not incapacitated nevertheless do not have the quality of health that is set as the goal for normal individuals. When health is considered as that quality of physical, mental, and emotional well-being that enables one to live effectively and enjoyably, it becomes apparent that many people regarded as being well actually do not possess a high quality of health. They may be free from disabilities and yet not possess an adequate level of well-being.

The health goal that the community health program seeks for every citizen is not only an absence of disabling defects and disorders, but also a vitality, buoyancy, and an abundance of energy that enables the individual to do the things he wants to do and reasonably expects to do, with a corresponding enjoyment and gratification in living. Not perfect health, but a high level of well-being in which an individual finds life stimulating, is a realistic goal for citizens of every community.

QUESTIONS AND EXERCISES

1. What are the advantages and disadvantages of a high degree of mobility in a population?
2. What constitutes the community in which you live?
3. What favorable characteristics would you look for in a community?
4. Make an analysis of the neighborhood in which you live.
5. Explain how one dramatic incident can unite a community in a common health cause.
6. Explain how one citizen can provide the spark necessary to deal with a long-existing, unresolved health problem.
7. Using an example, show how a particular industry attracts a particular type of people with particular health problems.
8. What are some obstacles to community health progress?
9. Analyze this statement: "It is impossible to eliminate community customs but not difficult to modify them."
10. Why should churches have an interest in community health?
11. To what extent does economics enter into community health promotion?
12. Evaluate this statement: "Transient families are community health liabilities."

REFERENCES

American Public Health Association: Health is a community affair, New York, 1970, The Association.

Bryant, J.: Health and the developing world, Ithaca, N.Y., 1969, Cornell University Press.

Conant, R. W.: Politics of community health, National Commission on Community Health Services, Washington, D.C., 1968, Public Affairs Press.

Engel, A.: Perspectives in health planning, New York, 1968, Oxford University Press, Inc.

Engelhart, N. L., Jr.: The school, neighborhood nucleus, Architectural Forum 79:89, 1943.

Fry, H. G., and associates: Educational manpower for community health, Pittsburgh, 1968, University of Pittsburgh Press.

Georke, L. S., and Stebbins, E. K.: Mustard's introduction to public health, ed. 5, New York, 1968, The Macmillan Co.

Ginzberg, E.: Urban health services: the case of New York, New York, 1970, Columbia University Press.

Hanlon, J. J.: Public health: administration and practice, ed. 6, St. Louis, 1974, The C. V. Mosby Co.

Henkle, O. B. M.: Introduction to community health, Boston, 1970, Allyn & Bacon, Inc.

Hobson, W., editor: Theory and practice of community health, ed. 3, New York, 1969, Oxford University Press, Inc.

Jones, B., editor: The health of Americans, Englewood Cliffs, N.J., 1970, Prentice-Hall, Inc.

Kosa, J., and associates: Poverty and health: a sociological analysis, Cambridge, Mass., 1969, Harvard University Press.

Laframboise, H. L.: Health policy: breaking it down into more manageable segments, Journal of the Canadian Medical Association 108:388-394, February 3, 1973.

Larimore, G.: Health planning, Archives of Environmental Health 20:128, 1970.

Meadows, P.: Public health in a new community, American Journal of Public Health 60:1980, 1970.

Medical and Research Association of New York: Poverty and health in the United States, a bibliography with abstracts, New York, 1967, The Association.

Michael, J.: A basic information system for health planning, Public Health Reports 83:21, 1968.

Morgan, L. S.: Community development: observation around the world, American Journal of Public Health 55:607, 1967.

A new perspective on the health of Canadians, a working document, Ottawa, Canada, April 1974, Canadian Department of Health and Welfare.

Paul, B. D.: Health, culture and community, New York, 1967, Russell Sage Foundation.

Prohansky, H.: Environmental psychology: man and his physical setting, New York, 1970, Holt, Rinehart & Winston, Inc.

Taugenhaus, L. J.: A division of community health services, Archives of Environmental Health 20:732, 1970.

Turner, C. E.: Personal and community health, ed. 14, St. Louis, 1971, The C. V. Mosby Co.

Zald, M. N., editor: Organizing for community welfare, Chicago, 1967, Quadrangle Books, Inc.

3 ▪ HUMAN ECOLOGY AND CONSERVATION OF HUMAN RESOURCES

I find the great thing in the world is not so much where we stand, as in what direction we are moving.

Oliver Wendell Holmes

The most important thing on earth is life, the most important form of life is human life, and the most important human life is one's own life. Man is born a biological being and inherent in the individual is a psycho-physiological pattern or matrix expressing the need and desire for survival. This pattern in man's makeup gives force and direction to the means he employs to promote his own well-being as well as to postpone death. The individual alone can do much to enhance his survival, but the society in which he lives, through collective action, can aid the individual in his desire to survive. In helping the individual to survive, society itself is benefited. Because society's greatest resource is its members, it is incumbent upon society for its own survival to carry forward measures for the conservation of human resources.

Man is widely dispersed over the face of the earth. Of all forms of life man possesses the greatest degree of adaptability. He can adjust to a greater variety of conditions than any other living form. He can be found in the arctic region as well as in the tropics. Most important of all, man has the great ability to bend nature to his will and to solve problems of survival created by environmental conditions. In solving one problem relating to survival, man frequently creates another problem. He finds survival a constant struggle in which he must look for other problems as soon as he has solved one. Basically, good public health is good ecology, and persons concerned with health planning must keep this principle constantly before them.

HUMAN ECOLOGY

Human ecology is the study of the relations between human beings and their environment. Man deals with an environment that is physical, chemical, biological, and behavioral-sociological. Man lives in an organic relationship with his environment, and a degree of interdependency exists. Just as the environment affects man, so too man alters the environment. Most of the time the human being alters the environment to his advantage, but at other times his alteration of the environment reacts to his disadvantage.

To understand his environment, man calls on many academic disciplines to study an array of factors with beneficial or adverse effects. Some problems of environment control cut across several disciplines, indicating that the field of human ecology is a collective discipline. In listing environmental factors and academic disciplines that are the concern of human ecology, it must be acknowledged that some factors could be listed under other headings than here indicated or could be listed under all three classifications. This

27

classification is somewhat arbitrary but does have value as an overview and in terms of organization.

The physical-chemical factors of man's environment include the following:

Climate	Noise
Food production	Debris
Air pollution	Soil
Radiation	

The biological factors of man's environment include the following:

Food production	Pathogens
Food conservation	Other parasitism
Nutrition	Vectors
Physiological effects	Water pollution
Poisons	Animal life

The behavioral-sociological factors of man's environment include the following:

Social structure	Leisure
Communication	Stress
Learning	Population imbal-
Economics	ance
Mobility	

This chapter will deal with those factors relating to the conservation of human resources and will leave discussions of other factors to subsequent chapters. Logically, human ecology should be woven into any discussion of community health.

HUSBANDING OF FACTORS AFFECTING LIFE

Man has not conquered nature and doubtless never will, for biological laws are always at work and ignoring these laws will not alter their certain, inevitable course. Man can modify the course of nature and alter conditions to aid in his own survival. He even makes it possible for the biologically weak to survive and thus benefit most those who have the least biological endowment. A common misconception prevails that this is artificial selection and is dysgenic in that it enables the "poorest" segments of our species to survive. Biologists recognize that there is no such thing as artificial selection, that it is just as much natural selection when the brain is used to aid survival as when legs and wings are used.

No acceptable evidence exists that man today is biologically inferior to man of previous centuries or that he is better endowed biologically. Mankind recognizes values other than biological endowment. Why should not the person with diabetes have the right to life? By making it possible for these people to survive, mankind in return has received the intellectual, artistic, and other benefits that the special gifts of many of these people have made possible.

A number of basic factors exist that affect man's life on earth and that man must conserve and convert to his survival and well-being. These are readily recognized as indispensable to man's survival. Equally apparent is what man must do about these factors. Conservation is not the hoarding but the wise use of facilities. The conservation of human resources means the husbanding and most effective use of the basic factors most essential to man's survival, his quality of well-being, and the extension of his prime of life. Conservation entails balancing future needs as well as present requirements. Conservation of human resources means giving consideration to climatic conditions, food supply, utilization of land and water, the birthrate, other living forms, technological developments, and other factors fundamental to the existence of the human species.

CLIMATIC EFFECT UPON HEALTH

People living in the temperate zones have a longer life expectancy than people living in the tropics. This holds true also for people who normally live in temperate zones but who migrate to the tropics and live there. In conditions of excessive heat, physical and mental activity decline, bodily functioning tends to become reduced, and resistance to infection is apparently less than under cooler temperatures. Standard aptitude and intelligence tests administered to college students reveal lower performances in the heat of summer than in the cool days of the winter months. Experiments with rats indicate reduced performance when the ambient temperature is increased.

Animal husbandmen have observed that twice as much time is required to grow a steer to a thousand-pound weight in Louisiana as is required in the northern states. They also report that the animal's maximum weight in Louisiana is considerably less than that of the animal raised in the northern states. Temperature has a general effect on human behavior. In the northern United States, Christmas is celebrated with a vigor and boisterousness that is not demonstrated in the southern states.

Temperature cycles of the world have had a significant influence not only on the health of the human species but also on the economy and general culture of nations. During the glory of Greece and the height of Rome, Europe was in the throes of a cold cycle that provided ideal temperatures for agriculture in the Mediterranean area. Culture flourished in those nations that enjoyed a thriving agriculture, but those nations in northern Europe that had prevailing temperatures too low for growing crops declined culturally as well as in other respects. During the period of low temperatures, the population of Ireland consisted of sheep, goat, and cattle herders and their families. Vegetable crops were almost nonexistent. Ireland's general culture declined with its economy.

During the Dark Ages, the thermometer had swung to the other extreme and reached its peak about A.D. 850. Grapes and other crops usually associated with the Mediterranean area grew abundantly in England. This was the period when the Norsemen were making their explorations to the North American continent and elsewhere. During this hot era, Greece experienced a steady decline as her agriculture and general economy faded. Ireland flourished and probably was the most cultured nation in Europe. This hot period was followed by a cooling period. Ice that formed in some of the northern nations during the year A.D. 1000 did not begin to melt until the onset of the present upward trend of temperature.

The most recent rising phase of the temperature cycle appears to have begun around 1880, but the rise in temperature was not appreciable until the period beginning in 1930. Since that time there appears to have been a gradual, somewhat irregular, but nonetheless measurable increase in the world's temperature. Glaciers are receding and objects and forms of life frozen in ice a thousand years ago are being exposed. How long this upward cycle will continue no one can predict accurately. Whether a predicted constant temperature rise during the next 200 years will materialize no one knows, but the rising increase in carbon dioxide is providing an atmospheric layer that holds heat next to the earth.

Man does not now possess technological knowledge to alter the world's temperature. He must, however, adapt to any temperature rise that may occur if he is to prosper and even survive. Certainly air conditioning, refrigeration, and other technical developments indicate that man has already attacked the problem of excessive heat. Changes in agricultural crops and procedures will be inevitable in man's continuing efforts toward survival if he finds he must live in constantly rising temperatures. New problems in parasitism and in human physiology will appear. Some nations may benefit from the warm centuries ahead and rise to positions of dominance in the world, whereas other nations may decline in relative importance in the world.

WORLD POPULATION

From 1910 to 1975 the world population increased from 1.5 to 4 billion. The rate of increase is such that, if maintained, the population will double in 40 years. However, the world birthrate declined from 34 per 1,000 in 1965 to 30 per 1,000 in 1974. During these years 128 countries, including the most populous, experienced decreases in birthrates that were greater than those noted in death rates. The net result has been a slowing of the rate of natural population increase (excess of births over deaths) (World Population Growth and Response, 1965-1975).

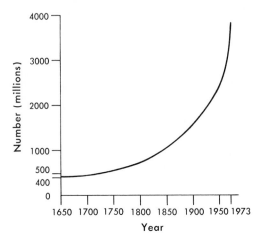

Fig. 3-1. World population.

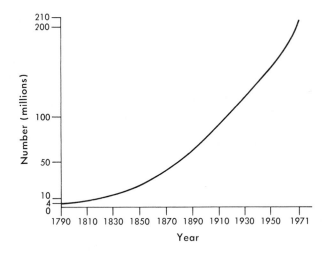

Fig. 3-2. Resident population, United States, 1790 to 1971.

Long-term predictions of population growth are very speculative, because many factors, including technological, legislative, climatic, and cultural, influence population growth.

At the present time, two-thirds of the people of the world do not have sufficient food. Where starvation exists, disease flourishes. The malnourished are more susceptible to infection than the well-nourished. Famines cause people to migrate and, by so doing, to spread infectious disease. Only if there are sufficient technological develop-

ments in the fields of agriculture and health, and only if these advances are made available to all nations, can the present rate of population increase be expected to continue during the present century.

BIOTIC POTENTIAL

Perhaps human population changes can best be understood by a consideration of the biotic potential of a nation as related to environmental resistance. The basic concept can be presented in the following equation form:

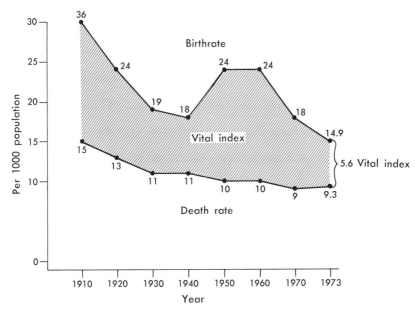

Fig. 3-3. Vital index, United States, 1910 to 1973.

$$\text{Population} = \frac{\text{Biotic potential}}{\text{Environmental resistance}}$$

$$\text{Biotic potential} = PZ_n(R^{n\,=\,1})$$

P = Number of females of child-bearing age
Z = Number of young
n = Number of generations
R = Proportion of females

Environmental resistance is expressed in parasitism, food supply, accidents, cold, heat, and other factors that may affect life adversely. The biotic potential of the human is generally thought of as a birthrate of 50 per thousand per year. This rate has been attained in the Ukraine over a 5-year period and in Bengal over a 10-year period. During the 10-year period from 1930 to 1940, the Warm Springs Indians of Oregon had an average birth rate of 50 per thousand per year. Perhaps scientific advances in the prevention and correction of human infertility and sterility could raise the present acknowledged maximum human birthrate, but until such time this maximum will have to be accepted. Governmental policies directly affect birthrates. A pronatal policy embodies inducements and rewards for large families, and the reverse is true of antinatal policy.

United States policy has been generally neutral in this regard. However, both the birthrate and the absolute number of births have been falling since 1957 (4,300,000) to 1976 (3,128,000)—a 27% decline.

To a certain extent, man can bend nature to his will and control his environment. The extent to which man will be able to control the factors of environmental resistance will be the important element in determining the direction of human population growth in the world in the immediate future as well as over the coming centuries. For an individual nation to survive it must have a positive vital index. By the vital index is meant the relation of births per thousand to deaths per thousand population (Fig. 3-3). If the United States has a birthrate of 14.9 per thousand and a death rate of 9.2 per thousand, it still has a healthy vital index of 5.6. When a nation's vital index begins to approach 2, that nation's population is becoming static. If deaths exceed births in a nation, that nation will have a negative vital index symptomatic of national decline.

In the United States the population increased at a rate of 0.6% per year in 1975. In terms of food supply there is no threat of a "population explosion." This nation can produce sufficient food for a population of 250,000,000 without being hard pressed. Distribution of food still poses a problem, but production is not likely to be a concern for some years to come. The two critical problems created by the present population increase are waste disposal and transportation. Satisfactory disposal of both solid and liquid wastes challenges the nation's economic means and technological know-how, and one does not have to be a traffic engineer to recognize the gross inadequacy of our transportation system, particularly around the metropolitan areas.

Zero population growth in the United States would mean reducing the birthrate to the level of about 10 per 1,000 people. This could be a deciding factor in solving the problems of waste disposal and transportation; however, there could be an adverse effect on the nation's economy. Throughout the history of the United States the nation's economy has been based on an anticipated increase in the number of consumers. Zero population growth would cause some problems, but this nation has encountered difficult problems before and has come up with the solutions. The benefits of a reduced population growth may outweigh the difficulties that would be created.

Pandemics

The term "pandemic" literally means "all people" and is used to denote a disease con-

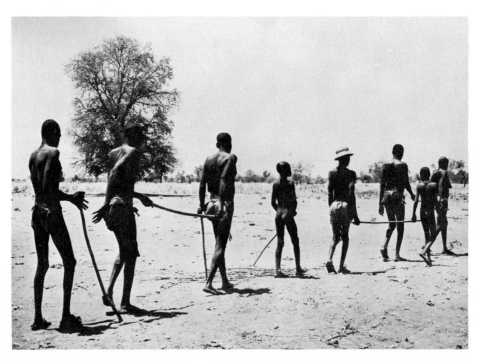

Fig. 3-4. Eyes in danger. Onchoceriasis, or river blindness, is widespread in Central America and in large stretches of central Africa. The disease is caused by a minute worm transmitted to man by the bite of infected flies. A multitude of these worms invading the eye causes ocular disturbances and sometimes blindness. In many communities blind adults must be led by the children. A WHO expert committee on onchoceriasis, which in 1953 studied the disease and possible means of prevention, reported infection rates of 80% to 100% in different countries of Africa and America. (Courtesy World Health Organization)

flagration over a considerable area. A state-wide outbreak of a disease may be regarded as a pandemic, but generally the term is used to denote a nationwide, continentwide, or worldwide outbreak. The past has seen devastating pandemics of bubonic plague, yellow fever, cholera, smallpox, typhus fever, and syphilis. The 1918-1919 influenza-pneumonia pandemic caused 400,000 deaths in the United States, 10 million deaths in India alone, and more than 20 million deaths throughout the world. In some of the underdeveloped nations of the world during the past decade pandemics of acute infectious diseases such as cholera have occurred. These outbreaks have usually been confined to a single nation or to a small group of nations. Even in the underdeveloped nations there is not likely to be a devastating pan-

demic of an acute infectious disease such as occurred in the past, but moderately severe outbreaks can be expected for decades to come. In the well-developed nations scientific advances in the field of epidemiology make even a moderate pandemic of an acute infectious disease highly unlikely.

Chronic infections still plague vast segments of the population in many nations of the world. At the present time there are more than 200 million malaria cases in the world, 260 million hookworm cases, 650 million people with ascarids, and 5 million cases of leprosy, of which 3 million are in Asia. Asia has 335 million people who harbor the parasitic ascarid. Each of these Asians will harbor between six and nine adult ascarids. The total weight of the worms thus carried by these 335 million Asians will be

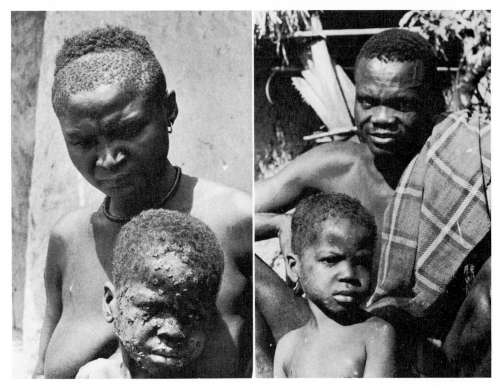

Fig. 3-5. A, Yaws: the affliction of this 5-year-old African boy. Yaws is a widespread disfiguring treponemal disease causing deep-seated infirmity if untreated. It can be cured by a single injection of long-acting penicillin. **B,** Yaws conquered: the same 5-year-old African boy, 10 days after receiving a single injection of penicillin. (Courtesy World Health Organization)

in the neighborhood of 37,500 tons and will consume as much food each day as a population of more than 40,000 people. The infant nation of Indonesia had 15 million cases of yaws before a staff of Indonesians trained by United Nations technologists and supplied with penicillin from the United Nations proceeded to wipe out the disease. One injection of penicillin usually cures yaws, so that virtually the entire Indonesian population is now free of the disease.

In America smallpox, diphtheria, influenza, meningitis, encephalitis, poliomyelitis, and other infectious diseases that conceivably could break out in pandemic form can be controlled effectively with the means at our command. A mutant pathogen of man may arise and challenge America's ability to control the spread of disease. However, America is armed with a variety of teams of specialists able to solve disease control problems that might arise. Advances in our knowledge of infection and its control will pay ample dividends in terms of protection for the future.

AGRICULTURAL CONSERVATION AND HEALTH

The relationship between the vitality of a nation's agriculture and the nation's health is readily recognized. The food supply of a nation not only determines the health of the people, but also the nature of its population growth. America's farm situation is undergoing some changes that are of interest in terms of the nation's health and its population. According to the records of the United States Bureau of the Census, the farm population declined from 34.7% of the total in 1910 to 4.8% of the total in 1970.

The number of farms also declined, but the average acreage of each increased from 138 to 390 acres. The total farmed acreage also increased to 1,121 million in 1970 from 879 million in 1910. Agricultural specialists report that it is desirable to shift 40 million acres of cropland acreage into other uses. They also report that 216 million acres could be shifted from grassland and woodland to cropland. About 280 million acres of productive land have been destroyed by neglect. However, at least 33 million acres of land not now in production could be reclaimed with adequate irrigation. Whenever we see topsoil washed away, we should remind ourselves that it takes from 2,000 to 5,000 years to build 1 inch of topsoil and that the average depth of topsoil in the United States is only about 8 inches.

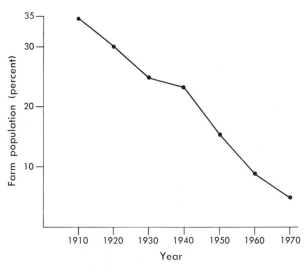

Fig. 3-6. Farm population as percentage of total United States population, 1910 to 1970.

The United States Department of Agriculture has reported that approximately 96% of America's farms are of the family type and that while 54% of our farms produce only 9% of the products, the remaining 46% produce the remaining 91% of the products of the farms.

From all these data it would appear that America's agriculture is in a healthy state and that adequate food is available for the entire population. Agricultural production has advanced at a rate faster than the rate of population increase. Certainly no immediate food shortage is discernible unless some unusual catastrophe should befall the nation. However, there are developments symbolic of problems that might conceivably plague the nation in the future. Los Angeles County serves as a classic example. Between 1909 and 1949, Los Angeles County led every county in the nation in farm wealth. The Research Council, Occidental and Pomona Colleges, has reported the following changes in Los Angeles County agriculture:

Los Angeles County

Year	Acres of oranges
1936	43,775
1957	12,092
1966	2,480

In adjoining Orange County

Year	Acres of oranges
1936	66,252
1957	36,407
1966	22,040

What has happened to agriculture in a spectacular manner in Los Angeles County is true to some extent throughout the nation. Every year thousands of acres of farmland are taken out of production for highways, airfields, golf courses, industrial plants, housing developments, and other purposes. The productivity of America's agriculture not only is basic to the nation's health and the extent of its population growth but is the key to its general cultural advancement. In a nation where less than 20% of the employed can supply its people with food, it is possible to have other workers available for industry, transportation, construction, education, music, painting, writing, entertainment, and the multitude of other pursuits that make possible a more fruitful and complete mode of living through the diversity of experiences and services that are made available.

FRUITS OF TECHNOLOGY

Population changes affect the economic, political, social, and cultural aspects of a nation. In the United States there seems to be an impelling fear that a population increase will have a disastrous effect on the economy of the nation as well as on the nation's health. We need to recall that in the 50 years extending from 1880 to 1930, the population of the United States increased two and one half times and that during the same period the output of coal increased 50 times, pig iron 50 times, cotton 20 times, and railroad mileage was extended 3,000 times. Population increases not only are aided by technological developments, but there seems to be a reciprocal action in which population increases promote technological advances. The public in general, and even population experts, have been inclined to be ultraconservative in the prediction of population increases.

In July 1938, The National Resources Committee, appointed by President Franklin D. Roosevelt, presented its report to the nation and predicted that the United States would attain a population peak of 158,335,000 in 1980. In the voluminous report to President Roosevelt the Committee stated that when the peak was reached in 1980 a gradual decline would follow. What the Committee failed to understand was not only the nation's fecundity but the technological advances that would appear in the years ahead.

In the United States in 1960, per capita consumption of resources was 18 tons, while that for the rest of the free world was 2 tons. The 18 tons consisted of 0.75 tons of food, 2.15 tons of agricultural supplies, 5.4 tons of building materials, 7.2 tons of fuel, and 2.55

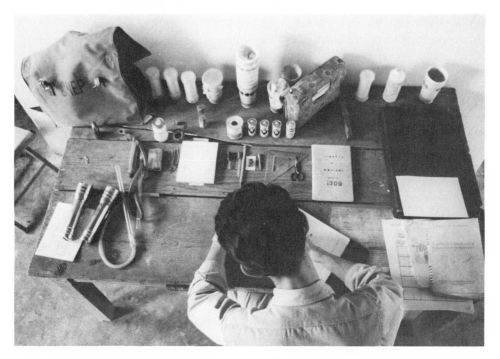

Fig. 3-7. Malaria field laboratory. Malaria, an important health hazard, has rendered vast fertile areas unfit for habitation and production. Through WHO programs thirty-five nations classified as malarious areas have eradicated the disease. (Courtesy World Health Organization)

tons of metallic ore. Of greatest significance in terms of national health and population growth is the efficiency in farm production and the outlook for the future. In 1860 an American farmer produced enough food for 5 other people; in 1900 this had risen to 8 others, in 1940 to 11 others, and in 1950 to 14 others. In 1972 efficiency had so increased that a farmer produced enough food for 46 others and in 1980 this figure doubtless will be more than 55 others. Mechanization of farming has led to fewer farm laborers and increased output. The mechanical revolution in agriculture has not terminated, yet it is already being overshadowed by the chemical revolution developing in America's agriculture.

The development of fertilizers by the chemical industry is leading to unbelievable production records. Fertilizer use has been instrumental in building up continuing food surpluses. In 1900 American farmers used less than 2 million tons of commercial fertilizer. In 1965 consumption of commercial fertilizer on American farms was over 30 million tons. Through the use of fertilizer some yields have been increased by as much as 100%.

The development of DDT, BHC, and other insecticides has been a milestone in man's battle with insects. Man has yet to conquer the insects, but never in history has he held them under such control as we do in American agriculture. The battle against weeds is yielding to technological developments. The use of 2,4-D, DNBP, and 2,45-T has reduced the amount of cultivation necessary on American farms. Experimentation yielding better seeds, better strains of plants and animals, and the addition of antibiotics to animal feeds has increased the productivity of the nation's farms. Improved methods of food processing, better refrigeration, improved packaging, and better methods of food preservation have reduced food wastes and thus contributed tangibly to the total food supply available to the American table.

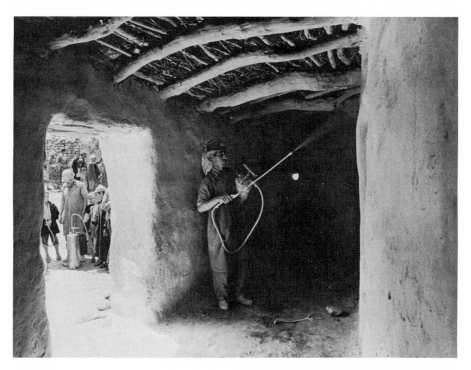

Fig. 3-8. Malaria eradication in a Moroccan village by spraying DDT. WHO started a malaria eradication program in 1955 and today the disease has disappeared from large parts of Southeast Asia, Europe, and the Americas. (Courtesy World Health Organization)

By 1980 America could double its 1970 food output per year if necessary. It is a safe prediction that many new technological developments will have a profound effect on agricultural production before 1980. The development of proteins through the propagation of chlorella, one of the algae, and the use of yeast living on a simple saw-dust medium are two fields of investigation now being pursued. The fruits of technology will add measurably to both the health and the general welfare of American citizens. Certainly technology will assure America of the qualitative and quantitative food supply that is necessary for a high level of national health.

SOCIAL ASPECTS OF HEALTH

A reciprocal relationship exists between health, agriculture, and the general social level of a nation. The promotion of health has a beneficial effect on the economy of a nation, which in turn will affect the nation's cultural and social advancement. Health promotion is not dysgenic. Clear up disease and people can feed themselves. At the termination of World War II, four out of every five people living in Greece had malaria. Led by the United States, an intensive program was instituted to eradicate the disease in Greece. With the use of DDT to eliminate the *Anopheles* mosquito and chemicals to treat the existing cases a near miracle was achieved, not only in terms of health but in terms of the nation's food supply. Agricultural production was increased by 40% so that more milk, poultry, olives, and other foods were available to the people. In Greece the social implications of good health and adequate food were already obvious.

At the base of the Himalayan Mountains lies the Terai Plain with its rich soil needed to feed the hungry mouths of India. Because of widespread malaria, only wild animals such as tigers and elephants were able to live there. In 1945 an intensive program was instituted to eliminate the *Anopheles* mosquito and by 1949, 35,000 acres were planted in wheat, rice, and fruits, and eleven industrial plants were in operation. It is the only event on record in which DDT eradicated tigers. In Africa the elimination of insect-borne diseases alone would make 4½ million square miles of land available for agricultural purposes. This is an area 50% greater than the 3,022,000 square miles of the United States.

APPRAISAL

It is to America's advantage to assist the underdeveloped nations in improving both their health and their economies. Pearl Buck has stated from firsthand observation: "Democracy cannot flower in the weeds of want and abject poverty." Prolonged poverty leads to lethargy, further famine, and disease. America's Point IV Program seeks to make her technological advancements available to the underdeveloped nations. Soil fertility, better seed, the use of fertilizers, agricultural mechanization, and parasite destruction are advancements that Americans can make available to those nations with teeming millions who are ill fed, ill housed, ill clothed, short lived, and exist under deplorable conditions.

Nations digressing from plenty to poverty become aggressive and even belligerent. Germany and Japan are classic examples. To maintain peace and promote its own welfare, America must contribute to the health and welfare of the peoples of other nations. Biological pressures are the principal roots of major wars; through health promotion, related to economic development, America can assist in removing biological pressures. If the United Nations survives it will be because the biological roots of man have been overcome. The greatest barrier to a solution to the present world situation is self-interest. Nations and people alike share with reluctance. Each clings to his resources. America must share its technical know-how in the field of health promotion for corollary to health promotion is to make available America's technical know-how in agricultural production. Better health for other nations will mean a more healthful and peaceful world in which America can live. What has a beneficial effect on the health of the people in other nations indirectly will have a health value for the people of our own nation.

Control of the birthrate is the other half of the population equation. Unless underprivileged nations take effective measures to bring their birthrates to an approximation to optimum food production, famine and disease will still stalk their people. The technological know-how of contraception should be made available to these nations, just as other knowledge has been given to them. Because of resistance from centuries-long traditions, religious dogma, and even ignorance, 50 years may elapse before a tangible balance is attained between population increase and food production. At the present time the world population is increasing at a rate of 2.0% a year compared with the population increase of 1.1% in the United States. For the United States, as well as the world, a goal of zero population growth is still a long way into the future.

QUESTIONS AND EXERCISES

1. Explain this statement: "Man is born a biologic being, he has to become a social being."
2. What evidence is there that the human being possesses an inherent drive to survive?
3. What evidence is there that the advances in health sciences have had a dysgenic effect on America's population?
4. What is meant by the conservation of human resources?
5. Analyze this statement: "Citizens of the southern states do not live as long as those in the northern states because of the south's excessive heat."
6. For the past 30 years the Alaskan glaciers have been reducing rapidly. What interpretation do you make of this and what is the significance of the phenomenon?
7. Speculate as to what effect a constantly rising world temperature will have upon life expectancy, health, the economy, and the general culture of the southern states, the northern states, Canada, Russia, the Scandinavian nations, and the Mediterranean nations.
8. In what type of nation does the Malthusean theory

hold and in what type of nation does it not hold?

9. Predict the world population for the year 2,000 and present the factors that were considered in arriving at your estimate.

10. What is meant by saying that man is able to push his population limit upward?

11. One county with a vital index of 16 has a neighboring county with a vital index of 4. What differences would you expect to find in the two counties?

12. Why should America make its technologic knowhow of disease control available to all nations?

13. Appraise the present practice of having "teams" of specialists in disease control programs.

14. What are the social and health implications in the decline in America's farm population?

15. What will be the health consequences of agricultural production advancing at a rate slower than the rate of population increase and when will this occur in the United States?

16. How do population changes affect the economic, political, social, and cultural life of a nation?

17. What has been the effect of the discovery of DDT on the health and culture of the world?

18. What has been the effect of advances in agricultural technology on the health and culture of the world?

19. Analyze this statement: "Clear up disease and you promote starvation because there will be more mouths to feed."

20. How does health conservation promote peace?

REFERENCES

Broughey, A. S.: Man and the environment: an introduction to human ecology, New York, 1971, The Macmillan Co.

Chute, R. M., editor: Environmental insight, New York, 1971, Harper & Row, Publishers.

Cox, G. W., editor: Readings in conservation ecology, New York, 1969, Appleton-Century-Crofts.

Darnell, R.: Ecology, Dubuque, Ia., 1972, William C. Brown Co., Publishers.

Hertzler, J. O.: The crisis in world populations, Lincoln, 1967, University of Nebraska Press.

Howe, E. E., and associates: An approach toward the solution of the world food problem with special emphasis upon protein supply, American Journal of Clinical Nutrition **20:**1134, 1967.

Lockley, R. M.: Man against nature, New York, 1971, International Publishers Co., Inc.

Odum, H. T.: Environment, power and society, New York, 1971, John Wiley & Sons, Inc.

Prohansky, H.: Environmental psychology: man and his physical setting, New York, 1970, Holt, Rinehart and Winston, Inc.

Regal, J. M.: Oakland's partnership for change, Oakland, Calif., 1967, City of Oakland Department of Human Resources.

Ridgeway, J.: Politics of ecology, New York, 1971, E. P. Dutton & Co., Inc.

Scott, J. M.: Rain—man's greatest gift; the story of water, San Bernardino, Cal., 1967, Culligan Book Co.

Shimkins, D. B.: Man, ecology, and health, Archives of Environmental Health **20:**111, 1970.

Stevens, K. M.: Ecology and etiology of human disease. Springfield, Ill., 1967, Charles C Thomas, Publisher.

World population growth and response, 1965-1975, Washington, D.C., April 1976, Population Reference Bureau, Inc.

4 ▪ LIFE EXTENSION

*Life is like a game of tables, the chances are
not in our power, but the playing is.*

Terence

How long we live is of concern to all of us. That more human beings survive to later years than in past generations is generally recognized in America. During the past half-century, man has been able to make spectacular gains in life expectancy and he is optimistic that he can continue his great strides in extending the average length of human life. Evidence presently available would seem to indicate that man's greatest advance in the extension of life on earth is behind him and that henceforth extending life expectancy will be a more difficult task and increases will proceed at a much slower rate. However, this statement is made on the assumption that our present conception of human life-span is valid and that knowledge of disease prevention and cure and of the nature of the aging process will not advance spectacularly beyond our present levels. Man will solve many of these problems and will continue to push the ceiling of life expectancy upward.

LIFE-SPAN AND LIFE EXPECTANCY

Life-span and life expectancy are two different phenomena. Life-span is the recognized biologic limit of life. Based on present knowledge, biologists tend to set the human life-span at 120 years. They recognize that with an increase in our knowledge of the biology of man, this figure may be projected upward, perhaps by even more than 30 years. However, the figure is now set at 120 years because scientists do not possess reliable data of any human being living beyond this age. The usual report of some person living beyond 120 years always emanates from primitive areas where unreliable records, or no records at all exist. Biologists acknowledge that in all probability even the person who lives to age 115 years has shortened his life by adverse health practices. Scientists recognize that improper dietary practices, infections, excessive fatigue, prolonged exposure, inadequate rest, and other factors may well have shortened the life of the person who lives to age 115. Obviously, not all people have a life-span of 120 years. Some people likely have a life-span considerably below 100 years. This is indicated by failure of any member in some lineages to reach the age of 60 years. Life-span is an inherited characteristic that is determined at the time of the fertilization of the ovum by the sperm. Man can do nothing to extend the span but he inadvertently does many things to prevent realization of his life-span.

By life expectancy is meant the average duration of time that individuals of a given age can expect to live, based on the longevity experience of the population. Expectancy is expressed as the average number of years an individual of a given age can expect to live. These averages are based on the assumption that the longevity experience of the immediately preceding years will prevail in the future. America's experience has been that future years likely will be favorable to an extension of longevity beyond what the immediate past years indicate. All averages on expectancy apply to the age group. Obviously individuals within a group will vary, some experiencing an expectancy considerably above the average and some below the average. Americans are prone to assume that they possess the greatest life expectancy of any people in the world. Data from the World Health Organization should cause Americans to reflect on their relative world position in terms of life expectancy. With all of America's medical, hospital, and other health facilities, along with her favorable economic position, it is natural to assume that she would lead the world in longevity.

Women in America have a very favorable life expectancy as compared with the women of other nations, but America's men do not fare so well. As Table 4-1 reveals, even at birth the American male has a shorter life expectation than the males of twenty-one other nations. However, even more disturbing is the fact that by the time the American male has reached the age of 40 years, his life expectancy is less than that of the men of nineteen other nations.

America's position is not altogether unfavorable. With the strides that she has made in her life extension during the past 65 years,

Table 4-1 ■ Expectation of life at birth in selected nations (indicated year in parenthesis); Demographic yearbook, 1975

Country	Male	Female
Sweden (1975)	72.1	77.5
Norway (1975)	71.3	77.6
Netherlands (1975)	71.2	77.2
Japan (1974)	71.2	76.3
Denmark (1974)	70.8	76.3
Iceland (1975)	70.7	76.3
Switzerland (1975)	70.3	76.2
Spain (1975)	69.7	75.0
Canada (1974)	69.3	76.3
Italy (1974)	69.1	74.9
England and Wales (1974)	68.9	75.1
Germany, East (1974)	68.8	74.2
France (1974)	68.6	76.4
New Zealand (European) (1974)	68.6	74.6
Iceland (1974)	68.6	72.3
Israel (1975)	68.5	72.8
United States (1975)	68.2	75.9
Belgium (1974)	67.8	74.2
Germany, West (1974)	67.6	74.1
Austria (1975)	67.4	74.7
Scotland (1975)	67.2	73.6
Hungary (1975)	66.9	72.6
Finland (1975)	66.6	74.9
Northern Ireland (1975)	65.0	73.6
Union of Soviet Socialist Republics (1975)	64.0	74.0
Mexico (1970-1975)	61.0	63.7
India (1973)	41.9	40.6

America has reason to feel confident that she can extend her life expectancy appreciably during the next 65 years. During the first 65 years of the present century, America extended her life expectation at birth by about 25 years. No recognized biometrist would predict that America will extend life expectation by an equal amount during the next 65 years, but the extension of life expectance at birth by as much as 10 years in the United States during the next 65 years is entirely possible.

Extension of life expectancy

In the United States during the period from 1900 to 1968, life expectancy at birth increased by 21 years for white males, 26 years for white females, 28 years for nonwhite males, and 34 years for nonwhite females. For nonwhite as well as white citizens, there has been a greater improvement in the life expectancy of the female than of the male.

The greatest gain in life expectancy during the first half of the twentieth century can

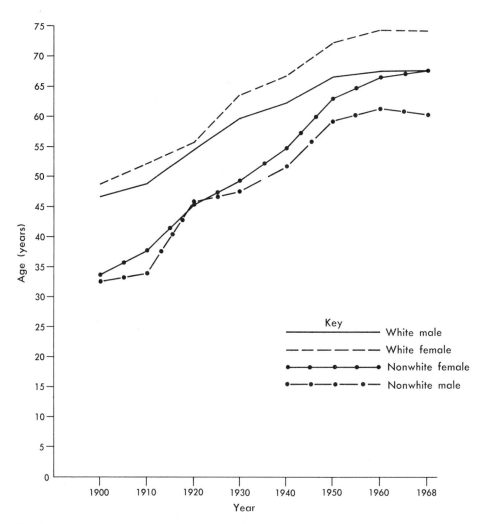

Fig. 4-1. Estimated average length of life in years at birth, United States, 1900 to 1968. (From reports of the National Centers for Health Statistics)

be attributed to the prevention of deaths in infancy and childhood. However, in recent years progress has been made in extending the length of life by the postponement of death in the later age brackets so that in 1968 life expectation of a person of 40 was actually more than 6 years greater than the life expectation of a person of 40 in the year 1900. However, this increase has become minimal and may well have leveled off.

Data on life expectation at birth are important, but equally significant are data on life expectancy at various ages. Studies indicate that college graduates have a greater life expectancy than that of the general population. Even noncollege graduates, by the application of sound health principles and the utilization of available medical and health facilities and services, can extend their life expectation considerably beyond the average if they possess a basic biological endowment or life-span of over 100 years.

A phenomenon of interest but without an adequate explanation is that the people of seven Midwestern states consistently have a greater life expectancy than that of the people of other states in the nation. Iowa, Kansas, Minnesota, Nebraska, North Dakota, Oklahoma, and South Dakota regularly exceed the national life expectation figures by at least 2 years and occasionally 3 years for both the male and the female. No acceptable explanation of this phenomenon has been made. The national origin of the population, economic means, climate, vocations, living practices, and other factors have been analyzed, but nothing has been discovered that distinguishes the population of these states from the population of other states.

FACTORS DETERMINING LIFE EXPECTATION

Longevity is a general term that incorporates a vast number of factors significant to individuals who are interested in appraising their own life expectancy. Fortunately, no one knows precisely what his or her life ex-

pectancy is, but it is possible to establish the approximate probable lifetime by considering the various factors that seem to determine how long one lives.

Race. Tables dealing with life expectation indicate that the racial factor is important in longevity. At the time of birth, in 1968, the white male in America had a life expectancy of 7.4 years greater than the nonwhite male, and the white female had an expectancy of 7.4 years greater than the nonwhite female. These data doubtless conceal some economic factors that are adverse to the nonwhite individual.

After age 74 years, however, there is a crossover in the white/nonwhite rates in both sexes. Whites enjoy lower mortality rates until age 74 years, when nonwhite rates become lower and remain so. Nonwhites who have surmounted the cultural barriers and environmental hazards to health may represent a hardier group of survivors compared with their white counterparts of similar age.

Inheritance. Long-lived parents tend to have long-lived offspring. What actually is transmitted is not the abstraction, long life, but rather the adequate body structure, the efficiently functioning organs and systems, resistance to diseases, the ability to recover from injury or disease, the capacity to produce the necessary body enzymes, and the various other attributes necessary for long life. Studies in England on the nobility and upper-class families, conducted by Karl Pearson and M. Beaton, demonstrated a marked consistency between the length of life of parents and their offspring. In a comparable study, S. J. Holmes obtained the same findings.

Dr. Raymond Pearl, the American biometrist, utilized a different approach to avoid errors common in studies based on genealogies. Dr. Pearl devised the method of "Total Immediate Ancestral Longevity" (TIAL), which is the sum of the ages at death of both parents and all four grandparents of a given individual. There is little likelihood that the TIAL will fall below 100 or will exceed 600. Dr. Pearl found that for all of his subjects 90 years of age or over, (longevous group), 45.8% had two long-lived parents, while in the unselected subjects (control group), only 11.9% had two long-lived parents. The significant difference in the two percentages doubtless represents inherited endowment. The possibility remains that biased factors exist. A study was made by Dr. L. I. Dublin and H. H. Marks of 118,000 white males, ages 20 to 64 years, granted life insurance between 1899 and 1939. At every age the lowest death rate occurred for those men who had both parents living when the insurance was granted. At the other end of the scale, the death rate was highest among those men whose parents were both dead at the time the insurance was issued.

In considering the influence of inheritance on the length of life, one should not overlook the fact that living in a long-lived family usually means certain environmental advantages that could be favorable to longevity. Having both parents living to look after his welfare should be an aid to an individual in obtaining the highest possible portion of his potential, both in quality of health and length of life. Certainly gains in the longevity of the general population must be attributed to environmental gains rather than genetic changes. Inherited longevity still has its advantages in determining one's length of life, but with modern advances perhaps these advantages are not as great as they were at the turn of the century.

Gender. At birth, the American white female has an expectancy at least 7 years greater than the male, and the nonwhite female has approximately a 6-year advantage over the nonwhite male. Though the differential between the life expectancy of the female and the male declines during the ensuing years, she tends to have an advantage all through life. A woman appears to inherit a better constitution in terms of long-wearing qualities. She has less bulky musculature and more flexible soft tissues. She is less prone to heart disorders and arteriosclerosis. She has lower blood pressure and a higher white cell count, both of which are to her advantage. She has an advantage in not being called upon to do heavy manual labor. She rarely engages in hazardous occupations, and her accidental death rate is much lower than that of the male. Perhaps as important as any factor is that she lives under less daily tension. The American male seems to shorten his life by the intensity of his daily living and the tension that he experiences in his vocational pursuits. Women seem to possess both the means and the social encouragement to give release to their emotions, a practice the male could emulate to his benefit.

With emancipation of the female, however, her advantage in longevity may decrease. Adolescent groups now contain the same proportion of female cigarette smokers as males, although females smoke fewer cigarettes and inhale less. Unfortunately, they find it more difficult to stop smoking than males, and recidivism is higher in females. The habit of cigarette smoking is equated with freedom and social advancement in the advertisements directed at females. Obesity is more prevalent in females than in males, particularly in the lower socioeconomic groups. As females achieve economic parity with males, the differential in mortality rates may decline.

Occupation. The general designation of occupation as a factor in longevity incorporates a number of variables such as the types of individuals who go into the different occupations, the hazards in the occupations, the economic position of different occupations, and the educational background of men in the various occupations. Longest lived are clergymen, lawyers, engineers, teachers, doctors, and farmers, essentially in this order. Next longest lived are business executives, white collar workers, and skilled tradesmen. Shortest lived are the unskilled workers, miners, quarrymen, and granite workers.

Income. Favorable living conditions, associated with income, have a definite influence on longevity. Families with a favorable income are able to avail themselves of the best medical care, proper nutrition, good housing, and other advantages that make a longer life possible. People living in cities with a high level of income live longer than those living in cities of low income. The advantage conferred by high income is no longer effective, however, in very old age groups, that is, those over 85 years. After this age, genetic endowment is totally dominant, and socioeconomic status is of no influence on further life expectancy.

Marital status. Married men live longer than single men. Many men in poor health prefer to remain single, which partially accounts for the shorter life expectancy of the single men. Doubtless the orderly life of the married man operates to his advantage in preserving his life. Among women, the picture of longevity varies. Up to the age of 40, married women have a greater life expectation than single women, but thereafter married women and unmarried women have the same life expectancy.

Body build. An individual inherits a particular type of body build that can be modified but little through nutrition or other means. While people of certain body builds live longer than those of other body types, no one is doomed to a short life expectation merely on the basis of his body build. People who are well built and of average height and weight tend to live longest. As a group, people of very large stature do not live as long as those who are smaller than average in height and weight. Extreme underweight during young adulthood has an adverse effect on length of life. Those who are somewhat underweight in later years tend to have a favorable life expectancy. Obesity, particularly in the later years of life, has an adverse effect on longevity. People more than 25% overweight have a 75% higher death rate than those in the average weight category.

Temperament and habits. Easygoing people outlive fast-paced and excitable individuals. Tension, overstrain, overeating, and general excessiveness associated with high-tension living tend to shorten life. Cigarette smoking and heavy drinking both reduce life expectation. Manual labor, even heavy manual labor, before the age of 40 does not appear to affect the length of life, but hard manual labor continued after the age of 40 years does appear to shorten life. Generally, people of a temperament that leads to a pattern of moderation in living reap benefits from their modes of life in terms of more years added to their lives.

Blood pressure. Low blood pressure, unless extremely low, favors longevity. The higher the blood pressure the shorter the life, partially resulting from the relationship of blood pressure to heart and kidney disorders and stroke. An unusually rapid or irregular pulse is usually associated with short life expectancy. Individuals with high blood pressure or with rapid pulse need not assume the fatalistic attitude that they are doomed to a short life and can do nothing to extend their expectation. Modern medical treatment and their own efforts can have a significant effect on postponing death.

INDIVIDUAL APPLICATIONS

Both the individual and the community can take effective measures to extend life expectancy. If each of us knew precisely what the cause of his death will be, it would be possible to concentrate our efforts on one specific problem in survival. Fortunately, no normal person can predict with accuracy what the cause of his death will be, but one can study the most likely causes of death. We know that more than 76% of all deaths this year will result from three causes: cardiovascular diseases, cancer, and accidents. Breaking these data down on the basis of age groups, we can be more specific in concentrating our attention on the most likely cause of our death. In addition, if the citizens of a community were informed on what they can do to promote their own quality of health and postpone death, life expectation could be extended appreciably in that community.

A community can contribute to life expectation through an effective program of health education that gives citizens a knowledge of what they as individuals can do to promote their present health. Individuals should be concerned about the condition of their heart, arteries, kidneys, lungs, and other vital structures. Periodic medical and dental examinations would give them an appraisal of the condition of these structures and warn them against the development of the various chronic disorders of adulthood. People need to adopt a positive health-oriented mode of behavior, emphasizing proper diet and rest, regular exercise, and avoidance of tobacco and alcohol. A life-style of moderation with a value system geared to health results in zestful living and longevity. A community program of adult health promotion that emphasizes the annual medical examination with a suitable follow-up should yield tangible results in extending the life expectancy of citizens.

Any community with adequate medical and health services and facilities is contributing to the life expectancy of its citizens. The extent to which these services and facilities actually contribute to the postponement of death will depend on the understanding that citizens have of these services and facilities and the extent to which they avail themselves of the medical and health services in their community.

Research and the understanding, prevention and control of heart disease, cancer, and other of the principal causes of death will largely determine the future extension of life expectancy. A single breakthrough on the problem of cancer may well have a marked influence on life expectation. New methods and techniques in heart surgery could increase life expectation at age 50 by several years. Inroads on the accidental death rate could have a profound effect on life expectation. A community might well visualize what the effect on the longevity of its citizens would be if deaths resulting from accidents were halved within the next year.

Promoting community health in virtually all spheres will have some influence on life expectation. Maternal, infant, and child health programs, adult health programs, prevention of disorders, communicable disease control measures, safety promotion, industrial hygiene programs, reduction of alcoholism, improved sanitation, programs to deal with disasters, and the extension of community health services, directly and indirectly, influence the length of life people of the community will enjoy. Because we know the specific leading causes of death, we have specific targets toward which to direct our efforts. Programs can be directed into channels leading to likely dividends. This holds true for a community program, and it is equally true for the individual. Knowing statistically what the causes of his death most likely will be, the wise person will utilize all of the measures, devices, and services available to aid in postponing his or her death. Perhaps a word to the wise is superfluous.

QUESTIONS AND EXERCISES

1. Identify some families that doubtless have a long life-span and some families that appear to have a short life-span.
2. Why does Sweden have a greater life expectation than the United States?
3. What factors probably account for the poor life expectancy of the American male at age 50?
4. What great discoveries would be instrumental in extending American life at least 10 years by the year 2000?
5. Why do females in the United States live longer than males?
6. Explain the paradox that a child born in the United States can expect to live a greater number of years after his first birthday anniversary than after the day on which he was born.
7. Why do college graduates have a greater life expectation at age 30 than people of the same age who have not attended college?
8. What is the role of economics in life expectancy?
9. Why may the early death of parents have an adverse effect upon the life expectancy of their offspring?
10. What is the social and the economic significance of the American wife outliving her husband by an average of 8 years?
11. What factors are favorable for a long life for clergymen?
12. Cigarette smoking markedly increases the risk for certain major diseases. List four.
13. Appraise your own present health status in terms of life expectancy.
14. Evaluate the attitude of people who do not want to know that they have a disability.

15. What can a community do to counteract this point of view?
16. Study the established health practices of five of your acquaintances who are more than 70 years of age. What did you learn of value to you?
17. How would you proceed to make this knowledge available to the citizens of your community?
18. Consider the program to educate our teen-agers not to smoke. How could this program be extended to include all factors that most threaten a long life?
19. To what degree is the extension of life expectancy a matter of community education?
20. Which is most important—a long life, an enjoyable life, or a productive life, and are the three incompatible for one individual?

REFERENCES

Bureau of the Census, U.S. Department of Commerce: Statistical abstract of the United States, Current, Washington, D.C., Bureau of the Census.

Cassedy, J. H.: Demography in early America: beginnings of the statistical mind, Cambridge, Mass., 1969, Harvard University Press.

Holder, L.: Education for health in a changing society, American Journal of Public Health **60:**2307, 1970.

National Vital Statistics Division: Vital statistics of the United States, Washington, D.C., Annual, Government Printing Office.

World Health Organization: Demographic yearbook, Geneva, Switzerland, Annual, World Health Organization.

PART II

Promoting community health

5 ▪ MATERNAL, INFANT, AND CHILD HEALTH

Their mother hearts beset with fears,
Their lives bound up in tender years.

Christina Rossetti

Promoting the health of a community means promoting the health of its citizens. A community health program should be organized on a basis that recognizes the special health needs and the different health problems of the various segments within the population. Health problems of the expectant mother, the infant, the child, the adult, and the aging have many things in common, but each category has special aspects of these common problems as well as unique problems. Community measures to promote the health of one group frequently will be applicable to the needs of other groups, but directing the community's attention to the specific needs of a particular population segment will assure the necessary measures to protect and promote the health and general well-being of that specific group.

PROGRESS IN MATERNAL HEALTH PROMOTION

At the turn of the century, when America's population was about 76 million, more than 20,000 women died in childbirth each year. Some 70 years later, with a population of more than 200 million, the yearly number of deaths of women resulting from complications of childbirth has been reduced to less than 500. The chances of a woman's surviving childbirth in America today are about 7,999 out of 8,000. This improvement in survival should continue.

Maternal mortality rates

Maternal deaths are those associated with deliveries and complications of pregnancy, childbirth, and puerperium. Rates are on a basis of 100,000 live births occurring in a given year to mothers of each age and racial group. Data from the National Center for Health Statistics indicated that the maternal death rate in the United States for 1971 was approximately 2.6% of what it was in 1915. For the white race, the maternal mortality rate in 1971 was only 1.9% of what it was in 1915. The maternal mortality rate for nonwhite mothers has also declined to 3.6% of the 1915 rate, but in 1971 the nonwhite rate was 3.5 times the white rate.

The causes of maternal mortality have altered, reflecting the relative decline of hemorrhage, infection, and toxemia. Anesthetic misadventures are relatively more common now as other causes have decreased and as the number of patients receiving anesthesia for childbirth has increased. Paradoxically, advances in medicine have provided challenges in obstetrics. Patients with congenital heart disease as well as juvenile diabetics are now able to become pregnant, and their safe delivery demands skill. The contributions of abortion to maternal mortality have dramatically decreased with safe legalized abortions in contrast to criminal septic abortions. Widespread availability of effective contraceptive technics has reduced the number of

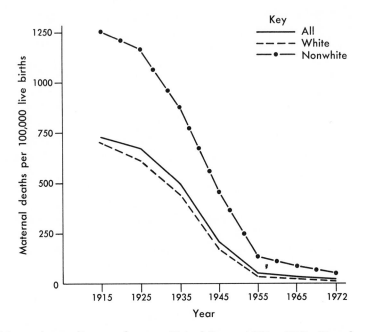

Fig. 5-1. Maternal mortality rates by race, United States, 1915 to 1972. (Data from Vital statistics of the United States, vol. 2, 1973)

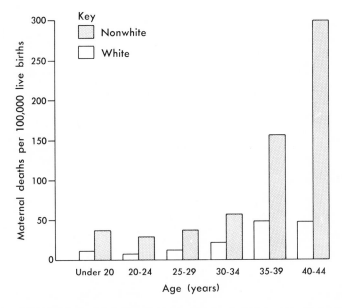

Fig. 5-2. Maternal mortality rates by age and race, United States, 1972. (Data from Vital statistics of the United States, vol. 2, 1973)

unwanted pregnancies, which in turn has reduced maternal mortality. The radical changes in abortion laws and contraceptive use are the result of societal pressures to which medicine has responded. In 1976 1 million pregnancies occurred in girls age 17 years or less, and 600,000 of these resulted in live births. This represented almost 20% of the total 3,128,000 live births in 1976. Society has adjusted to this fact by providing for continuation of schooling during and following pregnancy. Pregnancy is no longer the leading cause of school dropouts, which it was prior to 1975. Women now have choices available in planning children by means of contraception, terminating unwanted pregnancies by abortion, and antenatal services for safe delivery. The community role lies in making potential users of these options aware of them and counseling as to appropriate choice. Early and reliable preg-

nancy testing is now available. This is important since antenatal care should be sought early in pregnancy, during the first 3 months.

Legal abortions

Safety of abortions is closely correlated with the stage of pregnancy; abortion performed at less than 12 weeks of gestation, when suction curettage is used, is very safe, with a mortality rate of only one tenth of the low rate prevailing at term delivery.

Direct means for promoting maternal health

Antenatal care emphasizes early detection of abnormalities and identification of the high-risk mother and infant. At the first visit a complete medical, surgical, and obstetrical history is obtained, and a physical examination is performed. Routine laboratory data are obtained, including blood type and rhe-

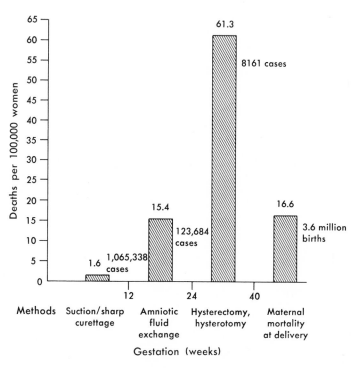

Fig. 5-3. Death-to-case ratio for legal abortions, by method, United States, 1972 to 1973. (From Center for Disease Control, MMWD Morbidity and Mortality Weekly Report, vol. 22, no. 53, Dec. 29, 1973)

sus factor determination; urinalysis; complete blood count; rubella titer; tests for syphilis, gonorrhea, and abnormalities of hemoglobin synthesis (sickle cell); and cervical smear. A social worker may interview the couple and discuss the community resources that are available. The antenatal visits provide an opportunity for education in health-related behavior, including dental care, avoidance or reduction of cigarette smoking, balanced exercise, and rest. A supportive, nonjudgmental, warm, sympathetic climate is maintained, so that communication and compliance is enhanced between patient and provider, and responsibility is shared. Precautions in the early stages of pregnancy include avoidance of infection, avoidance of exposure to irradiation, and avoidance of ingestion of drugs. These three factors contribute to congenital defects. Nutrition in pregnancy is most important, and the diet must contain adequate protein. Nutrition maintenance should be a continuum, with infancy, childhood, pregnancy, lactation, and geriatrics being special points along it. Women should be prepared for safe childbearing by adequate nutrition before pregnancy, rather than merely during it. Height of the mother is important, for taller women have larger pelvic bones, and as height falls below 5 feet the percentage of mothers experiencing difficulty in delivery resulting from pelvic problems increases sharply. Height is related to nutrition during the growth period, before the epiphyses close and bone growth ceases. Also important is nutrition in adolescence, after growth ceases but before pregnancy occurs, or preconception nutrition. Mothers who are normal or overweight have a better pregnancy outcome than those who are underweight.

High-risk pregnancies can be identified, and these are cared for in special clinics. Predictors are age, particularly under 15 or over 35 years; previous obstetrical difficulty such as unexplained stillbirths, premature deliveries, and abortions; and mothers who are under 60 inches in height or those who smoke a pack of cigarettes daily. Education for childbirth should start at school in human biology studies. During pregnancy the most effective education is in peer group sessions, when experienced mothers can lead others. The removal of fear is of greatest benefit, and attendance of fathers is of value in sharing. Visits to the delivery and newborn suites and meeting the staff are beneficial. Various groups endorse different plans of preparation

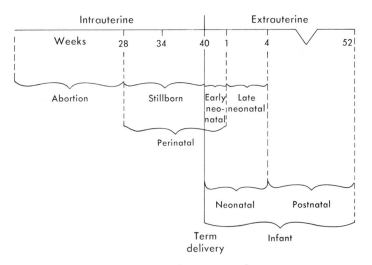

Fig. 5-4. Reproductive mortality rates.

and practices during childbirth, but the common thread is of open discussion, question and answer, and removal of fear. Couples in such programs will enjoy the emotional experience of pregnancy and delivery.

Perinatal mortality is the number of fetal deaths (stillbirths) from the twenty-eighth week of pregnancy plus the number of deaths in the first week of life per 1,000 live births. This reproductive index comprises both intrauterine and extrauterine deaths and is a measure of the efficiency of the obstetrical and neonatal services. Deaths that occur during this time span may be ascribed to haz-

ards of the birth process. Perinatal mortality is most heavily influenced by the prematurity rate, which is the percentage of all babies born who weigh 2,500 grams or less (5½ pounds). The survival of such infants is naturally lower than that of term-sized infants, mainly because the respiratory system of premature infants is not sufficiently mature to adapt to extrauterine life. Advances in neonatology, through the use of intensive care nurseries or prematurity centers, have been tremendous so that survival is improving for all birthweight ranges. The perinatal mortality rate is falling, but its decline is limited

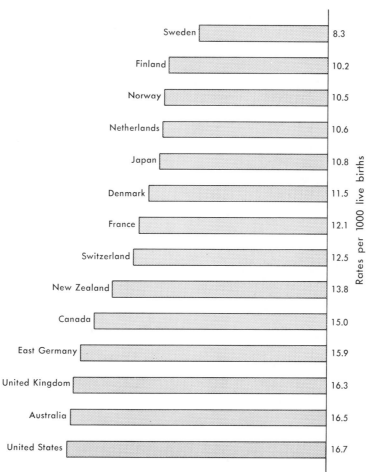

Fig. 5-5. Infant mortality, selected countries, 1975. (From World Health Organization: Demographic yearbook, Geneva, Switzerland, 1975, World Health Organization)

by the prematurity rate, which has remained constant since 1950. It was thought that the prematurity rate would fall in response to improved social conditions, but a complex interaction of factors has been operating. A high proportion of births now derive from adolescent mothers and those in lower socioeconomic strata, and both these groups have increased prematurity rates. Mothers aged less than 15 years had a prematurity rate of 15.8% in 1973 contrasted with an overall prematurity rate of 7.6% in that year. Risk factors for prematurity include (1) previous history of premature delivery, (2) age less than 15 years, (3) lower socioeconomic group, (4) height under 60 inches, (5) more than 15% underweight, and (6) a history of cigarette smoking. These factors are interrelated and are amenable to community influence in nutrition, in family planning, and in health education. There tends to be a continuum of pregnancy wastage, and it is necessary to break the cycle of poverty and deprivation.

Infant mortality is the number of deaths occurring under 1 year of age per 1,000 live births. It will be appreciated that deaths in the first week of life contribute both to perinatal and infant mortalities. International comparisons of infant mortalities are often made; however, it must be kept in mind that infant mortality in advanced countries is much influenced by deaths in the first month of life, which comprise 80% of the deaths in the first year. This high proportion results from the reduction in deaths caused by infectious causes, which earlier in this century contributed to the high infant mortality rate (Fig. 5-6). Reduction of infant mortality depends now on reducing deaths immediately following birth. This in turn means reducing the prematurity rate. Countries that have low infant mortalities, for example, Norway and Sweden, have prematurity rates of about 3% compared with 7.6% in the United States. Weight for weight, babies have a higher survival rate in the United States than in any other country because of our advanced neonatology. But in the United States we have to contend with relatively more low birthweight babies, which adversely affects our reproductive indices. Improvements will also stem from reduction in the needless waste of

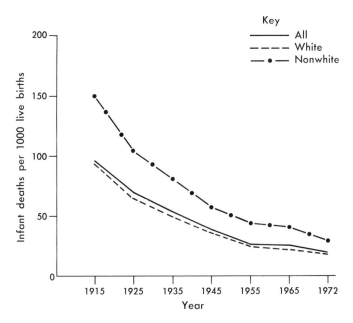

Fig. 5-6. Infant mortality rates per 1,000 live births, United States, 1915 to 1972. (Data from Vital statistics of the United States, vol. 2, 1973)

infant lives caused by accidents and by infectious diseases. Community action is effective here in providing a safe environment by legislation; immunization programs; reduction of burns, traffic accidents, alcoholism, and child abuse; and education of mothers to bring their children to a doctor early in illness, when infectious disease may be successfully treated. Adequate provision of community resources to provide alternate child care facilities for working mothers is imperative.

COMMUNITY HEALTH PROGRAMS FOR CHILDREN

Basic health services for the prevention of disease and the early identification of illness or disability should be available to all children. Well-child clinics providing assessment of growth and development, nutrition, nurturing and anticipatory guidance, and immunization for all children should be available. Well-child care at regular intervals may be performed by allied health personnel other than physicians. Competent pediat-

ric nurse practitioners, experienced public health nurses, and all physician's assistants working in tandem with psychologists and educators can assess the progress of a child, interpreting these steps and the next to be expected to the person caring for the child.

Fostering the mother-infant bonding and utilizing anticipatory guidance to prevent problems will enable the child to grow up in a healthy and well-structured atmosphere. Early recognition of social and psychological components will permit early and simple correction of adverse circumstances.

Basic health services with well-child clinics should also include an immunization program.

Active immunization procedures

Active immunization of infants and children provides an effective means of disease prevention and health maintenance. In its report the American Academy of Pediatrics Infectious Disease Committee recommends that no single set of considerations be applied

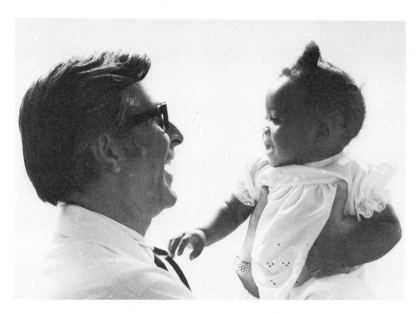

Fig. 5-7. Child health promotion. The health department medical and nursing staff conducts routine and special examinations of well children in ambulatory clinics. (Courtesy Johns Hopkins Medical Institutions)

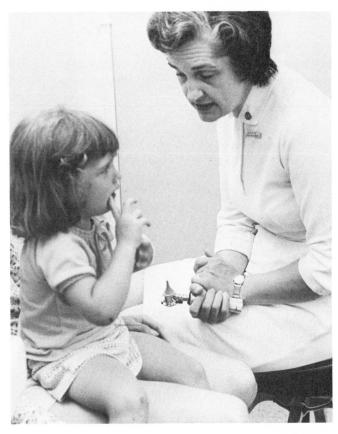

Fig. 5-8. Health education for parents and children. Clinical settings tend to maximize the quality but minimize the quantity of information effectively transmitted. (Courtesy Johns Hopkins Medical Institutions)

for the use of these vaccines in all situations in patients. A number of factors in each community must be considered in preparing a schedule for the active immunization of healthy infants and children. These factors include the following:

1. The current risk from the disease for which active immunization is available
2. The characteristics of the vaccines, particularly their efficacy and safety
3. The most efficient and expeditious ways to use the vaccine within the general framework and patterns of good health care for that community

The generally recommended age to begin routine immunizations is 2 months. The first vaccines given are diphtheria and tetanus toxoids combined with pertussis vaccine or DTP, in addition to trivalent oral poliovirus vaccine, TOPV. Measles vaccine for rubeola is most effective when given after 1 year of age because all maternal transplacental antibody has been catabolized by then. In some populations where natural measles occurs frequently in the first year of life, it is indicated to administer the rubeola vaccine as early as 6 months of age. If this is necessary in this community, a repeat dose of measles vaccine should then be given after the age of 1 year to immunize any infants whose earlier vaccine response had been blocked by passive immunity.

Neither the depot nor the "plain" triple antigens have been widely used on patients more than 6 years of age because of the possibility of reactions to either diphtheria or

Table 5-1 ■ Recommended schedule of active immunization of normal infants and children

Age	Vaccine	
2 months	DTP	TOPV
4 months	DTP	TOPV
6 months	DTP	TOPV
1 year	Measles Rubella	Tuberculin test Mumps
1½ years	DTP	TOPV
4-6 years	DTP	TOPV
14-16 years	Td* and thereafter every 10 years	

*Td-combined tetanus and diphtheria toxoids (adult type) for children more than 6 years of age in contrast to diphtheria and tetanus (DT), which contains a larger amount of diphtheria antigen.

Table 5-2 ■ Recommended schedule of active immunization of children 1 through 5 years of age

Time of inoculation	Vaccine
First visit	DTP, TOPV, tuberculin test
1 month later	Measles, rubella, mumps
2 months later	DTP, TOPV
4 months later	DTP, TOPV
6 to 12 months later or preschool	DTP, TOPV
14-16 years	Td—continue every 10 years

pertussis antigen. There is abundant evidence that untoward reactions to diphtheria antigen increase with age. The adult type of combined tetanus-diphtheria toxoid (Td) is the recommended product for children more than 6 years of age and for adults.

Interruption of the recommended schedule, with a delay between doses, does not interfere with the final immunity achieved, nor does it necessitate starting the series over again, regardless of the length of time elapsed. It is important that the family keep a personal immunization card to record a child's history. This record is valuable for public health agencies especially during epidemics, because it indicates readily which children are protected against the disease.

Primary immunization of children not immunized in infancy

Children less than 6 years may be immunized with depot triple antigen (DTP), using three doses intramuscularly at intervals of 4 to 8 weeks. This would be particularly important in the outbreak of one of the diseases. For children more than 6 years of age, adult type of tetanus-diphtheria (Td) toxoid is preferred. Pertussis vaccine at this age is not regularly recommended, but it may be used in special circumstances. Live attenuated measles, mumps, and rubella vaccines may be used in persons of any age if no contraindication exists. Similarly, live poliovirus vaccines may be used for older children and adolescents.

Immunization of children in institutions and day-care centers

Children in institutions and day-care centers may be exposed to communicable diseases; therefore, careful attention to immunization is advised for healthy, institutionalized children.

Selected screening programs

Screening for tuberculosis prior to rubeola vaccine should be performed routinely. In addition a hematocrit for anemia during the

Table 5-3 ■ Recommended schedule of active immunization of children 6 years of age and over

Time of inoculation	Vaccine
First visit	Td, TOPV, tuberculin test
1 month later	Measles, rubella, mumps
2 months later	Td, TOPV
6 to 12 months later	Td, TOPV
14-16 years	Td—continue every 10 years

first 6 months of life should be done on all children. This is particularly important in the small birth weight infant who has grown quickly.

Other diseases to be screened for depend on the community and the population at risk. Thus screening for sickle cell anemia, Tay-Sachs disease, thalassemia, etc. should be done if the population is of the appropriate ethnic origin.

Screening should be carefully performed for illness prior to placement in day-care centers or prenursery school situations. It should be repeated again for the preschool physical examination, and hearing, speech, and eye examinations should be performed. Routine screening for these conditions can be performed by trained paramedical personnel. Dental evaluation and fluoride therapy for the prevention of caries are also necessary.

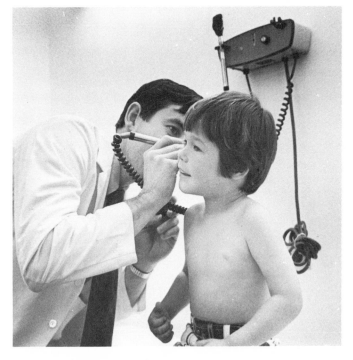

Fig. 5-9. Child health promotion. The health department medical staff conducts routine and special examinations of children. (Courtesy Marion County, Oregon, Health Department)

Table 5-4 ■ Federal programs for children

Program	Office	Comments
Maternal and Child Health (MCH)	DHEW, Health Services Administration (PHS)	Financial support to extend and improve services for reducing infant mortality and improvement of the health of mothers and children; special projects of national significance
Crippled Children's Services (CC)	DHEW, Health Services Administration (PHS)	Financial support to the states to improve medical-related services to crippled children and for special projects contributing to services for crippled children
Developmental Disabilities (DD)	DHEW, Social and Rehabilitation Service	A comprehensive plan for the administration and distribution of federal resources for the developmentally disabled
Early and Periodic Screening, Diagnosis and Treatment (EPSDT)	DHEW, Social and Rehabilitation Service	Assistance to states to provide EPSDT services to Medicaid children under age 21 years
Sudden Infant Death Syndrome (SIDS)	DHEW, Maternal and Child Health (PHS)	
Child Abuse	DHEW, Assistant Secretary for Human Development	
Immunization Program	DHEW, Center for Disease Control	
Sexually Transmitted Diseases	DHEW, Center for Disease Control	
Title I—Education/Health	DHEW, Office of Education	Formula grants to local educational agencies to expand and improve the educational programs to meet the special needs of educationally deprived children
Head Start	DHEW, Assistant Secretary for Human Development	Project grants and research contracts to provide educational, nutritional, and social services to preschool children of the poor and their families so that the child enters school on equal terms with less deprived classmates
Vocational Rehabilitation	DHEW, Social and Rehabilitation Service	
Mental Health	DHEW, Alcohol, Drug Abuse and Mental Health Service (PHS)	Funds authorized on a matching basis for initial staffing of facilities offering mental health services for children

*From MacQueen, J. C.: The provision of contemporary child health services through community child centers, Iowa City, Iowa, October 1976.

Continued.

Table 5-4 ■ Federal programs for children—cont'd

Program	Office	Comments
Day Care	DHEW, Social and Rehabilitation Service	Funding to state welfare agencies to provide child care and supportive services to WIN registrants and participants in WIN employment and training programs
Women, Infants, Children (WIC) Food Program	Department of Agriculture, Food and Nutritional Service	Assistance to provide nutritious food to participants identified as nutritional risks
Migrant Program	DHEW, Office of Education	Formula grants to expand and improve educational programs for children of migratory agricultural workers

School health education programs

Educational programs within the school setting aimed at preparing children for parenthood as well as their personal hygiene, nutrition, and sexuality should be instituted on a community-wide basis. The cooperation of the schools should be sought since children are a captive audience during their school hours. Furthermore, attendance of parents at school functions enables an extension of health education to the family.

Health services for chronic disease and disorders

Special health services for chronic disease and disorders such as cerebral palsy, epilepsy, congenital malformations, etc. require careful planning within the community. Different health professionals need to be involved, and continuity as well as comprehensiveness of care are essential to prepare the child for the best quality of life possible. Much of the care may be provided by nonmedical providers, particularly in the educational setting in other areas in the community. Unfortunately, because of the large number of programs that provide services for different problems, obtaining care may reveal a frustrating maze. Many programs provide only parts of the full care needs for each child, and each program may have different eligibility rules as well as a separate point of entry that is often difficult to locate.

In complicated congenital deformities such as meningomyelocele, children frequently require the services of more than one program and/or need a service that is not provided within the community in which they live. There is no greater deterrent to the effective and efficient provision of health services for children with chronic disease than the fragmentation of services as a result of the creation of categorical programs.

Clinics that are aimed at the physically handicapped, with all the related physiotherapy and educational needs provided for in that particular child, may not be adaptable for children with straightforward educational problems lacking the physical components.

Habilitation programs for an orthopedic deformity may not be available for children damaged by trauma. Again, the fusing eligibility and elimination rules may result in children slipping between the cracks of programs that are narrowly categorical.

During the past 40 years in the United States many programs have been developed by the federal government and by the states to provide some health services for children. These programs have had a major role in improving the health of the nation's children. There is general agreement that for a number of reasons some of them are now less effective. The federal Maternal and Child Health

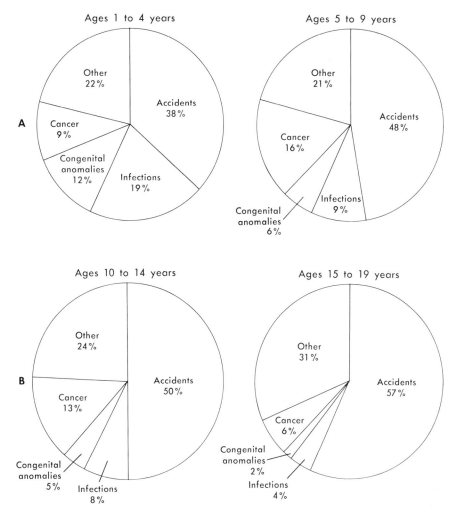

Fig. 5-10. Five leading causes of mortality for children, United States, 1971. (Data from Vital statistics of the United States, vol. 2, 1973)

(MCH) and Crippled Children's (CC) programs of Title V of the Social Security Act were created to provide national leadership in the field of maternal health and child health and to direct the state Maternal and Child Health and state Crippled Children's programs. Thus the state Maternal and Child Health programs remain the major providers of basic health services for mothers and children, and the state Crippled Children's programs remain the major public system for providing services for children who require special health services for chronic diseases and disorders. The legislation that created these programs did not relate them to community health programs as needed to provide a direct patient service. Other categorical programs created by Congress have independent organizational structure at the federal, state, and community level, that is, Title I programs, the Developmental Disabilities program, and the Early and Periodic Screening, Diagnosis and Treatment (EPSDT) program. Some of these function at the national, state, and community level parallel to, or even in open competition with, each other and with the MCH and CC programs. The result is a duplication of services, inefficiencies in administration, and increased costs. More importantly, the fragmentation of service results in some children receiving suboptimal care or not receiving needed services.

Mental retardation and mental health programs

Different states and different communities have tried to approach the mental retardation programs with special units for the identification and care of such children. Mental health programs frequently dovetail into the adult services and may function through the schools.

Health-related services

Psychological services may be obtained through mental health programs or the school system. It is the responsibility of each community to determine the organization of its community child center. The services offered in such a center should be strongly influenced by national and state goals, but services offered should be determined by the community after careful study of that community's needs. The organization of the community child center should be the responsibility of the community itself. Thus the number and type of health services provided in such centers will vary a great deal. Services, for example, for the protection of the juvenile, the management of teenage pregnancy and abortion counseling, VD programs, etc. should be available for all children who need them.

Child death rates

Death rates of children do not tell the entire story of child health, but certainly a knowledge of what causes deaths at the various ages of childhood should be of benefit in any community health program. Specific death rates point out where specific emphasis must be placed if we are to save the lives of our children. Tables for one particular year do not necessarily represent the exact pic-

ture for all years, yet the 1971 experience of the United States is fairly typical of the years from 1950 to the present. While the rates from year to year shift slightly, the general relative positions of the various causes of death remain quite constant.

To say that all of these deaths could have been prevented would be unrealistic, but to say that at least half of them could have been prevented with our present knowledge and means would be a reasonable appraisal. Certainly accidental deaths, which loom so prominently in the statistics of childhood, can be reduced materially. Deaths from infectious diseases can be controlled better than is indicated in the statistics. Age group 10 to 14 years has the lowest single death rate of any age group in the entire population. Yet the death rate for this group and the other three should be reduced.

QUESTIONS AND EXERCISES

1. Why is death from puerperal sepsis virtually inexcusable at the present time?
2. Appraise this statement: "The maternal health program is a phase of the general, overall community health program and not an independent program isolated from all other health measures."
3. Why is it desirable for a woman to have a premarital medical examination to determine her capacity for childbearing?
4. What is the reciprocal obligation of the expectant mother and society?
5. Why is the American maternal mortality rate higher than New Zealand's even though obstetrics is just as far advanced in America as it is in New Zealand?
6. To what extent is legislation of benefit in maternal health promotion?
7. Appraise the economic factors in your community that are significant in maternal health.
8. Consider one of the leading causes of infant deaths and propose measures for reducing the number of infant deaths from this cause.
9. Where in the field of infant hygiene could time and funds for research be best invested?
10. Make an analysis of the causes of infant deaths in your county during the past 5 years and propose measures to improve the situation.
11. What are contributions of voluntary agencies to the infant health program in your community?
12. Propose a 5-year community program to educate parents in the advisability of taking apparently healthy children to their family physician or pediatrician for a checkup at regular intervals.
13. What resources are available in your community

for obtaining the correction of a defect in a child whose parents cannot afford the necessary services?

14. Evaluate this statement: "The school assumes the role of the parent when it concerns itself with the pupil's health."
15. What official agencies are available in your community for helping a family with a child needing orthopedic services?
16. What nonofficial agencies are available in your community for helping a family with a child needing orthopedic services?
17. What are some of the special social and mental health problems associated with disability in childhood, and what is a community's responsibility in dealing with these by-products?

REFERENCES

American Academy of Pediatrics: The report of the Committee on Infectious Diseases, ed. 17, Evanston, Ill., 1974.

Ames, L. B.: Child care and development, ed. 6, Philadelphia, 1970, J. B. Lippincott Co.

Chase, H. C.: Perinatal and infant mortality in the United States and six West European countries, American Journal of Public Health **57:**1735, 1967.

Comprehensive health care for children and families, Sixth Bi-Regional Conference, University of Minnesota and the University of Michigan, Ann Arbor, 1967, University of Michigan School of Public Health.

Crawford, C. O.: Health and the family, New York, 1971, The Macmillan Co.

Deutach, M., and associates: The disadvantaged child, New York, 1967, Basic Books, Inc., Publishers.

Ellis, R. W. B., and Mitchell, R. G.: Diseases in infancy and childhood, ed. 6, Baltimore, 1968, The Williams & Wilkins Co.

Fraser, G. R., and Friedmann, A. I.: Causes of blindness in childhood, Baltimore, 1968, The Johns Hopkins Press.

Freud, A.: Normality and pathology in childhood, New York, 1967, International University Press.

Geertinger, P.: Sudden death in infancy, Springfield, Ill., 1968, Charles C Thomas, Publisher.

Jolly, H.: Diseases of children, Philadelphia, 1967, F. A. Davis Co.

Krugman, S., Ward, R., and Katz, S. L.: Infectious diseases of children, ed. 6, St. Louis, 1977, The C. V. Mosby Co.

Levine, M. I., and Seligman, J. H.: Your overweight child, New York, 1970, Hawthorn Books, Inc.

MacQueen, J. C.: The provision of contemporary child health services through community child centers, Iowa City, Iowa, October 1976.

Shapiro, S., and associates: Infant, perinatal, maternal and childhood mortality in the United States, Cambridge, Mass., 1968, Harvard University Press.

Shepard, K. S.: Care of the well baby, ed. 2, Philadelphia, 1968, J. B. Lippincott Co.

U.S. Department of Health, Education and Welfare, Public Health Service: Morbidity and Mortality Weekly Report **24**(3):27, January 18, 1975.

Wiedenback, E.: Family-centered maternity nursing, New York, 1967, G. P. Putnam's Sons.

6 ▪ ADULT HEALTH

He who hath good health is young.

H. G. Bohn

It is interesting to observe the cycle that public health is in the process of completing. At the turn of the century, when the attention of the health profession was directed toward the prevention and control of communicable diseases, major emphasis was directed toward the child of school age. It soon became apparent that for proper control measures it would be necessary to go back to the preschool child. It then became obvious that the infant could not be neglected, and the child under the age of 1 year became the object of an intensive program of communicable disease prevention and control that soon expanded into an interest in all aspects of infant health. If everything possible was to be done for the infant, it would be necessary to consider prenatal factors, and this logically led to intensified efforts in the field of maternal health.

With the great advances in communicable disease control and the prevention of death in the early years of life, a greater proportion of the population not only survived to adulthood but lived into the categories of late adulthood and even old age. Now the organic diseases, usually most prevalent in adulthood, became the leading cause of death and the principal factor in disability. This directed the attention of the health profession to the health of the adult population and those citizens in the late years of life.

AGE DISTRIBUTION OF THE POPULATION

Human beings actually do not live longer than they did in 1900. At the turn of the century, some citizens attained the age of 100 years. Today, a much greater proportion reach the age of 100. At the present time over 15,000 of our population are over 100 years of age. Today, over 10% of our population is over 64 years of age, contrasted with 3.4% in 1880.

Fig. 6-1 shows the fall in age-adjusted death rates (such rates express most directly the probability of dying) from 1900 to 1973. The rate of fall is decreasing, particularly in those aged over 55 years. This is a result of the difficulty in preventing deaths caused by heart disease, cancer, and stroke.

Even with the advance in postponing death and extending life expectation, we are still a relatively young nation. According to the nineteenth United States Census for 1970, the median age in the United States was 28 years.

There is an excess of females over males, which is becoming more pronounced, and in 1970 the United States had 5 million more women than men. This excess is particularly noticeable in the older age groups so that among those over 64 there are only 722 males per 1,000 females. This discrepancy is the result of the higher death rates suffered by males in three of the leading causes of death —heart diseases, cancer, and accident.

Certain economic, social, medical, and community health problems are inherent in

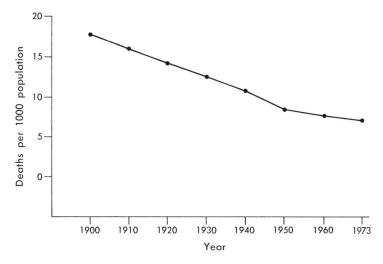

Fig. 6-1. Age-adjusted death rates, United States, 1900 to 1973. (From Vital statistics of the United States, vol. 2, 1973.)

the changes in the nation's population age distribution and sex composition. From statistics on the causes of death and the incidence of various diseases of the adult group, we have a guide to the direction an effective adult health program should logically take.

PRINCIPAL CAUSES OF DEATH

According to the data in Table 6-1, the four leading causes of death account for 73% of all deaths; over half of those are a result of cardiovascular disease. The 1973 list contrasts with causes of death prevailing in 1900, when influenza and pneumonia ranked first, tuberculosis second, heart disease third, and gastroenteritis fourth. The leading cause in 1900 is now relegated to fifth place, contributing but 3% of total deaths, as opposed to 55% in 1900.

Significant as the decline in the general death rate for adults has been, of more immediate interest and value is an analysis of the principal causes of death at the present time. Such an analysis will be an aid in pointing up the particular health problems that exist in the adult age groups in America and the areas where special emphasis must be placed (Table 6-1).

Table 6-1 ■ Proportionate mortality rates from twelve leading causes of death: United States, 1973

Rank order	Cause of death	Percent of total deaths
1	Diseases of heart	38.4
2	Malignant neoplasms	17.8
3	Cerebrovascular disease	10.9
4	Accidents	5.9
5	Influenza and pneumonia	3.2
6	Diabetes mellitus	1.9
7	Cirrhosis of liver	1.7
8	Arteriosclerosis	1.7
9	Certain causes of mortality in early infancy	1.5
10	Bronchitis, emphysema, and asthma	1.5
11	Suicide	1.3
12	Homicide	1.0
All other causes		13.2

(From Vital statistics of the United States, vol. 2, 1973.)

Cardiovascular disease

Deaths in the United States in 1973 totaled 1,973,003, and 1,037,492 of them were caused by cardiovascular causes, a rate of 494 per 100,000 population. This rate appears to have peaked in 1963 and is now decreasing. Coronary (ischemic) heart disease is the greatest contributor, with two-thirds of the cases, and stroke is responsible for one-fifth. The common underlying pathological factor is atherosclerosis, a disorder of the blood vessels where the caliber of the vessel is narrowed and the elasticity is decreased. This process is associated with aging, but the rapidity and the extent of involvement is extremely variable among different people. The resulting disease depends on which organ system is chiefly affected and how severely it is affected.

Coronary heart disease

Normal function of heart muscle is dependent on an adequate blood supply, which is provided by the coronary arteries. Narrowing of the caliber of these vessels is caused by deposits of cholesterol and fat beneath their inner lining. As the blood flow is consequently reduced, the patient may notice chest pain on exertion (angina pectoris). This condition may progress to fibrosis of the heart muscle, reduction of cardiac function, and, ultimately, death. The narrowing of the coronary vessels may become so acute as to permit a blood clot (thrombus) to form, thus suddenly arresting the blood supply to a portion of the heart muscle. This is called a myocardial infarction, or heart attack, and results in the sudden death (within 2 hours) of the patient in almost one-fourth of the cases. Two-thirds of all heart attack victims survive their first attack, but of the fatalities 70% occur outside the hospital (that is, before the patient can reach the hospital).

Risk factors. Risk factors may be divided into modifiable (that is, those we can do something about) and nonmodifiable. Among the latter are age, sex, family history, and personality type.

1. Age. The incidence of heart attacks rises steeply from age 35 to 55 years and then falls as those susceptible to the disease are eliminated.

2. Sex. Males below 50 years of age are afflicted in a ratio of 4:1 compared to females. After 50 years of age the male excess is markedly reduced but still persists. This suggests some hormonal factor in etiology.

3. Family history. There is a strong familial tendency toward coronary heart disease, particularly on the male side. Families share many habits and customs of exercise, diet, and life-style; thus it is not clear whether this familial predisposition reflects a genetic or environmental cause.

4. Personality type. This is included as a nonmodifiable risk factor, for it has not been proved that it can be changed. People of a striving, time-conscious pattern are labeled type A personality. They are involved in a chronic struggle against time or another person. There is no limit to the number of events these persons squeeze into a day. They have an intrinsic drive toward some goal that gives status and personality enhancement, and the achievement of this goal is opposed by time, persons, and things. Consequently, persons with type A personality often suffer frustration, are constantly in a hurry, and have free-floating hostility. Type A behavior is not characterized by worry but by overanxiety or hysteria. The converse of the type A personality is the type B personality, expressed by tranquility. Persons with type A personalities suffer higher rates of heart attack than those with type B.

Modifiable factors. Three factors—high serum cholesterol levels, high blood pressure, and cigarette smoking—have been identified as being positively correlated with increased rates of heart attack. Nations whose citizens have high serum cholesterol levels, chiefly the westernized countries, have heart attack rates much higher than countries such as Japan, whose people have low cholesterol levels. Cholesterol levels are closely related to the percentage of saturated animal fats in the diet. Alteration of the national diet is the most promising avenue to reduction of coronary mortality. High blood pressure is associated with increased risk of heart disease, and reduction of the pressure by diet and drug therapy reduces the risk. Cigarette smokers have an increased risk of heart disease; this is similarly reduced when they abandon the habit. These three modifiable risk factors act in a synergistic fashion. Other variables, particularly stress and sedentary habit, have been named as possible risk factors. Stress is very difficult to measure, since it may be considered as a form of emotional tension. A period of severe stress or overfatigue is commonly identified as preceding a heart attack. Sedentary habit, or lack of exercise, is alleged to predispose to heart attacks. The evidence is inconclusive, except that in those who practice regular exercise the outcome of a heart attack is more favorable than in those who do not. The benefits of regular exercise are many and may include a reduced rate of heart attack, but this is not proved. Obesity is associated with increased frequency of heart attacks, particularly in the markedly obese. The difficulty is that such patients are frequently hypertensive, of sedentary habit, or diabetic, and it is difficult to identify which is the operative factor in the web of causation.

In summary, coronary heart disease is multifactorial in origin. Atherosclerosis is usually present, together with elevated cholesterol, sometimes accompanied by other risk factors.

HYPERTENSION

Hypertension is a common community problem. Surveys have found that about 15% of the adult white population and 30% of the adult black population are affected, representing over 20 million hypertensive people in the United States. Of all hypertensive persons in the community approximately one-third are undiagnosed, and one-third are

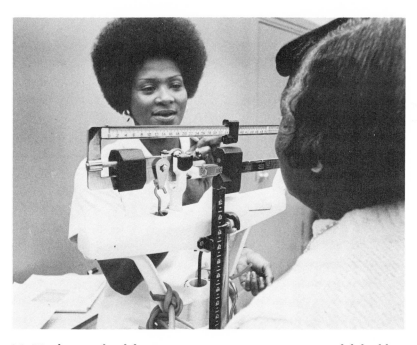

Fig. 6-2. Weight control and diet management are major strategies in adult health promotion, especially for patients with diabetes, hypertension, and heart disease. Public health nurses, nutritionists, physicians, and community health educators participate in these programs. (Courtesy Johns Hopkins Medical Institutions)

inadequately controlled. The natural course of hypertension spans some 15 to 20 years, starting on the average around age 35 years and often ending in premature death around age 50 years. The duration of the disease is for the most part (75%) asymptomatic. When symptoms do occur they are manifested by damage to the following organs—heart, brain, kidney, and fundus of the eye. Hypertension is the single most important risk factor for strokes, both hemorrhagic and thrombotic, and is a very important risk factor for heart disease. The cause of hypertension is unknown in 95% of cases. There is often a family history of hypertension, and relatives of hypertensive persons have been shown to be more likely to be hypertensive (especially children of two hypertensive parents). Obesity and salt consumption are correlated with hypertension, and both of these factors are modifiable. Smoking and high blood cholesterol are not associated with the development of hypertension, but the prognosis in hypertensive persons who smoke or have hypercholesterolemia is reduced. A great advance has been made in the treatment of hypertension with the introduction of effective drug therapy. Hypertension lends itself well to community control, because community surveys can be performed to identify people who are hypertensive and do not know it. People can visit centers that have been set

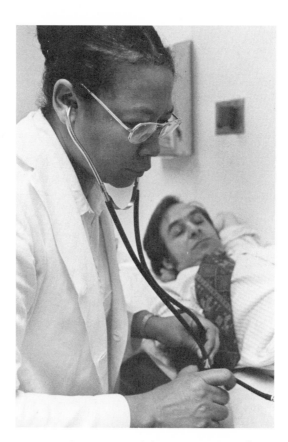

Fig. 6-3. Blood pressure control. Patients with hypertension must be assisted by community agencies to maintain a lifelong regimen of diet and medicine to prevent strokes and other cardiovascular complications. (Courtesy Johns Hopkins Medical Institutions)

up in their community and have their blood pressure recorded, after which they can be referred for treatment if needed. Once the cases are identified the problem then lies in effecting compliance in taking the drug and maintaining normal levels of pressure. The benefits from the increasing number of hypertensive persons who have been brought under control because of efficient drug therapy will be demonstrated by reduced mortality and morbidity. This reduction will stem both from a decrease in the number of heart attacks in which hypertension was a factor and also, more importantly, in reduction of the number of cerebrovascular accidents, or strokes, particularly of the hemorrhagic variety.

STROKE

This is the third ranking cause of mortality, following heart disease and cancer and preceding accidents. Stroke is essentially the result of interference with the blood supply to the brain, which may be either gradual or abrupt. An artery of the brain may rupture, usually one with preexisting damage, the result of atherosclerosis. This is particularly likely if the patient has high blood pressure— the weakened vessel is inadequate to withstand the higher pressure. Such hemorrhagic strokes have a high fatality rate and are usually found among older people. A blood clot may form in the artery either because of an obstruction resulting from atheroma in a similar way to that which occurs in the coronary artery of the heart. Alternatively, the clot may be formed elsewhere, such as in the heart itself, if there is a damaged valve there. In either event the clot blocks the cerebral artery and deprives the brain tissue of oxygen. This type of stroke is termed thromboembolic and occurs in younger patients, possibly without such fatal results. Many people recover from the initial stroke, but they are often left with some residual disability. Despite devoted efforts of therapists and the perseverance of patients, complete recovery after stroke is uncommon. Particu-

larly in older people stroke is a major source of morbidity. The hope lies in prevention, chiefly by controlling hypertension.

CANCER

Cancer is a group of diseases found in all races and ages of man and all other animal species. It is a cellular disorder in which there is uncontrolled and disordered growth of abnormal cells, which if unchecked will cause death. Cancer cells grow for no reason. They displace or destroy normal cells and, if not stopped, spread to other parts of the body. Thus cancer has two hallmarks—reproduction and invasion. Reproduction of cells is, of course, a normal biological function in growth and repair of tissues. Cancer cells, however, have a higher rate of cell growth than the normal tissues from which they are derived as well as a microscopic appearance that suggests a resemblance to immature rather than mature tissues. Cancer cells invade by three main mechanisms. The first is by direct spread or extension, growing into surrounding tissues and failing to respect the boundaries from which they are derived. Cancer cells may also invade lymph channels and be carried to distant parts of the body. Lymph is a clear transparent fluid that is collected from the tissues throughout the body, flows in channels, and is eventually added to the blood circulation. The lymph channels meet at points such as the axilla or the groin where there are lymph nodes or local enlargements. The cancer cells are carried in the lymph channels from their original site to the first group of lymph nodes. There the cancer cells may enlarge and grow. This gives rise to the term "positive nodes," which signifies spread of the tumor to such lymph nodes. The cancer cells may also be carried directly in the bloodstream, which enables them to reach distant parts of the body where they grow, attempting to reproduce the tissue of their origin. This new or secondary tumor is called a metastasis. The original tumor may be silent, that is, without symptoms such as pain or bleeding early in its life, and it may spread quickly. These factors make some cancers difficult to treat successfully and emphasize the necessity of early diagnosis.

In 1973 there were 351,055 deaths from cancer—17.8% of the total deaths. Both the number of cancer deaths and the proportion of total mortality in the United States accounted for by cancer have been increasing. In 1976 675,000 new cases of cancer occurred (this excludes skin cancer and in situ cancers, that is, those cancers that have not yet invaded other tissue). Cancer deaths during 1976 were somewhat over half of the number of new cases. Cancer is predominantly a disease of middle and old age; it is rare in children and young adults. Persons around age 70 years account for a higher number of cases than any other age group. The risk of developing cancer increases with age. The male death rate exceeds that of the female. At the present time the chance of a person who is less than 20 years old developing cancer sometime during his or her lifetime is about one in four for males and slightly higher for females. The most common site in males is the lung, followed by the prostate. In females breast cancer is the most common, followed by colon and rectal cancer, which is the third most common site in males. Surveys conducted in 1947 and 1969 reveal that cancer of all sites has increased most rapidly in black males, with a 36% increase over this 22-year time span. White males suffered a 7% increase, whereas females of both races showed a 14% decrease in cancer incidence of all sites. Cancer of the stomach has decreased in both sexes and both races, as has cancer of the cervix in females. Lung cancer rates have increased 133% in white males and 233% in black males over the time span considered, with similar increases in females, 108% for white and 213% for black, though from a much lower base. Since lung cancer is caused by tobacco smoking, the increase in smoking noted among females will produce an increasing rate of lung cancer among women in the future.

The cause of cancer is unknown, but risk factors affecting various groups have been identified. There is a familial tendency for the development of cancer, especially of breast, stomach, and large intestine. However, it is not known at the present time to what extent this is truly a genetic factor or whether it is caused by environmental factors such as diet, life-style, or occupation, which may remain similar from one generation to the next.

Repeated infections, particularly viral, are associated with cancer of the cervix. Virus infection may be but one element in a chain of causation, and tumor induction may require the triggering of latent viruses in the cell by an external physical or chemical agent.

Radiation may also be a cause, stemming from industrial and medical uses of x-rays and radioactive devices. Older radiologists have been shown to have an excess mortality from leukemia. Uranium mine workers have been found to develop lung cancer at higher rates than does the general population. The atomic bomb survivers in Japan have experienced excessive mortality from leukemia.

The factor most clearly related to development of cancer is cigarette smoking. All the tissues in smokers that are exposed to the carcinogens in tobacco smoke have higher rates of cancer. These include the larynx, oral cavity, esophagus, lung, and urinary bladder. The impact of cigarette smoking is very large, both because of the prevalence of the habit (about 40% of adults in the United States are smokers) and because of the high relative risk of lung cancer that accompanies cigarette smoking.

Specific occupational exposures, such as to asbestos, result in higher cancer rates. The contribution of air pollution is difficult to evaluate because of the long latent period for many cancers (20 to 40 years) between exposure and diagnosis of the cancer combined with the confounding effect of cigarette smoking.

Treatment and survival of cancer patients

A cancer patient may be treated by surgery, irradiation, and drugs. Surgery may range from simple local excision of the tumor to radical surgical exenteration of the tumor, the surrounding tissues, and the lymph nodes, so that the whole tumor area is excised. This may involve diversion of the urinary or alimentary tract. Irradiation may proceed or follow surgery and may be applied by different emitters. Drug therapy may involve altering hormonal status if the tumor is hormonal dependent, and chemotherapy involves use of cytotoxic and antimetabolite drugs. The type of treatment used depends on many factors, such as the organ or origin of the tumor, the extent of invasion, the microscopic appearance, and the age and general health of the patient. Often a combination of two or more treatment methods are used, and a second or third course of treatment is frequently helpful. The dominant factor in the prognosis for cancer patients is the stage at which treatment is first begun. Cancers may be divided into those that are still localized, that is, confined to the organ of origin, and those that have spread to the neighboring lymph glands or distant organs of the body. In every case the outlook is markedly improved if the cancer is treated when it is still localized. Some examples of the superior 5-year survival rates for localized tumors compared with those that have spread are listed in Table 6-2. This table demonstrates that if the number of cases diagnosed and treated in the localized form is increased, overall survival will increase. Of the cancers listed in Table 6-2 those diagnosed in a localized, or early, stage in 1971 were as follows: lung, 17%; colon/rectum, 42%; breast, 45%; uterine cervix, 75%; and prostate, 65%.

Early detection of cancer

The most promising method of early detection is screening people who have no symptoms but who, by reason of their age, sex, occupation, or life-style, may be in a high-risk group. The validity of screening methods varies. Some have proved most effective, the outstanding example of which is the Papanicolaou smear. Cervical cytology —the Pap smear—is both sensitive and specific in detecting precancerous changes in the cervix. The test is reliable, painless, inexpensive, and lacks morbidity; as a result it has achieved wide popularity among health providers and patients. Between 1964 and 1969 the proportion of women with cervical cancer diagnosed in the earliest stage rose from one-third to three-fourths. The 5-year survival rate in the earliest, precancerous stage, of cervical cancer is 100%. Virtually all women can be saved if the diagnosis is made at this point, which can be done by the cervical smear technic. The community problem is that certain groups of women, including the old, the poorly educated, and those who are not assimilated into the com-

---

Table 6-2 ■ Cancer 5-year survival rates percent for cancers treated between 1965 and 1969 (adjusted for normal life expectancy)

	All cancers	Lung	Colon/rectum	Breast	Uterine/cervix	Prostate
All stages	40%	8%	45%	64%	64%	56%
Local	67%	30%	70%	84%	80%	68%
Regional	34%	7%	35%	56%	42%	50%

From American Cancer Society: CA—Cancer Journal for Clinicians **27**(1):40-41, January/February 1977.

munity, do not seek out the screening test. Community efforts can be directed toward identifying these women and encouraging them to avail themselves of this protection.

The picture in breast cancer is not as promising, but two methods can be employed on a community basis. The most important is that of breast self-examination, which can be used by all women, examining their own breasts every month. The method is simple to learn and can be taught by demonstration, films, television programs, and printed material. Community health leaders can make everyone aware of this method. Soft tissue x-rays or mammography holds great promise of identifying early tumors that are too small or inaccessible to palpate. Mammography has reduced mortality from breast cancer in women over 50 years of age.

The gloomy outlook in lung cancer is slowly improving. Although we can identify persons of high risk, namely males over 45 years of age who smoke more than one pack of cigarettes daily, it is still difficult to detect lung cancer early. This is because x-ray changes occur late and lung cancer cells are difficult to produce and interpret microscopically. Not all tumors exfoliate cells that may be coughed up and recognized as cancer cells under the microscope. Periodic lung cytology examinations in high-risk groups will become a community program if the present research trials prove the method feasible.

Colon and rectal cancers may be detected by the presence of blood in the stools. Although this is frequently not caused by cancer, sigmoidoscopy (direct vision of the lower bowel) and an x-ray examination of the lower bowel are indicated if blood is present. Tablets may be developed, which, when dropped into the toilet bowl, will give a characteristic color if blood is present in the stool. Such a mass screening program offers the best hope of early detection of colon and rectal cancers at present.

Cancer research

Cancer research has the following three thrusts: (1) to discover the etiology of the cancer so that preventive methods may be taken, (2) to pioneer new screening programs for early detection, and (3) to improve results of treatment for persons with cancer. The public should not be persuaded to believe that if sufficient money is spent the threat of cancer will be removed. The unfortunate fact is that, in cancers in which the cause has been discovered, the number of cases has actually increased. Lung cancer is the classic example, the cause being cigarette smoking, but prevention involves altering behavior, which is difficult to achieve. Many cancers may be prevented by modification of life-style to avoid known hazardous habits and customs and by using early detection methods already available. The community effort must be directed toward making people aware of this, rather than making them dependent on research results or cures at some future date. Persons must be made aware of the fact that the gift of health lies in their own hands.

CHRONIC DISEASES

Chronic diseases that have an impact on the community through morbidity rather than mortality are led by diabetes and arthritis.

Diabetes

Much is known about diabetes, but the basic pathogenesis is not understood. One percent of the population of the United States, 2 million persons, have diabetes and are aware of this fact. An additional 1% have diabetes and do not know it. Ninety-five percent of diabetic persons suffer the disease after the age of 40 years—maturity-onset diabetes. Diabetes should be viewed as a vascular disease as well as a metabolic disorder with altered carbohydrate metabolism. The morbidity of diabetes is caused by its vascular complications. Coronary heart disease rates are increased in diabetes, as are those for renal disease, and, if the retinal arteries are involved, diabetic retinopathy and blindness ensue. Blood supply to the limbs is decreased, usually in the foot and calf, and gangrene with resulting amputation is common. Diabetes is associated with obesity, hypertension, and atherosclerosis.

Half of all diabetic persons may be treated by diet alone—one that is low in calories and fat. The remainder require insulin or oral hypoglycemic drugs. Community efforts are needed, for the prognosis in diabetes is related to the resources of the patients, their families, and the communities in which they live. Diabetics who are old, poor, or live alone do poorly. The duties of the community toward persons with diabetes are similar to those with hypertension. Screening programs to uncover the disease early, before it is symptomatic, are of prime importance. After having identified the patients, the importance of following both the diet and drug regimen must be explained.

Arthritis

Arthritis and rheumatic diseases are the most common cause of lost work days annually in the United States, although the respiratory diseases account for the greatest number of episodes of sickness. It is difficult to determine the prevalence of arthritides because of the range of symptom complex and the variability of diagnostic standards. If major mobility limitations are used, National Health Survey figures show 210,000 disabled, yet the prevalence of some arthritic symptoms is 3%, or 6,300,000 persons. Rheumatoid arthritis is a systemic inflammatory disease with local joint manifestations, in which the small joints of the hands are often affected early. The disease pursues a chronic course marked by relapses and remissions. The sex ratio shows an excess of females, 2.5 to 1. Risk factors include lower socioeconomic status, infections, trauma, winter season, and social stress. The age of onset is young, between 20 and 45 years, commonly 30 to 40 years. In contrast, osteoarthritis affects older persons exclusively and occurs in larger, weight-bearing joints, hips, and knees. Trauma and obesity are antecedent factors. The community role includes employers providing work for those arthritic persons who are able to work, a surprisingly high proportion. Transport services from home to treatment facilities, home visits, and meals on wheels services are all vital to these patients.

Prevention of chronic disease

The influence of medical treatment on established chronic disease is minimal in general. The thrust must be toward earlier diagnosis, and patients, health professionals, and the community all have a role in this. Tuberculosis, hypertension, diabetes, syphilis, and gonorrhea can all be diagnosed early by simple tests and treated or controlled successfully. Screening tests are available for many diseases, such as cervical, breast, and colon cancers. The American Cancer Society has set a fine example in health education with the following seven danger signals:

1. Any sore that does not heal
2. A lump or thickening in the breast or elsewhere
3. Unusual bleeding or discharge
4. Any change in a wart or mole
5. Persistent hoarseness or cough
6. Persistent indigestion or difficulty in swallowing
7. Any change in normal bowel habits

Patients suffering from certain diseases have been forming activist groups to aid others in a similar predicament. Parents of children with multiple handicaps have organized in various communities to identify community resources that may be available. Groups such as these remove fear and stigmata of the disease and raise morale and achievement.

PROMOTION OF ADULT HEALTH

People must be educated into positive health-oriented behavior. Their health lies in their own hands, and diseases reflect lifestyles.

In addition to the regular, annual health inventory, there are a number of other contributions that individual citizens can make to their own health. The promotion of cir-

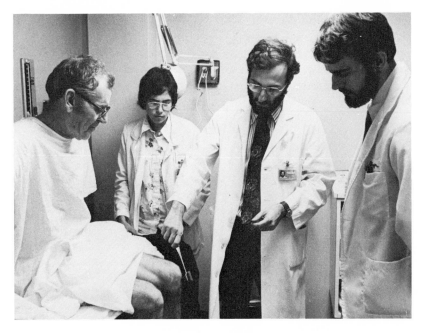

Fig. 6-4. Physical examination. The periodic health examination can yield early detection of conditions for which later recognition could mean death or serious disability. (Courtesy Johns Hopkins Medical Institutions)

culatory efficiency through physical activity adapted to one's capacity, regularity in living, relaxation, rest, proper nutrition, avoidance of extreme fatigue, avoidance of unnecessary exposure, avoidance of harmful substances, prevention of disease, immediate treatment of disease and disability that do occur, promotion of wholesome life interests, and attainment of emotional stability are all important in the promotion of a high level of health, the extension of the prime of life, and a greater life expectancy. Time and effort devoted to health promotion is well invested. They are wise adults who appreciate the quality of health they have. They are wiser adults who protect and maintain their most valuable physical asset—health.

Basic to a community program of adult health promotion is health education. This includes education of the person who is a patient, which is the responsibility of the attending physician; it includes family education, which is the joint responsibility of the physician and the public health department;

and it includes community health education, for which the public health department has primary responsibility.

To be health-informed is not enough. Adults must be health-educated in terms of having a fundamental understanding of health that they identify with themselves and apply to themselves. This means citizens who value the health that they now possess, seek to understand how they can preserve and promote that health, and put into practice those measures that will assure them of the highest level of health their native endowment will provide.

A community health education program must be organized under the direction of a competent health educator working from a community health center supervised by the community health department. No program of public health education could be highly effective without the cooperation and support of the medical profession. All program planning should include representatives of the medical society. The practicing physician has an invaluable contribution to make to the health education phase of a community's adult health promotion program.

Health education must utilize all forms of communication—speaking, writing, demonstrations, radio, and television. It must recruit all people who may have a contribution to make. It must enlist the services of all organizations—official health agencies, the medical profession, voluntary health agencies, service clubs, church groups, labor unions, parent organizations, neighborhood units, and other organized groups. A community health council composed of representatives from various community organizations can be a productive force in a community health education program. Such a council is an unofficial body reflecting community interests and needs. The council serves as a coordinating and catalytic agency in the community. Its function is to cooperate in the program, not to operate it.

The health education program must concentrate on specific health problems and at the same time must promote general health education. It must deal with the present but must project itself into a continuing program for future needs.

QUESTIONS AND EXERCISES

1. Why is the quest for health seemingly an endless journey?
2. How would the conquest of infection affect the incidence of the degenerative disease?
3. What is meant by a nondegenerative, organic disease?
4. Why is it important that effort be extended toward research in the treatment as well as in the prevention of the degenerative diseases?
5. What indications exist that the American adult is taking a more objective attitude toward diseases of the circulatory system, and what American in the last 15 years unintentionally contributed most to this change of attitude?
6. Why is the death rate from vascular lesions affecting the central nervous system higher among females than among males although men have a higher incidence of arteriosclerosis and hypertension?
7. Why does the United States not invest more money in research related to circulation in the human?
8. In the United States in 1900, nephritis ranked sixth as a cause of death with a specific rate of 88.6 per 100,000. Now more than half a century later, the rate is about 4 per 100,000. To what do you attribute the decline in this specific death rate?
9. Propose a program for your community to decrease the incidence of cancer of the respiratory tract.
10. Why is it preferable to teach a respect for cancer rather than a fear of cancer?
11. Using only local funds and resources, set up a community program designed to obtain early discovery of cancer through the regular medical examination of virtually all adults.
12. What additional services and facilities are needed by your community for an adequate cancer control program?
13. Propose a program designed to discover all cases of diabetes mellitus in your community.
14. Survey the services and facilities available in your community for the diagnosis and treatment of arthritis.
15. What additional services and facilities are needed by your community for an adequate arthritis program?

REFERENCES

Baldry, P. E.: Battle against heart disease, New York, 1971, Cambridge University Press.

Bennett-England, R.: As young as you look, New York, 1971, Fernhill House, Ltd.

Blumenfeld, A.: Heart attack: are you a candidate?, New York, 1971, Pyramid Publications.

Blumenthal, H. T.: Cowdry's arteriosclerosis, ed. 2, Springfield, Ill., 1967, Charles C Thomas, Publisher.

Epstein, F. H.: Predicting coronary disease, Journal of the American Medical Association **201:**795, 1967.

Facts on the major killing and crippling diseases in the United States today, New York, 1967, National Health Education Committee, Inc.

Gomez, J.: How not to die young, New York, 1971, Stein & Day Publishers.

Homola, S.: Secrets of naturally youthful health and vitality, Englewood Cliffs, N.J., 1971, Prentice-Hall, Inc.

Jones, B., editor: The health of Americans, Englewood Cliffs, N.J., 1970, Prentice-Hall, Inc.

Levin, D., Devesa, S., Goodwin, J. D., and Silverman, D. T.: Cancer rates and risks, Washington, D.C., 1974, U.S. Department of Health, Education, and Welfare, Public Health Service, National Institutes of Health.

Lewis, F. C.: Doctor looks at heart trouble, Garden City, N.Y., 1970, Doubleday & Co., Inc.

Lowman, J.: Why grow old?, New York, 1971, Grosset & Dunlap, Inc.

McKegney, F. P.: Treatment of chronic illness—home or nursing home? Journal of the American Medical Association **210:**1060, 1967.

Marston, R. Q.: Cancer research—a study of man and his environment, American Journal of Public Health **59:**1589, 1969.

Mead, S.: How to stay medium-young practically forever, New York, 1971, Simon & Schuster, Inc.

Mihich, E.: Immunity, cancer and chemotherapy, New York, 1967, Academic Press, Inc.

National Advisory Cancer Council: Progress against cancer 1970, U.S. Department of Health, Education, and Welfare, Public Health Service, National Institutes of Health.

Schneider, D. E.: Psychoanalysis of heart attack, New York, 1967, The Dial Press.

Seidman, H., Silverberg, E., and Holleb, A.: Cancer statistics, 1976—a comparison of white and black population, New York, 1976, American Cancer Society, Professional Education Publications.

Shapiro, S., Strax, P., and Vener, L.: Periodic breast cancer screening: the first two years of screening, Archives of Environmental Health 15:547, 1967.

Stamler, J., and associates: Epidemiology of hypertension, New York, 1967, Grune & Stratton, Inc.

Sutton, M.: Cancer explained: symptoms, signs and early diagnosis, New York, 1967, Hart Publishing Co., Inc.

White, P. D., and Donovan, H.: Hearts: the long follow-up, Philadelphia, 1967, W. B. Saunders Co.

7 ▪ COMMUNITY GERIATRICS

It is too late! Ah nothing is too late.
Till the tired heart shall cease to palpitate.
Cato learned Greek at eighty; Sophocles
Wrote his grand Oedipus, and Simonides
Bore off the prize for verse from his compeers,
When each had numbered more than four-score years.
And Theophrastus, at four-score and ten
Had but begun his Characters of Men.
Chaucer at Woodstock with the nightingales,
At sixty wrote the Canterbury Tales.
Goethe at Weimar, toiling to the last
Completed Faust when eighty years were past.
These are indeed exceptions; but they show
How far the gulf-stream of our youth may flow
Into the arctic regions of our lives ----
For Age is Opportunity No Less
Than Youth Itself! Though In Another Dress,
And as the evening twilight fades away
The sky is filled with stars, invisible by day.

from *Morituri Salutamus*
H. W. Longfellow

Like other minority groups, the aged are subject to misunderstanding and discrimination by the majority. Just as many of the health problems of the poor are related to problems of racism and class and as some problems of women are related to sexism, so too are major problems of the aged related to "ageism." A community approach to the health of the elderly therefore must concern itself with public and professional attitudes toward aging and stereotypes about the aged. Institutional prejudice against age also exists to the extent that our community services and institutions discriminate against the aged in ways that threaten their access to preventive and health care resources. Community health programs attempt to adjust resources and organizational arrangements to meet the special needs of older people.

Gerontology and geriatrics both study the aging process including biological, psychological, and social change. Gerontology concerns itself with the natural aging process and with pathological aging. Geriatrics deals with the care of the aged and concerns itself primarily with enabling old people to live productively and enjoyably. The research health scientist finds gerontology of special interest but is not indifferent to the problems of geriatrics. The applied field of community health will deal more with geriatrics than with gerontology; hence, this chapter will be concerned with health as an aspect of geriatrics.

It must be recognized at the outset that health cannot be isolated from the total life of the citizen. Of necessity, aspects of living indirectly related to health must be considered. Aging could be thought of as a process that begins with conception. In practice, aging is regarded as that phase in life when bodily functioning begins to decline. Technically, then, it would be in order to describe everyone over the age of 30 as aging. The problem here is with the particular health factors that are of special importance at a given age. Because the age of retirement is usually accepted as 65, it is customary to think of anyone beyond this age as being in the classification of "aged." Yet a person of chronological age 55 could be older physiologically than another individual of age 75 (Quirk and Skinner, 1973). The arbitrary age of 65 is accepted in health circles as marking off a segment of America's population that has health needs different from those of other segments. This is accepted even though it is acknowledged that many of the health problems that exist in the individual over age 65 began at younger ages.

Chronic diseases and aging are not synonymous. Many of the elderly are in excellent health. Those who are not seen by physicians and welfare agencies tend to be overlooked in the evaluation of the general health of older citizens. Approximately half the nation's senior citizens do suffer impairments that may mean limited activity. According to the Council of State Governments, 17% of America's citizens over age 65 are disabled with an impairment sufficiently severe to make them homebound or unable to work.

AMERICA'S AGING POPULATION

That the age distribution of America's population is shifting toward the older group is general knowledge. The number of people in the nation over age 65 has more than quadrupled since the year 1900. Today there are over 22 million people in this age category, and the number is increasing at the rate of about 400,000 a year. Approximately 1 out of every 10 people is in the senior citizen category. Because of the rapidly dropping birthrate, the U.S. age pyramid, as shown in

Fig. 7-1, is shrinking at the bottom and growing wider at the top. By 1980 the percentage of the population 65 and older will increase from 10% to 25% if the birthrate continues its downward trend. These people merit an organized community program for the promotion of their health. Actually, concern for the health of the older age segment of the population is not a new interest. It is a concern of long standing that has been intensified by the rapid increase in the number of older people.

Every community has its segment of elderly people. Some communities have a greater percentage because of the tendency of younger people to migrate to other sections of the nation where there are better economic or other opportunities. Newly developed communities tend to have a small proportion of elderly people because the pioneering that the development of a new community requires tends to appeal to the young rather than to the old. Regardless of whether a community has a high or a low proportion of elderly people, every community has the challenge of providing for the health needs of its aging population.

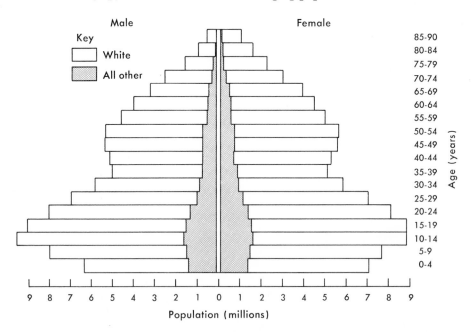

Fig. 7-1. Age-sex distribution of population by color, United States, July 1, 1973.

FACTORS IN AGING

Aging is a natural process with a number of physiological changes, many of them merely a decline in the rate of functioning. A reduction in the metabolic rate of about 7% occurs every 10 years after the age of 30. There is a retardation of the rate of cell division, cell growth, and cell repair. Tissues, including their cells, tend to dry out. A fatty infiltration usually occurs with cellular atrophy, and a decrease in the speed of muscular response and a decline in muscular strength occur. With a reduction in the efficiency of circulation, endurance is adversely affected. Connective tissues suffer a decrease in elasticity, bones become more brittle as the amount of organic material becomes reduced, teeth lose their structural integrity, and functioning of the digestive system declines so that digestion proceeds at a much slower rate. Many people over age 65 produce no hydrochloric acid in their stomach. Some of the nutritional deficiency in the older individual can be attributed to poor digestion and inadequate absorption rather than a poor diet. There is a general decline in the functioning of the nervous system and special sense organs. Because of a delayed response to infection or any other disorder, illness tends to be extended in the older person.

The principal concern of health science, however, is with pathological aging, which means a hastening of the aging process by adverse factors affecting body functioning. Repeated insults to the body leave their toll. The prime of life, as we know it, could be extended greatly and thus aging could be delayed if all factors that produce pathological aging could be prevented or dealt with summarily. Unfortunately, we do not know all of the factors that contribute to pathological aging, but evidence indicates that certain factors are significant.

Low-grade infection, particularly of a chronic nature, takes a toll. Toxins from the environment also hasten the aging process. Extended critical illness from which an individual recovers nevertheless hastens aging. Deteriorating diseases such as hypertension and diseases such as arthritis and rheumatism tend to produce premature aging. Chronic tension, worry, and fatigue, associated with an inability to relax, can hasten the aging process. The stress syndrome masks a disturbance of biochemical functioning that can take a considerable toll in terms of premature aging. Irregularity in the mode of living can have a harmful effect on the prime of life as well as on later health.

In the early years of life, indiscretion and prolonged stress may seem to have little effect on the general quality of the individual's well-being, but the toll will be collected in the later years of the person's life. Inactivity can be a factor in producing pathological aging. The level of effectiveness that the circulatory system attains is dependent on regular activity to challenge the circulatory system and on the native endowment one may possess in the way of a circulatory system. Marked nutritional deficiency that results in emaciation over an extended period of time has a recognized adverse effect on the retention of the prime of life. Nutritional deficiency such as one observes in some of the underdeveloped nations of the world would be rather rare in America; yet malnutrition to a lesser extent, such as we find in America, can have some effect on the aging process. Inadequacy of vitamins, proteins, and minerals in the diet can have an effect in producing premature aging. Cigarettes and alcohol are the most clearly isolated agents contributing to more rapid degeneration today.

CHARACTERISTICS OF ELDERLY PEOPLE

Every individual is unique, as much among the elderly as among the individuals of other age categories. Yet there are certain characteristics that distinguish the elderly, and these characteristics will be found in varying degrees in most senior citizens. It would be inaccurate to speak of a typical elderly person, although it would not be inaccurate to say that one could expect to find in most, if not all, older people the following characteristics: (1) loss of status and an increased uncertainty about personal worth, (2) an insecurity associated with a feeling of inability to meet the demands of life, (3) apprehension about health, (4) difficulty in adjusting from a work routine to one of retirement, (5) an inability to find avenues of service that will provide personal gratification, (6) difficulty in meeting stresses created by social change, and (7) limited incentive for social participation. Elderly people are eager to be useful in some capacity. Women make the transition into retirement more easily than men, partially because they have been preparing for the later years of life and usually have experienced a gradual transition into that phase (Lewis and Butler, 1972). They have developed interests and associations that provide opportunity for useful service. Men, on the other hand, may find retirement an entirely new way of life and may find themselves floundering helplessly in an attempt to find some social grounds on which to tread. Life soon loses its objectivity for one who finds no purpose in day-to-day living. Preparation for retirement has become as important in America as preparation for employment (Thurnher, 1974).

STATUS OF THE ELDERLY PERSON

Each day the community sees its elderly people and may assume that they are living more enjoyably and effectively or more unhappily than they really are. Yet each community should make a critical appraisal of the status of its elderly citizens. Retirement provisions in America are still inadequate but are being improved rapidly. The Office of Research and Statistics, Social Security Administration, Department of Health, Education and Welfare, reports that of citizens 65 years and older, 39% are retired (30% Social Security, 6% railroad retirement, 3% private pensions), 4% are living on veteran's benefits, 5% are on public assistance, 33% are living on the income of their employment, 15% are living on investment income, and 5% are supported by relatives.

As the provisions of the Social Security program are broadened, a greater percentage of citizens over age 65 will receive old age and survivors insurance benefits, and a smaller percentage will be employed. Socioeconomic factors may even produce a retirement age of 60 for the general population. The earlier retirement age will pose additional problems unless better programs are promoted for preparing people for retirement (Streib and Schneider, 1971).

Approximately half the men over age 65 are potential members of the labor force, and many of them prefer to work. Frequently it is not possible for them to continue in the type of work they were pursuing before retirement and it is necessary to learn a new type of work. Some find that their skills and trades have become obsolete and for this reason have to find new types of employment. Many of these individuals have an adequate physical capacity as well as an adequate learning capacity to take up new jobs, but industries are reluctant to employ elderly workers because they tend to be slower and have a high accident rate and a higher rate of absenteeism. However, the older worker is generally meticulous in work, produces work of a high quality, and is extremely reliable. There is a need to lower work barriers for the elderly who are physically and mentally capable. Employment opportunities need to be increased for those elderly citizens capable of contributing to the community's economy. Part-time jobs have their merit, particularly when the elderly person supplements work with other community services and activities.

Personal adjustment is the key to satisfactory retirement. Workers must alter their lives when retirement is reached. Preparation for successful old age should begin at about age 40, with the development of a wide range of interests and channels of community service. The individual who begins preparing for old age a quarter of a century in advance will find the tansition into retirement very natural and not at all difficult. Elderly persons must be able to accept change, cultivate a range of interest, maintain a willingness to learn, and participate actively in community affairs.

HEALTH PROBLEMS CREATED BY LONGEVITY

Table 7-1 reveals that many of the disorders causing death in the later years had their genesis long before the victims reached 65 years of age. With these particular causes of death, such as diseases of the heart, arteriosclerosis, and other degenerative diseases, primary prevention is too late in these advanced years of life. The main problem becomes that of proper medical supervision for the afflicted individual. Primary prevention is still in order for certain infectious diseases, such as influenza and pneumonia, and for accidental deaths. Early detection and treatment of malignant neoplasms and hypertension could give these older citizens several additional years of life. Even indi-

viduals over age 65 who appear to be in excellent health should have a thorough medical examination once every 2 years (Anderson, 1974). Certainly, those who obviously are not well should have periodic checkups more frequently (Ellwood and Oakes, 1975).

Several disorders not commonly a cause of death nevertheless represent important problems for the aged. Arthritis and rheumatism, two of the principal causes of disability in the aged, can usually be treated to relieve patients of much of their pain and enable them to extend their activities. Disorders of vision are common among the aged. Some degree of correction is usually possible even though the individual's vision with glasses is not normal. When the loss of vision has progressed to a state where the individual is no longer able to read, records are available that enable the blind or near blind to enjoy hearing the literature or feature articles of the day that they would normally read. Loss

Table 7-1 ■ Death rates for selected causes, United States in 1925, 1950, and 1973 for persons ages 75 to 84 years

Cause of death	Rate per 100,000 in age group 75 to 84 years		
	1925	1950	1973
Diseases of the heart	3,225	4,311	3,609
Malignant neoplasms (cancer)	1,027	1,153	1,188
Cerebral hemorrhage and other vascular lesions affecting central nervous system (strokes)	1,867	1,500	1,234
Influenza and pneumonia	1,072	297	296
General arteriosclerosis (artery disease)	520*	392	191
Accidents	443	316	160
Diabetes mellitus	162	167	180
Cirrhosis of liver	72	37	29
Other bronchopulmonic diseases (lung)	<30*	30	126
Hypertension without mention of heart	5*	110	37
All causes	11,929	9,331	7,932

National Center for Health Statistics: Vital statistics for the United States, vol. II, Mortality, selected years (Health, United States, 1975, p. 553).

*Estimates for period before statistics were recorded on this category.

of hearing in the later years of life is common. Hearing aids have been developed to the point where a much higher percentage of the hard of hearing are aided to hear adequately for customary needs. Deafness produces a feeling of loneliness. This increases the need to develop programs to provide whatever hearing can be obtained.

Mental disorders are usually not recorded as a cause of death, but mental disturbance is a health problem among longevous citizens. Mild senile psychosis may produce such symptoms as confusion, disorientation, inability to identify familiar people and places, slovenliness, suspicion, and even abusiveness.

Elderly persons may not appear to be as alert as they were in their earlier life and yet can be highly effective for the needs of life. One needs but to recall the late Oliver Wendell Holmes, Associate Justice of the United States Supreme Court, who was writing brilliant judicial opinions at age 90.

In considering the health of an elderly person, it is realistic to set different standards than one would set for an individual of age 40. An appraisal should be made of the health assets as well as health liabilities possessed by the person. Based on this appraisal, a program of health promotion for the individual should be formulated. It is wiser to set a lower realistic goal that can be attained than a goal that will result in disappointment and loss of self-esteem.

MEETING THE GERIATRICS PROBLEM

The health of the older age groups in the population has become recognized officially as a public health problem. The National Institute of Aging of the United States Public Health Service has been established to support research in gerontology and demonstrations in geriatrics. Plans and programs must originate with communities. Many state health departments have agencies for the promotion of the health of older citizens.

California, Connecticut, Indiana, Massachusetts, and New York have set up special administrative agencies to promote a statewide program directed toward the promotion of the health of the aged. In 1945 the Indiana State Health Department established a Division of Adult Hygiene and Geriatrics. The objectives of the Division are: (1) to study the factors of life that are related to senescence and senility as they are influenced by age, environment, heredity, and the diseases and disabilities associated with advancing years; (2) to help the public to know that senescence is normal, that senility is not a necessary part of age, and that through better understanding and cooperation, much of the premature deterioration of aging can be prevented; (3) to have the public informed on all helpful preventive knowledge concerning diseases and disabilities and advancing years, and to encourage the medical profession, both in teaching and practice, to be interested in the problem of aging, particularly in the anticipation of preventable diseases of increasing years; (4) to cooperate with and assist so far as possible the public and medical profession, as well as the public officials and others, in a full appreciation of the economic, social, and functional value and usefulness of men and women who, by reason of years and experience, constitute an increasingly important part of our population; and (5) to be interested in all laws, regulations, and facilities that affect the care and well-being and usefulness of elderly people, and to seek the improvement of such laws, regulations, and facilities as may affect elderly people adversely.

Community programs

It is on the community level that functional programs must be formulated, because at higher levels the program will fail to touch individual elderly citizens and their families. Of necessity, the state program will be far removed from the individual who needs health services. Yet the objectives of this particular state division are also the objectives of any community program.

In this field the problem of a community is basically threefold: (1) public education in

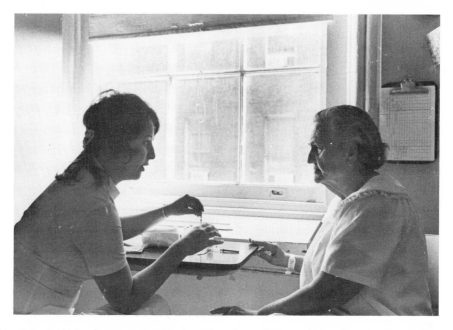

Fig. 7-2. Patient education for elderly. Chronic conditions require long-term maintenance and self-care. To be highly effective, education must be individualized at some point in the process. (Courtesy Johns Hopkins Medical Institutions)

the field of adult health, (2) integration of all services and forces in the community that have a service to offer elderly persons, and (3) the acquisition and provision of necessary services that the community does not now have available. A community health council can be an important agency in helping to determine the needs in the area of old age health promotion and the approaches that should be utilized. The official community health center may not provide medical service, but may serve as an information, coordinating, and program promotion center. Medical services generally are provided on a private basis by private practitioners. A community health program undertaken without the full approval and support of the local medical profession is unlikely to flourish.

Primary emphasis in the community program must be placed on public health education. The public needs to understand the nature of aging and the phenomena associated with advancing years. The public should understand what can be done to prevent some of the premature deterioration of aging and should have an understanding of measures for the prevention of diseases and disabilities of the advancing years. The public needs to be informed of the importance of medical supervision and the contribution that various individuals and agencies have to make to the elderly citizens of the community. Perhaps most important, the public needs to adjust its unrealistic perceptions of the aged themselves (Neugarten, 1973).

A community program to promote the health of elderly people must include attempts to provide the various services required for the treatment, hospitalization, and rehabilitation of those elderly people who have some disability. It must include provisions for activities that elderly people can enjoy through participation. For elderly people who are unable to pay for professional services the program should provide some means through which they may receive the professional services required.

Perhaps the greatest contribution such a

program can make is to give the elderly a feeling that someone is concerned with their problems and that there is an agency in the community to which they can turn for guidance and assistance. Most elderly people in a community are self-sufficient or have members of their immediate family who can provide any advice or assistance that may be needed, but some have no such source of aid. These individuals would be greatly benefited by an effective community health program for the elderly.

HEALTH PRACTICES

Most elderly individuals follow a normal course of living, though perhaps in second gear rather than in high gear and with modification of some of the established health practices. The particular routine of living adopted by each of these individuals should be adjusted to his or her capacities, past mode of living, present needs, and life interests. Certain factors are common to virtually all.

Nutrition. While the quantity of food required by the person in the later years of life is not as great as in the earlier years, the qualitative needs are just as important. Diversity of proteins, a sufficiency of vitamins, and adequate minerals should be included in each day's diet. Food should be attractive because the sense of taste becomes dulled with age. In the later years of life the output of digestive enzymes is reduced and the rate of digestion is much slower. For this reason, many elderly people find that eating more frequently and eating less at each meal is a highly satisfactory practice. Self-medication of the digestive system and supplementary vitamins should be used only on the advice of a physician (Crisp and Stonehill, 1976).

Activity. Unless a supervising physician advises otherwise, moderate activity is highly desirable for the normal elderly person. The general tone of body functioning that activity produces can be beneficial in producing a level of functioning near the maximum for the individual. Some degree of

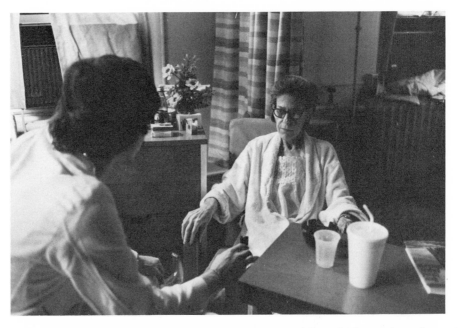

Fig. 7-3. Nutrition counseling. Before patients are discharged from the hospital, professional staff may lay the groundwork for follow-up home visits to assist patients. (Courtesy Johns Hopkins Medical Institutions)

fatigue during the day is normal, but excessive fatigue can be harmful. Activity can be purposeful, such as tending a garden or performing other simple tasks, and can be productive. Not rigorous activity, but moderately paced exertion, can be rewarding physically, emotionally, and socially.

Rest and sleep. Intervals of rest during the day should be coordinated with the tasks or activities requiring physical exertion. A midmorning, noon, and midafternoon rest period will be adequate for some, but others may need more frequent rest periods. Some elderly individuals do very well without any particular rest periods. This is true of the somewhat restless individual who prefers to be occupied with some task (Crisp and Stonehill, 1976).

Generally, as people get older they tend to sleep longer each day. The tendency is for the elderly person to go to bed earlier and to rise earlier than is the custom of the general adult population. Some seem to require less sleep than they did in earlier years. Each person in the old age group seems to adjust sleep to individual needs.

Safety. Physical injury and accidental death are high among people in the old age groups. Slowed reaction time, poor vision, and the inability to adjust readily to changing situations make the old person more accident prone than younger individuals. Conditions in the home should be made as safe as possible (Alvarez, 1973). Living on one floor is an effective safety measure, because falls on stairs constitute a frequent cause of death for old people. Having well-lighted rooms and hallways, and even the use of continuous dim light through the night, can be effective safety measures. Old people have a high fatality rate in motor vehicle-pedestrian accidents. Many elderly people object to being squired or guided. Such objections may have to be overruled when special hazards exist and when the individual appears to have difficulty in adjusting to the tempo of traffic (Alvarez, 1973).

Bathing. Bodily cleanliness has an important psychological value for the elderly. Yet it is frequently necessary to remind them of the need for a bath. A well-established living routine that includes bathing is a health asset for the elderly person. Because the old person's sensitivity to heat is reduced, it is sometimes desirable that a younger person test the temperature of the water in the tub or of the shower. Many old people have been severely scalded by bath water that they were not able to recognize as too hot until they had been badly burned. Bathing should contribute to a general feeling of well-being as well as to the health and esthetic life of the elderly (Coyle, 1972).

Clothing. Clean clothing adapted to the season and needs perhaps represents a factor in mental health more than in physical health. Extremely important for the elderly is a feeling of pride, status, or worth. Dress can be used to advantage in creating the state of mind that a person is important. Personal appearance can do much to give the elderly person the spark necessary for effective and enjoyable living.

Health practices of the elderly should be directed as much toward their mental and emotional needs as their physiological needs. Through health practices, it is possible to create in elderly persons the feeling that they are still very much a part of the community and that they have a significant, even important, role to play (Butler and Lewis, 1977).

MEDICAL SERVICES

Most communities can provide the variety of medical skills necessary for the more complex problems of the aged by calling on the services of the various specialists available in the area. Interest in the health aspects of geriatrics has been rising steadily, but the question is still unanswered whether a new specialty is needed. Many physicians and other professionals are members of the American Geriatrics Society or the Gerontological Society. The membership of these two organizations has increased tenfold since 1950. Unfortunately, medical and nursing students have shown resistance to working with geriatric patients (Kayser and Minnigerode, 1975).

Special geriatrics clinics have been established. Their goal has been to offer coordinated medical and social services to the independent, working, elderly group in order to aid them in retaining their independence. Clinics in Wakefield, Rhode Island, and at the Peter Bent Brigham Hospital, Boston, have demonstrated the value of coordinated medical and social service. In addition to providing important diagnostic service to the elderly group, the geriatrics clinic is able to formulate and supervise a continuing program of health supervision for its clients. Other geriatrics clinics are being organized, particularly in the larger population centers. Out of these pioneering efforts to provide organized health supervision for elderly citizens may well evolve the type of community programs needed to deal with the growing problem of providing for the health needs of the aged. The special demonstration project of the Kips Bay-Yorkville Health District in New York illustrates the experimental efforts under way to gain an understanding of what might be done in providing for the health needs of the aged. Other examples are the Home for the Aged and Infirm Hebrews and the Beth Israel Hospital in New York, the Brooklyn Hebrew Home and Hospital for the Aged, and the Waxter Center for Senior Citizens in Baltimore.

These efforts and special projects are most laudable, but as yet most communities rely on the general hospital and medical services that are already available. Older people require proportionately more medical services than the general population. In 1973 people 65 years and over had an average of 4.3 days in general hospitals, whereas those 45 to 64 years had only 1.7 days per person and those under 45 years had less than 1 day per year in short-stay hospitals (Health, United States 1975, p. 309). The National Center for Health Statistics (1975) reports that in a year, one out of every six citizens 65 years or older can expect to be hospitalized in a general, short-stay hospital with an average stay of 12 days.

NURSING HOMES

Nursing homes play an increasingly important role in the care of elderly persons. In 1973 the United States had 14,873 nursing homes and 6,961 personal care homes. These 21,834 homes had a total of 1,327,704 beds.

Although it may be saddening to note that more than a million aged people are in nursing homes, it is at the same time encouraging to note that over 19 million are not. Most of the geriatric concern has been with the 5% who are institutionalized. This has tended to bias popular and professional perceptions of what old age is like. We are guilty in the United States of "ageism" in our abandonment of many to nursing homes (Butler and Lewis, 1977).

Public health departments have been lax in licensing nursing homes. While all fifty states have licensing laws, the requirements are below the minimum standards recommended by the Committee on Aging of the National Social Welfare Assembly. The National Association of Registered Nursing Homes has made laudable contributions to the improvement of standards, and the efforts of this organization should be supported and encouraged. The present situation still calls for legal action for providing desirable standards through licensing of nursing homes (Kosberg, 1975).

Nursing homes should be affiliated with general hospitals and should cooperate with general hospitals. In such an arrangement, physicians will have elderly patients moved from the general hospital to the less expensive nursing home, where they know the chronically ill can receive the necessary nursing care. Such an arrangement also means a greater likelihood that the majority of the patients in the nursing home will be under medical supervision.

Physicians, nurses, occupational therapists, and social workers agree that the aging who are ill should be cared for in their own homes as long as possible. Obviously, there are situations that make this impossible or undesirable, but when home conditions are acceptable, some chronically ill can be as well taken care of in the home as in the nursing home or the hospital. Visiting nursing services can be utilized to good advantage, especially when only part-time nursing service is necessary (Warren, 1974).

REHABILITATION

The ill or disabled elderly person needs more than custodial care. Chronic disease hospitals are not the answer, because they tend to create the conception of lifelong disability. When hospitalization is necessary for an aged person, the general hospital can usually provide all of the services necessary for the care and treatment of the patient, without creating the impression of cold-storage institutionalization. In the general hospital elderly patients should have a combination of medical care and rehabilitation to prepare them for their mode of living after they are discharged from the hospital. Both nursing and social service are necessary before patients are transferred home. Perhaps

here the elderly person may need some supervision until a reasonable adjustment is made in terms of normal living routine. Even when the elderly person is in a domicile with other members of his family, social work services can be of value in aiding all concerned to understand what the needs of the elderly person are and how these needs are to be met (Tobin, 1975).

RELIGIOUS ACTIVITIES

The high percentage of church members in the United States who are over age 60 is evidence that the elderly person can find religious activities an avenue for gratification and the attainment of status. Even those who have not been churchgoers during their early years of life find church attendance and participation in the activities of the church both gratifying and challenging. The church performs a service for these individuals by providing them with opportunities for service. The regular churchgoers who attain the

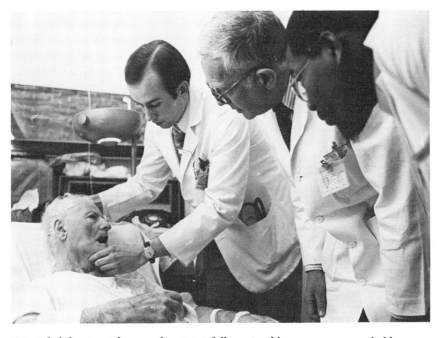

Fig. 7-4. Rehabilitation. The complications of illness in old age are compounded by economic loss and separation from family. Home-care programs sponsored by community agencies have proved their value in relieving some of these problems. (Courtesy Johns Hopkins Medical Institutions)

age of retirement now find additional time to serve in various capacities for the church, and participation in church functions becomes an extremely important part of their interest in daily life. Some enter into religion as an escape mechanism, but proper guidance from clergy and others can be helpful in preventing this.

Radio and television have brought religious services into the home for elderly shut-ins, and this has been one of the finest services of these two media. However, this should be supplemented by the churches providing additional, more personal, services to the shut-ins. These personalized services need not be of a strictly religious nature. Church people are in a strategic position to give the type of personal service that will help the elderly shut-in to attain and maintain the frame of mind and general well-being so essential to physical as well as mental health.

LEISURE-TIME ACTIVITIES

The value of recreation and social participation for mankind is generally acknowledged, but for no group are these of greater health value than for the aged (see Chapter 9). With a great deal of newly found time on their hands, the elderly need activities that will occupy them profitably and enjoyably. Some have business interests, trade skills, voluntary association memberships, or a garden to occupy their attention and time, but many are in need of help in developing satisfying leisure-time activities. Most of the elderly seek and enjoy the companionship of others (Nystrom, 1974). A community can provide for individual instruction for recreation purposes, but provision for instruction and supervision on a group basis is usually more practical.

Small groups of elderly people can take up arts and crafts, music, dramatics, poetry, and creative writing. The mutual encouragement, the sociability, and the general elation that come from such participation can do more for many of these elderly people than can the physician or the hospital. On the other hand, participation in social activities and associations cannot be offered as a substitute for health care (Bull and Aucoin, 1975).

On a large group basis, concerts, lectures, dancing, parties, excursions, and outings can be highly important in the lives of the elderly and can contribute measurably to their outlook. Checkers, chess, cards, and shuffleboard are popular games that can be organized and promoted among the elderly. Zest for living is extremely important in the health of these persons. Social action groups such as the Grey Panthers provide a vehicle for productive participation, but in communities without such organizations the community should provide avenues for the development and promotion of a zest for living. This aids elderly citizens in their feeling of security, which is a primary need of every person, but it also brings returns to the community in the continuing participation of the aged in community life.

APPRAISAL

Community responsibility for the health of the senior citizen encompasses concern for the citizen's total living. Included in the program are medical services, hospital facilities, nursing home provisions, housing conditions, health education, health counseling, recreation programs, and provision of opportunities for individual and group participation in productive and enjoyable activities. The community health department alone cannot carry the whole program, but it can be the agency that integrates all community resources having a contribution for the elderly. As an established official agency, the health department can initiate action necessary for the promotion of the well-being of the aged.

QUESTIONS AND EXERCISES

1. What are some signs of "ageism" in your community?
2. Why must gerontology concern itself with social and psychological aging as well as with physiological aging?
3. In 1883 Chancellor Bismarck of Germany set 65 as the age of retirement. Appraise the current use of age 65 as the landmark for the classification of "aged."

4. List twenty persons of your acquaintance who are over 65 years of age. What percentage have good health, what percentage have fair health, what percentage are ill but up and around, and what percentage are disabled?

5. What percentage of this twenty have health impairments that could be corrected or at least reduced?

6. To what extent do changes in the economy affect the population age distribution of a county or a state?

7. What factors are essential if an individual is to be relatively "young" at age 75?

8. What is the general social status of the elderly people of your community and what is the significance of their social status in terms of their health?

9. To what extent is the community health program for the aged primarily a program of curing illness rather than health?

10. What does your state health department have in the way of an agency and a program for the promotion of the health of the aged?

11. What special activities in the interest of better health for the aged are carried on by your official community health department?

12. What are the voluntary health agencies of your community doing in behalf of the health of elderly citizens?

13. What are the contributions of other institutions such as churches of your community to the health and general well-being of the senior citizen?

14. How interested and how well informed is the general public in your community about matters relating to the health of elderly people?

15. What would be a good routine of daily living for a man or woman of age 70 without impairments?

16. Why are health practices recommended for elderly people usually directed more to their psychological needs than to their physiological needs?

17. State the reasons for and against establishing a special geriatrics clinic in your community.

18. To provide ideally for the health needs of its elderly citizens, what should your community provide in the way of medical and other services and in the way of hospital and other facilities?

19. In terms of community geriatrics, evaluate the role of the state certified nursing home, affiliated with a general hospital, and staffed with registered nurses.

20. What organized leisure-time activities for the aged are now available in your community and what additional provisions should be made?

REFERENCES

Alvarez, W. C.: Hazards leading to accidents, Geriatrics **28**:76, 1973.

Anderson, H. C.: Newton's geriatric nursing, ed. 5, St. Louis, 1971, The C. V. Mosby Co.

Anderson, W. F.: Practical management of the elderly, Philadelphia, 1967, F. A. Davis Co.

Anderson, W. F.: Preventive aspects of geriatric medicine. Journal of the American Geriatrics Society **22**: 385, 1974.

Blenkner, M.: Environmental change and the aging individual, Gerontologist **7**:101, 1967.

Botwinick, J.: Cognitive processes in maturity and old age, New York, 1967, Springer Publishing Co., Inc.

Bull, C. N., and Aucoin, J. B.: Voluntary association participation and life satisfaction: a replication note, Journal of Gerontology **30**:73, 1975.

Butler, R. N.: Why survive? Being old in America, New York, 1975, Harper & Row, Publishers, Inc.

Butler, R. N., and Lewis, M. I.: Aging and mental health: positive psychosocial approaches, ed. 2, St. Louis, 1977, The C. V. Mosby Co.

Coyle, M. G.: Gynecological disorders of old age, Practitioner (London) **208**(1246):480, 1972.

Crisp, A. H., and Stonehill, E.: Sleep, nutrition and mood, New York, 1976, John Wiley & Sons, Inc.

Eisdorfer, C., editor: The psychology of adult development and aging, Washington, D.C., 1973, American Psychological Association.

Ellwood, T. W., and Oakes, T. W.: Failure by a group of elderly men to use a preventive health service, Journal of the American Geriatrics Society **23**:74, 1975.

Field, M., editor: Depth and extent of the geriatric problem: authoritative original contributions, Springfield, Ill., 1970, Charles C Thomas, Publisher.

Hazell, K.: Social and medical problems of the elderly, ed. 2, Springfield, Ill., 1966, Charles C Thomas, Publisher.

Health, United States, 1975, Rockville, Md., 1976, Health Resources Administration, Public Health Service, DHEW Publication No. (HRA) 76-1232.

Howell, T.: Student's guide to geriatrics, ed. 2, Springfield, Ill., 1970, Charles C Thomas, Publisher.

Isaac, B.: Introduction to geriatrics, Baltimore, 1966, The Williams & Wilkins Co.

Kayser, J. S., and Minnigerode, F. A.: Increasing nursing students' interest in working with aged patients, Nursing Research **24**:23, 1975.

Knowles, L.: Maintaining a high level of wellness in older years, Gainesville, 1965, University of Florida Press.

Kosberg, J. I.: Methods for community surveillance of geriatric institutions, Public Health Reports **90**:144, 1975.

Lewis, M. I., and Butler, R. N.: Why is women's lib ignoring old women? Aging and Human Development **3**(3):223, 1972.

Loether, H. J.: Problems of aging, Belmont, Calif., 1967, Wadsworth Publishing Co., Inc.

Marmor, T. R.: The politics of Medicare, Chicago, 1973, Aldine Publishing Co.

Mathieu, R.: Hospital and nursing home management, Philadelphia, 1971, W. B. Saunders Co.

Merrill, T.: Activities for the aged and infirm: a handbook for the untrained worker, Springfield, Ill., 1967, Charles C Thomas, Publisher.

National Center for Health Statistics: Current estimates from the Health Interview Survey No. 95, DHEW Publication No. (HRA) 75-1522.

National Institute of Child Health and Human Development: Research directions toward reduction of injury in the young and old, Bethesda, 1973, DHEW Publication No. (NIH) 73-124.

Neugarten, B. L.: Patterns of aging: past, present, and future, The Social Service Review 47:571, 1973.

Nystrom, E. P.: Activity patterns and leisure concepts among the elderly, American Journal of Occupational Therapy 28:337, 1974.

Quirk, D. A., and Skinner, J. H.: IHCS: physical capacity, age and employment, Industrial Gerontologist 19:49, 1973.

Rudd, J. L., and Margolin, R. J.: Maintenance therapy for the geriatric patient, Springfield, Ill., 1967, Charles C Thomas, Publisher.

Sigel, M. M., and Good, R. A., editors: Tolerance, autoimmunity and aging, Springfield, Ill., 1971, Charles C Thomas, Publisher.

Steinberg, F. U., editor: Cowdry's the care of the geriatric patient, ed. 5, St. Louis, 1976, The C. V. Mosby Co.

Sterne, R. S., Phillips, J. E., and Rabushka, A.: The urban elderly poor: racial and bureaucratic conflict, Lexington, Mass., 1974, Lexington Books.

Strauss, A. L.: Chronic illness and the quality of life, St. Louis, 1975, The C. V. Mosby Co.

Streib, G. C., and Schneider, C. J.: Retirement in American society: impact and process, Ithaca, N.Y., 1971, Cornell University Press.

Streicher, D., and Levinsohn, F.: Doctor talks to older patients, Chicago, 1967, The Budlong Press.

Thurnher, M.: Goals, values, and life evaluations at preretirement stage, Journal of Gerontology 29:85, 1974.

Tobin, S. S.: Social and health services for the future aged, Gerontologist 15:32, 1975.

Vedder, C. B., and Lefkowitz, A. S.: Problems of the aged, Springfield, Ill., 1965, Charles C Thomas, Publisher.

Warren, H. H.: Self-perception of independence among urban elderly, American Journal of Occupational Therapy 28:329, 1974.

Zax, M., and Spector, G. A.: An introduction to community psychology, New York, 1974, John Wiley & Sons, Inc.

8 ▪ COMMUNITY MENTAL HEALTH

Sweet are the thoughts that savor of content;
The quiet mind is richer than a crown—
A mind content both crown and kingdom is.

Robert Greene

If we include drug and alcohol abuse, no phase of the community health program is receiving more attention than mental health (Steinhart, 1973). Much of this attention arises from a widespread interest in mental disorder. Yet there has developed during recent years a very wholesome interest in the mental health of the normal citizen. Fortunately, mental disorder and mental health are no longer approached with trepidation and apprehension. More and more, America has learned to deal objectively with mental health and mental disorder. Many of the social movements of the 1970s, such as Women's Liberation, have as one of their main concerns mental health.

Knowledge in the field of mental health and mental disorder is grossly inadequate, but an understanding of this field is advancing rapidly through the extension of research into the diversity of facets inherent in mental health and mental disorder. Though more knowledge in this field is needed, if all of the knowledge now available were properly utilized, a highly effective community mental health program could be promoted. Such a program would concern itself with many phases of mental health—the mental health of the normal citizen, promotion of mental health, epidemiology of mental illness, mental disorder as a phase of social pathology, the various types of mental disorder present in the population, medical and hospital resources available, and provisions for rehabil-

itation of those who have been mentally ill. The community aspects of alcohol and drug abuse will be considered in Chapter 12.

CONCEPT OF MENTAL HEALTH

For practical reasons, the term "mental health" is used to include emotional and social well-being as well as the mental state of the individual. Emotions are intense feelings with physiological as well as psychological components. A person is not just angry mentally. He or she also experiences certain physiological changes as an aspect of anger. Yet all of it must, in the final analysis, be appraised in terms of the mental state experienced by the individual. Social adjustment perhaps represents a phase of mental health rather than an independent entity. It must be acknowledged that some individuals of normal mental health live extremely limited social lives and perhaps have an adequate level of mental health. Nevertheless, to attain a high level of mental health in today's pattern of life, social relationships can be a major factor.

Mental health must be evaluated in terms of the individual's productive and enjoyable living. This, perhaps, is best expressed by a statement of Dr. Karl Menninger:

Let us define mental health as the adjustment of human beings to each other and to the world about them with a maximum of effectiveness and happiness. Not just efficiency, or just contentment —or the grace of playing the rules of the game cheerfully. It is all of these together. It is the ability to maintain an even temper, an alert intelligence, socially considerate behavior and a happy disposition. This I think is a healthy mind. [Menninger, 1953.]

No one lives perfectly efficiently, nor does any normal individual experience continuous happiness. The best that the normal individual can do is attain happiness occasionally, and then only for short periods. Nor would it be fair to label an occasional lapse of "socially considerate behavior" a mental disorder. Imperfect people in an imperfect world means that even the highest level of mental health is not perfect health. We deal here with a relative matter with varying degrees of mental health.

MENTAL HEALTH OF THE NORMAL POPULATION

By "normal" is meant that which is accepted as the usual and must be regarded as within a range. No two individuals are alike. Each is unique. Yet most of us, in terms of mental health, fit within the overall pattern or range accepted as the usual. This allows for the wide span of individual differences to be found among persons whose conduct is regarded as within accepted patterns. Within this range of normal mental health we find various degrees or levels. Some individuals function efficiently on a high level and derive unusual enjoyment in their living. They encounter frustration, disappointment, and failure, but with a minimum of friction. They freely and effectively use their abilities in harmony with life's demands and gain a maximum of personal satisfaction and enjoyment in their accomplishments.

Another group of individuals adjusts to frustration, disappointment, and failure quite readily and experiences but a moderate amount of disturbance in the friction they encounter in life. This is a very commendable quality of mental health and perhaps should be rated as good mental health. Doubtless, many of the individuals in this group could attain an excellent level of mental health with a better understanding of mental health and an organized effort in self-improvement.

A third group constitutes the majority of people in our normal population. These individuals are not mentally disordered, although they do experience occasional or even more frequent emotional upsets. Their distinguishing characteristic is that at no time do they seem to attain a dynamic level of adjustment in which they attain considerable accomplishment with an accompanying great amount of enjoyment. They tend to operate in second gear and live rather uninteresting, uninspired, and passive lives. They drag through life, getting a half-measure of what life really has to offer. These individuals possess a fair level of mental health. Many of them, through proper understanding and application, could elevate their mental health level to the good and even to the excellent status.

Few individuals attain anything like 100% of their mental health possibilities. A few attain perhaps 90% of their mental health potential, but many individuals with normal mental health nevertheless have attained little more than 50% of their actual potential in mental health. To improve one's mental health, one must understand what motivates human conduct, the nature of emotional maturation, and the attributes of a well-adjusted personality. Persons need to understand why they do certain things, what gives rise to certain emotions, what they need to do to adjust to their emotional responses, and what personality qualities they need to fortify or develop. This is the area in which a community mental health program can provide its greatest service to the normal citizen. People of the community need a better understanding of mental health. This education can be provided through the various methods and devices available to community health personnel. Citizens need the benefit of mental health counseling by qualified mental hygienists. Some need guidance in special health problems they may encounter. Normal citizens in the community have a need for mental health services just as they have a need for services that promote physical health.

Disintegration of personality. No normal individual possesses all of the qualities of personality integration to a perfect or even near-perfect degree. Indeed, every normal person experiences emotional upsets and personality disturbances. Disease, pain, and fatigue are common causes of personality disintegration. Personal disaster such as the loss of an election, family disaster such as serious injury or death, and the mounting tensions of modern living may produce personality upsets even in the best integrated personality. The well-integrated personality tends to recover quickly from any disturbance. The poorly integrated individual not only is upset more easily but requires a longer time to recover even from a moderate disturbance. There are two good indications of the degree of personality integration. The first is the ability to meet challenging situations effectively and without disturbance, and the second is the ability to recover quickly from an upset.

STATE MENTAL HEALTH PROGRAM

In the past a question has been raised as to whether mental health is a community public health problem, and some lay and professional people still ask the question. A health matter becomes a public health problem when it is amenable to solution through public action. Many aspects of the mental health problem can be dealt with most effectively through public action. Psychiatrists are not always cordial to the concept that mental hygiene is a public health responsibility. Some psychiatrists feel that state hospital staffs should be responsible for all mental hygiene in the state. However, the psychiatric hospital is isolated from the community, and the hospital staff has neither the organization nor the experience to deal with integrated community action. Generally, psychiatric hospitalization is not a function of the state health department but is administered by a separate administrative agency such as a hospital commission. If public health departments were to administer hospitals for the mentally disordered, this function would soon dwarf other activities. Mental health promotion is a function of the state health department; mental disorders and

care of the mentally ill are the functions of psychiatrists and the hospitals for the mentally ill.

If mental health promotion in the community is a public health function, why are these programs not better and more extensively developed than at the present time? Mental health begins with people thinking of their own needs, then extending this consideration to those within the family circle, and finally, to those in the community at large. While thinking in terms of the community at large is at the end of the chain, nevertheless, leadership, organization, administration, and education can develop an effective, broad program of mental health on the state level as well as on the community level (Felix, 1967).

Many states, such as California, Minnesota, New Jersey, New York, and Vermont, have passed a Community Mental Health Services Act. Other states that have not enacted a specific mental health services act nevertheless have provided for the establishment of a statewide mental health program. A few states promote mental health as a component of existing programs, such as in the maternal and child health division of the state health department. However, an identifiable state mental hygiene agency within the state department of public health provides recognition of the importance of mental hygiene as a phase of public health service. Maryland gives prominence to the mental health program by naming the state public health agency the Department of Health and Mental Hygiene.

The division of mental hygiene, or some similarly designated agency, is charged with the primary responsibility for mental health promotion in many states. This division serves as the coordinating agency in the state for all statewide forces concerned with the promotion of the mental health of the general population. It cooperates with the various voluntary agencies and official agencies in the state that are engaged in some phase of mental health. It cooperates with the state department of education, the prisons, hospital commissions, and the hospitals. While its major concern is with the mental health of the normal individual, it does provide certain services directed toward assistance for the maladjusted—the mental health of the alcoholic, the narcotics addict, the delinquent, the criminal, the physically handicapped, the aged, and other segments in the population having special mental health problems. The division of mental hygiene may sponsor or support legislation on the subject of mental health, make statistical studies, provide library facilities, make mental health education materials available in other respects, provide consulting service to agencies or communities, set up workshops and seminars for professional personnel, sponsor special programs of mental health promotion, establish and promote mental health facilities, and otherwise serve as a general mental health resource for the people of the state.

Voluntary agencies such as the state mental health association play an important role in providing leadership for those groups and individuals in the state who have an understanding of the general problem of mental health and a sincere interest in mental health promotion. Various professional organizations whose members deal professionally with services and problems having mental health aspects have been of particular value in pointing out the need for greater services in the mental health field and have provided leadership and support necessary for its attainment on a statewide basis. Frequently, it is a movement initiated by groups such as these that give rise to the establishment of an official mental health agency in the state devoted to the promotion of the mental health of the general public.

COMMUNITY MENTAL HEALTH PROMOTION

Most communities have provisions for institutionalizing the mentally ill, although facilities for early diagnosis and care are frequently inadequate or totally absent. However, very few communities have a well-organized, well-functioning program for the promotion of the mental health of the normal citizen. Large portions of the community's population have a vital interest in mental health promotion as it relates to their community, their neighborhood, their family, and themselves. Yet few want to see a mental health facility located in their neighborhood. Establishing a community mental health program means developing community support. Leadership can come from the local mental health association, from the community health council, and from other sources. Productive action usually requires long-range planning rather than a high-pressure "crash" program. Lay leadership is important, even though primary responsibility must rest with the official community public health agency. Interagency cooperation is necessary for the success of a program such as one in mental health, and full cooperation can be obtained only with public understanding, public interest, and public support (Broskowski and Baker, 1974).

Mental health needs. A survey of the specific mental health needs of a particular community would be essential to the determination of what the mental health program should be in that particular community. There are certain factors and certain mental health needs that are common to most communities, but within the community, specific factors that influence the mental health of individuals must be recognized and evaluated. Socioeconomic, neighborhood, and ethnic backgrounds, family relationships, child-rearing practices, community norms, and cultural values all represent factors determining the soil in which the mental health program is to be planted (Dohrenwend, 1975).

Adult mental health needs, as well as the special or difficult problems for which adults have a need for special assistance, are in the province of normal, everyday adjustment. Individual and family counseling services, marriage counseling, sessions for expectant parents, child study groups, parent discussions, guidance services for elderly citizens,

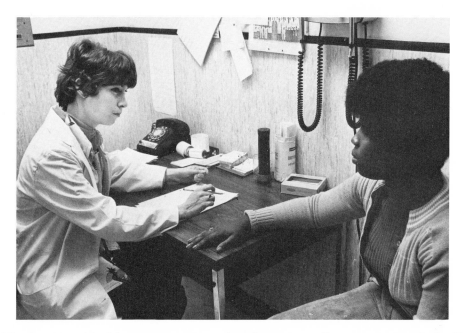

Fig. 8-1. Mental health promotion. Every clinical encounter offers opportunities for health workers to assist patients in coping with health problems and other sources of stress. (Courtesy Johns Hopkins Medical Institutions)

promotion of cultural interests, recreation programs, and general health information services all represent desirable needs in a community. No one agency will necessarily provide all of the services to satisfy these needs, but by means of an integrated community mental health program, some agency or individual will provide for each of the various needs. While a major portion of a community health program is directed toward normal people in the normal walks of life, there will be mentally disturbed people in hospitals, patients under physicians' care, patients who have been released from psychiatric hospitals and are in the process of rehabilitation, and individuals who have come to the attention of community agencies and are under the direction of these agencies.

Child and youth mental health services will be provided largely through the schools. Most communities have other agencies that will provide for some of the mental health needs of children and youth (Halpern and Kissel, 1976). These needs may not appear to be extensive, but they are extremely important. They include psychological testing and diagnostic services, counseling services for children, consulting services for parents of the youngsters, mental health guidance services for youth, remedial programs in the school, an inservice mental health training program for teachers, mental health instruction as a phase of the basic hygiene program, and family life education. An effective coordinated community-school mental health program should devote its major attention to the mental health of the normal youngster but must also provide for the mental health needs of the delinquent, the emotionally disturbed, the mentally retarded, the academically handicapped, and the youngsters who are having adjustment difficulties (Ross, 1976).

Organization and administration. The effectiveness of any community mental health program will depend to a considerable extent on its planning, organization, and direction.

A community may possess many resources for dealing with its manifold mental health needs, but unless some central agency exists that will crystallize the various services available, many needs that could be fulfilled will be neglected, many services will be inadequately provided, and there will be unnecessary duplication and even conflict in function. Setting up a central administrative agency does not mean that the various individuals, agencies, and services in the community will be hampered or otherwise obstructed in their functioning. Rather, it will mean an understanding of what services are available and the role of the various agencies and individuals in the total program. This will help reduce duplication and fragmentation of services.

In a given community, a considerable number of people may have a contribution to make to the community's mental health program. However, it is imperative that only those who are professionally qualified should participate in the community's organized mental health program. Individuals with a smattering of knowledge or with a morbid curiosity about mental health may be willing volunteers or even persistent participants, but the public is entitled to protection from the charlatans and the incompetent in mental health as well as in other areas of health.

Community mental health center. The Community Mental Health Centers Act of 1963 (U.S. Congress, 1963) authorized $150 million for fiscal years 1965, 1966, and 1967 for the construction of community mental health centers, which form the core of the national program. Allotments to states have continued to rise to $233 million in 1977, based on population, financial need, and the need for community mental health centers. Funds are provided on a matching basis. The centers are expected to include the following:

Inpatient services
Outpatient services
Partial hospitalization, including day, night, and weekend care

Community services, including consultation with community agencies and professional personnel
Diagnostic services
Rehabilitation services, including vocational and educational programs
Precare and aftercare community services, including foster home placement, home visiting, and halfway houses
Training
Research and evaluation

Congress appropriated an additional $8 million for grants to aid in the preparation of statewide plans for comprehensive mental health programs (National Institute of Mental Health, 1970).

Community health department mental health programs. Many county and city health departments have had a mental health division or section. Indeed, this has become a standard unit in the modern local health department. Frequently, this unit is organized as a clinic with a staff consisting of one or more psychiatrists, clinical psychologists, psychiatric social workers, and mental health nurse consultants. The staff provides consulting services for citizens who are normal, citizens who are mentally ill, and those who may be borderline cases. This service is extended to children as well as to adults. Marriage counseling and family counseling are frequently included in the services.

The staff provides diagnosis and recommends treatment. A limited amount of treatment may be provided, but the program is not designed for complete treatment. In some instances the mental health staff advises courts on matters relating to mental competence of people before the court. The staff may recommend rehospitalization and may assist in rehabilitation of a patient who has been released from a mental hospital.

The importance of a mental health unit in the community health department lies in its value as a resource for citizens who have a need for mental health consultation services. This gives citizens of the community a certain degree of security in the knowledge that competent mental health personnel are available when needed.

Logically, the community public health department can serve as the vital center of the overall community mental health program. The community health council that serves as the general sounding board for community health generally can serve as the connecting link between the general public and the health department. The council's function is basically advisory and in this respect is essentially an expression of community thinking and community needs. Certainly, most, if not all, of the mental health agencies of the community should have representation on such a council. Consumers should have at least equal representation. There may be merit in having a special mental health council, but the American tendency to overorganize frequently has an adverse effect on health promotion. The community's voluntary mental health association can serve as a valuable resource for the public health department without functioning as a specially recognized health council (Ruiz and Behrens, 1973).

The value of the service provided by each agency in the community would appear to depend on the freedom each agency has to do its best work within the general community mental health program or organized mental health plan. The work of the general medical practitioner or the psychiatrist should be regarded as a part of the total community mental health program, but these professional practitioners obviously need to pursue their professional services with minimal interference. Psychiatric clinics supervised by professional psychiatrists and staffed by other personnel will continue to be vital to the mental health needs of the community (Nash, 1975).

In addition to acting as the coordinating agency, the community public health department can point out mental health needs in the community that are not being met. It can assume the role of leader in obtaining the necessary services to fulfill the recognized needs. It can provide for the fullest use of voluntary services that are available in the community. It can serve as the liaison between segments of the public and the special mental health services these various segments of the public need. It can keep the community informed on matters of mental health, particularly in terms of services available, and how these services may be utilized.

Practicing physicians obviously have an important role in the mental health of the community. About 50% of general medical and surgical patients are estimated to have some kind of emotional disorder (Hanlon, 1974). Further evidence that patients who come with physical ailments to their family physicians are in need of mental health guidance is reported by the National Association for Mental Health: of all patients who go to general hospitals for physical ailments annually, 6 million are suffering from serious mental and emotional illnesses that are partly responsible for their physical complaints. Many individuals who would be classified as having normal mental health nevertheless have minor or moderate mental health problems and look to their family physician as their consultant in dealing with these mental and emotional disturbances. A citizen with a neurosis—under the supervision of a family physician, who understands the patient's total background—can usually adjust reasonably well to his or her situation and live a virtually normal life. In addition, the family physician is frequently the first person consulted when a family suspects that one of its members is suffering from mental disturbance. General medical practitioners, although they do not profess to be specialists in psychiatry, nevertheless have an adequate background to be an important resource in the community mental health program if continuing education programs are made available (National Institute of Mental Health, Alcohol, Drug Abuse, and Mental Health Administration, 1974).

Sociologists and social workers usually have a background that gives them an understanding of the field of mental health, the mental health program, and their place and contribution in the field. Working in cooperation with psychiatrists, family physicians, psychologists, and other professional people, sociologists and social case workers can make constructive contributions to community mental health through their understanding of various factors operating in the community and of the resources that can be drawn on to help the individual, the family, or the neighborhood (Wax, 1974).

Many small communities with limited professional mental health resources can draw on the facilities available in a large neighboring community. A reasonably well-organized mental health program, even in a small community, will have complete information on facilities available in nearby communities so that citizens in the smaller community can have the benefit of the highly trained psychiatrist and other specialists who are most likely to be practicing in larger cities.

EDUCATION FOR MENTAL HEALTH

People today frequently find themselves incapable of making the necessary adjustments to the kaleidoscope of modern life without assistance. The base of the pyramid we term the community mental health program is community education in mental health. Such a program is directed primarily to the mental health needs of the normal individual and is positive in its approach. Its objectives are to promote wholesome attitudes toward the whole field of mental health, to help people understand themselves as normal human beings, and to keep the community informed of the various mental health services and facilities that are available and how those services and facilities are best used.

A community mental health education program will function more effectively under the direction of an individual professionally prepared in the field of public health education. An important function of the program director is that of enlisting and utilizing the services of all qualified people or organizations in the community who can contribute to mental health education. This means organizing and administering a continuous program that provides for the mental health education needs of the various segments of the population. Resourcefulness and ingenuity are demanded, particularly when necessary resource people or organizations are not available.

As in other categorical programs, the function of health education in community mental health is to identify behaviors requiring development or change, to analyze the factors influencing these behaviors, and then to select or develop communications, community organization, and training methods to influence these factors. Examples of specific behaviors to which mental health education can be addressed are coping (Green and associates, 1976) and clinic dropouts (Kline and King, 1973). It is estimated that approximately one-third of the patients of community mental health centers drop out of treatment without staff approval or recommendation.

Community mental health education programs utilize discussion groups, pamphlets, radio, television, films, posters, newspapers, journals, institutes, and other materials and aids. Personal contacts between the health department and individual citizens are somewhat confined to public health nurses for purposes of conveying information or suggestions or advising the individual where certain information or services may be obtained. This service thus is not a consulting service, but rather an information service.

The development and utilization of clinical facilities in most communities for temporary hospitalization and care of mentally ill patients require public education even though the community relies on the state hospital facilities for its mentally ill who are in need of extended hospitalization. A developing trend is the establishment of long-term community care for the mentally ill. This could develop to a point where state hospitals will play a minor role or be abandoned. Most states have proprietary hospitals or sanitoriums that specialize in the care of the mentally ill, but these facilities are utilized by a small and declining percentage of mentally ill patients. Again, the supervision of clinical services for the mentally ill is the province of the medical profession, but the necessary funds for the construction and maintenance of adequate community facilities depend on the understanding and the interest of the general public. The proper utilization of such facilities similarly requires public education.

MENTAL ILLNESS

In the minds of a considerable proportion of the general population, the term "mental hygiene" refers exclusively to mental disorder of a major type. It is essential that the public recognize that major mental illness is an important consideration in the mental hygiene program but that equally important is the mental health of normal individuals. After all, most people in a community are normal, although they have their mental upsets and emotional disturbances and obviously do not have perfect mental health. Others in the community have mental and emotional deviations sufficiently severe to be disturbing but not constituting frank mental illness. Both the normal individual and the one with minor mental disturbances need consulting services of professional mental hygienists. The severely mentally ill are in need of special medical and hospital services, and this is the province of the psychiatrist or the medical practitioner. Psychiatry is that discipline or profession that concerns itself with the prevention, diagnosis, treatment, and cure of mental disorder. While others as well as psychiatrists may concern themselves with normal individuals, mental illness is the province of the psychiatrist.

The present psychosomatic approach indicates that the physical and psychological are interrelated and that mental disorders can have their genesis in a physiological disturbance. Mental illness, which was once regarded as primarily a problem of custodial care, is now regarded as a problem in medical care. This change has come about because

of the development of specific medication in the treatment of mental disorder and the concept that a mental hospital is a place where one can go for a short time for treatment. Cold-storage institutionalization has become obsolete, and today mental illness is regarded as truly remediable. Mental illness remains one of the five major health problems in America, but advances in the last decade indicate that a major breakthrough in the treatment and care of mental disorder has occurred and that the problem is yielding to the united efforts of the many disciplines attacking the problem. The general public is not yet aware that the success of chemotherapy in dealing with mental illness represents a landmark in the march of medicine as important as the use of artificial immunization against infectious disease.

Epidemiology of mental illness

Epidemiology concerns itself with the occurrence of phenomena affecting human health and welfare. It is a discipline that deals with population-based rates, with the incidence and prevalence of a specific condition, with age distribution, and with changes in the occurrence of phenomena.

Admissions to mental facilities. In 1965 the total of 144,090 first admissions to state and county mental hospitals was 14,392 more than the total number of first admissions in 1962. In 1969 state and county mental hospitals had 163,984 first admissions of mental and mentally retarded patients. Admissions to all psychiatric services in 1971 totaled 2.5 million, with 1.2 million in inpatient and 1.3 million in outpatient services. Males had higher admission rates to inpatient services, whereas females had higher outpatient utilization rates. The rates of admission by age groups are of interest (Table 8-1). If the present rate of admissions continues, more than 15 million people living in the United States will be admitted to a state or county mental hospital as patients.

Data on admission of patients by diagnosis give an indication of the principal causes of mental disorder afflicting the public (Table 8-2) and where people seek help for these conditions.

Whether mental disorder is on the increase in the United States is difficult to assess. More facilities are available, and people today are more inclined to use professional

Table 8-1 ■ Admission rates per 100,000 population to all inpatient and outpatient psychiatric services, by age, 1971

Age (years)	Rate of admissions
Under 18	626.8
18-24	1936.0
25-44	1982.2
45-64	1315.7
65 and over	615.2
All ages	1238.5

Table 8-2 ■ Admission rates per 100,000 population to all inpatient and outpatient psychiatric services, by diagnosis, 1971

Diagnosis	Rate of admissions	
	In-patient	Out-patient
Alcohol disorders	94.0	33.9
Depressive disorders	134.3	82.6
Brain syndromes	37.6	17.3
Schizophrenia	161.1	96.9
Drug abuse disorders	30.2	12.9
Other psychoses	9.8	9.1
Mental retardation	7.4	21.5
All other diagnoses	110.9	290.2
Undiagnosed	11.5	77.4
All diagnoses	596.8	641.8

Table 8-3 ■ Patients in state and county mental hospitals, United States, per 100,000, 1880 to 1971

Year	Rate per 100,000
1880	32
1920	230
1940	364
1955	390
1958	363
1960	343
1963	311
1965	287
1971	151

Table 8-4 ■ Patients in state and county mental hospitals, 1935 to 1971

Year	Number of patients at the end of the year
1935	389,000
1940	434,000
1945	463,000
1950	513,000
1955	559,000
1958	545,000
1960	536,000
1963	505,000
1965	476,000
1971	308,024

From National Institutes of Health: Utilization of mental health facilities, 1971, DHEW Publication No. (NIH) 74-657.

services and facilities. Chemotherapy has not reduced admissions significantly but does shorten the length of hosptial stay and increases outpatient utilization.

Population of mental hospitals. From 1880 to 1955 there had been a steady increase in the average number of patients in state and county mental hospitals per 100,000 people in the United States. Since 1955 there has been a steady decline (Table 8-3). In 1955 the average daily census of the state and county mental hospitals for mental disease in the United States was 559,000—54% of patients in all hospitals. In 1956 for the first time in the history of the United States, there was a reduction in the number of resident patients in the state and county mental hospitals. On December 31, 1956, there were about 7,000 fewer patients in these hospitals than on December 31, 1955. This was the result of the successful use of chemo-

therapy in the treatment of mental disorder. The decline was particularly significant when one considers that between the years 1945 and 1955 there was an average increase of 10,000 patients per year in these mental hospitals. Each year since 1956 there has been a further decrease in the year-end census of patients in mental hospitals (Table 8-4). In 1971 the census of patients (308,024) was a 30,568 (9%) decline over the previous year.

The incidence of the various mental disorders of patients in the state and county mental hospitals is portrayed in a report of the National Institute of Mental Health (Table 8-5). This report classifies 272,869 patients in state and county mental hospitals in 1972. It represents the prevailing distribution of various types of mental disorders in the mental hospital population.

The epidemiology of mental illness extends

Table 8-5 ■ Mental disorders of patients in state and county mental hospitals, 1972 estimate, by diagnosis and age

Mental disorders	Total	Percent
All patients	272,869	100
By diagnosis		
Schizophrenic reactions	110,469	40.4
Manic depressive reactions	8,240	3.0
Other psychotic disorders	7,612	2.7
Chronic brain syndrome	5,438	2.0
Senility diseases	27,674	10.0
Psychoneurotic reactions	7,944	3.0
Personality disorders	10,056	4.0
Alcoholism	17,538	6.3
Mental deficiency	23,440	8.6
All other diagnoses	54,458	20.0
By age (years)		
Under 25	34,376	12.6
25 to 34	29,792	10.9
35 to 44	34,209	12.5
45 to 54	42,947	15.7
55 to 64	60,027	22.0
Over 64	71,518	26.2

beyond hospitalized patients. A considerable number of people being treated through outpatient clinics are mentally ill. Nationwide records indicate that 2,500,000 men, women, and children are treated each year in mental hospitals, in psychiatric clinics, or by private psychiatrists. As will be indicated later, the number of patients served through outpatient clinics will be increased substantially as new methods of treatment are developed.

Available records indicate that about 200,000 children are brought to mental health clinics each year. Obviously, not all of these youngsters are mentally ill. Many are poorly adjusted and can benefit by counseling of the mental hygienist but would not be diagnosed as psychotic or even neurotic. The Department of Psychiatry, Columbia University, reports that 10% of public school children are in need of mental health guidance. This is not to be interpreted to mean that all of these children represent cases of mental disorder. Many people not classified as mentally ill nevertheless are in need of the services of mental health specialists.

Cost of mental illness

In 1945 the cost per patient in mental hospitals was $1.06 per day. In 1956 this figure had risen to $3.26 per day. In 1960 the cost had risen to $4.91, and in 1971 the cost per patient per day was $17.59. The financial burden of caring for the ill is considerable, but the price paid in other respects is even greater. Patients, their family, their neighborhood, their community, their employer, and the nation as a whole can be affected. Mental illness casts its shadow over all of us and makes prevention an attractive course for national policy (Harper and Balch, 1975).

Mental disorder and social pathology

Many factors contribute to the social pathology of a community, but most seem to relate to a failure in human adjustment. In some instances psychosis, in some cases a neurosis, and in other cases inadequate adjustment of an otherwise normal individual is fundamental to a particular social pathology. Mental disorder does not account for all crime, delinquency, alcoholism, narcotic addictions, divorce, and suicide. Indeed, the greatest portion is caused by people who are regarded as normal. Yet these individuals, regarded as normal, are generally people with explosive tempers, exaggerated feelings of inadequacy, marked feelings of persecution, or people who are asocial or antisocial, highly suspicious, overly sensitive, impulsive, overly emotional, unstable, or unable to obtain self-gratification through the normal avenues of life.

A review of the extent of social pathology gives us some indication of the magnitude of the problem. Approximately one out of every four marriages results in divorce. America has more than 2 million serious crimes each year. About 300,000 children between the ages of 11 and 17 appear in court in a year. Over 22,000 suicides are recorded each year. Mental health implications are obvious.

Factors in divorce. A successful marriage is basically a matter of personality adjustment. The individual who finds difficulty in adjusting to single life is ill-prepared to adjust to the complexities of married life. One needs but go over the complaints of wives and husbands in divorce actions to recognize the extent to which inadequate personal adjustment is the basic factor. A husband's complaints in divorce actions are revealing —wife's feelings are too easily hurt, wife criticizes me, wife is too nervous and emotional, lack of freedom in the home, wife is quick-tempered, wife nags, wife tries to improve me, wife complains too much, wife is not affectionate, wife is too argumentative, we cannot agree on choice of friends. Wives, on the other hand, offer these complaints— husband is nervous and impatient, husband criticizes me, husband is argumentative, husband is quick-tempered, husband doesn't talk things over, husband is selfish and inconsiderate, husband is touchy, husband doesn't show affection, husband is too demanding, our marriage is too confining, husband criticizes my choice of friends. These complaints, obtained from complaints filed in divorce proceedings, are an indication that personality, maturity, and adjustment are basic factors in marital stability.

Marriage counselors can provide a valuable service to a community for those individuals in marriage who are having difficulty in making an adequate marriage adjustment. More important is a community health service that assists people in problems of mental health before these people are married. Not all people in a community are in need of mental health counseling, and not all married couples need the services of a marriage counselor. A community health department that provides mental health counseling for normal people who do need such services will contribute not only to the general level of mental health but to the prevention of a great deal of social pathology in the form of broken families.

Factors in suicide. Most information on the mental state of people who attempt to take their own lives is obtained from those people who failed in a suicide attempt. There is one successful suicide for every three attempts, and about 5% of those who fail are repeaters. The rate among men is more than three times that among women. The suicide rate is low among certain groups. The rate is especially low among Mormons and Roman Catholics, and blacks rarely take their own lives. These data would indicate that the suicide rate can be influenced by conditioning in the individual's life. Studies indicate that perhaps 30% of those who take their own lives are actually mentally disordered. The remainder of suicides are largely the result of a decision that death is the best solution to a situation. For many of these there were coping possibilities that were not adequately explored. When life has lost its purpose or when the individual is badly frustrated, has lost self-esteem, or is depressed, an individual who lacks good personality integration may attempt to escape

from reality by self-destruction (Resnick and Hawthorne, 1973).

Helping individuals over the immediate crisis, together with counseling that helps them to see the problem and its solution, will not only prevent a present attempt but will prevent further attempts at self-destruction. People who threaten suicide often carry out their threats. That persons threaten to take their own life is an indication of disturbance and of the need for assistance. Most suicides can be prevented if people recognize that the individuals are disturbed, take action to protect the individuals against themselves, and assist them in understanding and solving the situation. Persons who suffer marked depression are particularly in need of guidance during the period of depression. Highly sensitive persons may take their own life in order to hurt others. These individuals simply are too "thin-skinned" and sensitive for the rugged world in which they live. For these individuals, mental health counseling is long past due. If a community has adequate mental health counseling and a considerable number of citizens who recognize the various factors that indicate that a person is likely to attempt to take his or her own life, it can be predicted conservatively that suicide could be cut to one-third of its present rate (Welu, 1972).

Mental illness among criminals. The first American study made of the incidence of mental illness among criminals was conducted more than a quarter of a century ago by Dr. Bernard Glueck, who conducted the first penal psychiatric clinic at Sing Sing Prison. Dr. Glueck's examination of incoming prisoners revealed that 12% were frankly psychotic and that 19% were borderline cases. A subsequent study by the National Association for Mental Health in eleven state penitentiaries of 8,581 consecutive admissions revealed that 25.4% were psychotic and that 14.1% were borderline cases. An early recognition of mental illness might have prevented some of the crimes in which these individuals were involved. It is in this respect that informed citizens of a community could be of service in recognizing abnormal behavior that could be associated with violence (Matthews, 1967).

Individuals who have a tendency toward violent outbursts of temper, who are overly suspicious, who have delusions of persecution, who are antisocial, or who are quarrelsome should be recognized as people who are more likely to be involved in actions of violence and destruction. Behind the wheels of automobiles a community will find people who are frankly psychotic, as well as borderline cases. Antisocial individuals behind the wheel of a motor vehicle have little respect for the rights or welfare of others. They not only will inconvenience others, but their recklessness, impatience, carelessness, excitability, and lack of responsibility can be important factors in causing motor vehicle accidents. In terms of accident prevention, a motor vehicle driver's personality mold is more important than a mechanical ability to handle the car. This may force communities eventually to deny a motor vehicle operator's license to an individual because of a personality deficiency as well as because of driving deficiencies (Williams, Henderson, and Mills, 1974).

After a crime has been committed, courts properly refer a prisoner to a psychiatrist for determination of the prisoner's level of mental responsibility. This is a procedure with which most responsible citizens will agree. A corollary of this program is an effort to determine irresponsibility in individuals before they become involved in serious crimes. It is not possible to predict all people who may engage in crime, but repeaters have identified themselves as possible chronic criminals and have indicated the need to determine whether they are mentally ill. Others who show marked deviation in their behavior pattern should also be examined to determine the degree of mental and emotional responsibility they possess. Unfortunately, the legal machinery is frequently cumbersome, and threats to civil rights can be so great that people in the professional

social field are hesitant to initiate any action to provide for the psychiatric examination and counseling of citizens who could be possible threats to the people of the community. It is possible to protect the rights of the individual whose conduct appears to deviate markedly from the normal and at the same time protect the welfare of the children and adults in the community (Kocher, 1976). This would truly be a program of prevention, both in terms of mental health and in terms of community protection.

PUBLIC RESPONSIBILITY IN MENTAL DISORDERS

The diagnosis of mental disorder is the province and the responsibility of qualified professionals. Unfortunately, the physician or psychologist frequently does not see the patient with a mental disorder until the condition is very far advanced or some crisis with serious consequences has occurred. There is a need in every community to provide the means by which people showing indications of mental disorder will be directed to professional sources for diagnosis, treatment, and care. This can be provided by having responsible people in the community informed on the early indications of mental disturbance or possible mental illness. The popular misconception that a mentally disordered person dresses oddly, has weird mannerisms, is likely to be maniacal, or talks foolishly must be displaced by a more realistic conception of the indications of mental disturbance. People in the parahealth fields could be trained to recognize some of the early indications of mental disorder. When this nucleus of professional workers coming in daily contact with the public is aided by other reliable citizens having an understanding of the early indications of mental disturbance, then a community possesses a valuable means by which individuals likely in need of diagnostic services and counsel are directed to services at an early stage when constructive and even preventive measures can be taken. In addition such a group of informed citizens in a community can be the means by which tragedies can be prevented (Jones, 1974).

Informed citizens can give responsible support to necessary programs for providing hospital clinics and other services necessary for the proper care and treatment of the mentally disordered. Well-informed people can lend the essential support to desirable legislation to promote an effective mental health program. They can also support the necessary official agencies, including courts, in their programs to deal with the mentally disturbed (Ruiz and Behrens, 1973).

MEDICAL RESOURCES

This year in the United States, about 2,500,000 men, women, and children will be treated for mental health problems in mental hospitals, in community mental health centers, or by private physicians. An appraisal of available medical resources in mental health must include clinics and professional personnel available to the general public, as well as psychiatrists, nurses, and other personnel available in psychiatric hospitals. An accurate accounting of all mental health services available to the general public is extremely difficult because of the number of medical physicians who devote but a limited portion of their practice to the mentally disordered but who contribute a very important service. Most studies are limited to those clinics and practitioners primarily concerned with the mentally ill.

Community mental health centers are playing an increasingly important role in the treatment of mental illness. With the development of effective alkaloids for treating specific types of mental disorder, about one-third of the patients now treated in clinics would have been hospital patients but are now able to remain at home. In addition many patients hospitalized for chronic disorders can now be released to return to their communities under the supervision of a clinic or a physician. More than half of these clinics were located in the northeastern United

States, which has about one-fourth of the population. Qualified authorities maintain that there should be one psychiatric clinic for every 50,000 people, a standard that would require nearly doubling the full-time clinics in the United States.

Psychiatrists and other professional personnel, both for general psychiatric needs and for mental hospital needs, are in short supply. In 1973 25,063 psychiatrists were in active practice, but only 12,773 were in private practice. Less than 10% of psychiatrists devote their practice to child psychiatry (American Medical Association, 1974). Psychiatric hospitals have a staff deficiency in most categories. In 1973 there were 27,000 active psychologists, a large proportion of whom today are employed in academic and other nonclinical activities, and many others are unemployed (National Center for Health Statistics, 1974). Progress is being made in personnel increases, even though a deficiency still exists. In 1945 state and county mental hospitals had only one full-time employee for every 6.8 patients. In 1956 they had one full-time employee for every 3.6 patients, and in 1968 one for every 1.6 patients. Estimated and projected full-time equivalent positions in community mental health centers are as follows:

	1968	1970	1980
Community mental health centers known and estimated to exist	125	300	2,000
Discipline			
Psychiatrists	747	1,740	11,600
Psychologists	383	918	6,120
Social workers	742	1,710	11,400
Professional nurses	852	2,040	13,600
Practical nurses	413	990	6,600
Attendants and aides	1,707	4,080	27,200
Other professionals	485	1,140	7,600
Other mental health workers	303	720	4,800
Total	5,757	13,638	90,920

With more successful treatment of the mentally ill and a declining population in our psychiatric hospitals, the need for hospital staff becomes less, but the need for community workers becomes greater.

Employment of clinical psychologists for the care of the mentally ill is a more recent development, but the service that has been given by clinical psychologists indicates that there will be an expansion of this service in the future. In 1968 somewhat more than 6,400 *clinical* psychologists practiced in hospitals, clinics, or similar medical settings. About 2,300 *counseling* psychologists worked in schools, industry, and community agencies to forestall mental illness. With the expanding concept of community service in mental health, clinical psychologists should become increasingly important as the value of their services becomes better appreciated (Autor and Zide, 1974; Shochet, 1974).

HOSPITAL FACILITIES

In 1973 there were 338,574 psychiatric beds in the United States representing 23% of all hospital beds. State and county hospitals accounted for 293,103 of these psychiatric beds. Veterans Administration, neuropsychiatric hospitals, private mental hospitals, treatment centers for children, and general hospitals provided the remaining beds. Many hospitals for mental patients do not merit approval of the American Psychiatric Association, but these hospitals gradually phase out. In the past decade there has been a pronounced decline in the number of mental hospitals and the average number of patients in these hospitals. An increasing number of mental patients are being cared for locally in general hospitals and under clinical supervision at community mental health centers.

REHABILITATION

Rehabilitation is the restoration to the fullest physical, mental, social, vocational, and economic usefulness of which an individual is capable. Total rehabilitation of persons who have recovered from mental illness may require only the services of their family physician or may require the well-

integrated program of a rehabilitation team consisting of psychiatrist, psychologist, psychiatric social worker, nurse, occupational therapist, rehabilitation therapist, and family counselor.

The success of chemotherapy in the treatment of mental disorder is relieving the overcrowding in mental hospitals in the United States but is increasing the need for rehabilitation services. With specific measures for the treatment of mental disorder, a mental hospital has become a place where one can go for a short time for treatment. This revolution in the treatment of mental disease means that custodial care is being replaced by medical treatment. A patient who has been hospitalized for several years has a social adjustment to make as well as a medical recovery. As the medication is effective in improving the patient's mental illness, the patient is permitted to visit a neighboring community under the guidance of a hospital attendant. After several escorted visits and observable improvement in adjustment to society, the patient is permitted to visit the community unescorted. When the patient's social adjustment and mental adjustment appear to be sufficiently advanced, the patient is permitted to return to his or her home and community, but only when adequate supervision is available. This means that both medical and social supervision must be provided.

A family physician may accept responsibility for the continuation of the treatment the patient has been receiving. Medical supervision may be arranged through a psychiatric clinic in the patient's community. Rehabilitation services also are needed to assist the recovered or recuperating individual to make the necessary social, economic, and other adjustments that normal living requires. Getting a job, finding social groups and interests, adjusting to the tempo of community living, and finding leisure-time activities may require the services of specially prepared people. Statewide clinic systems are emerging from the community mental health centers. State hospitals that presently have a rehabilitation service are establishing links with centers throughout the state where former patients in need of assistance may obtain rehabilitation services conveniently and promptly.

RESEARCH

It would be incorrect to say that research is the greatest need in the mental health field because hospital facilities, medical services, and other types of professional services are indispensable. Research has not received the attention in mental health that it has in most other areas of health. The fifty states, which properly provide millions of dollars for mental hospitals for the care of the mentally ill, appropriate for research only 1.5% of their total mental hospital budget. State mental health officials contend that from 4% to 7% of a state's annual budget for mental health should be allotted to research.

On a national scale the research program in the field of mental health is more encouraging, but the amount appropriated is still inadequate to do the job that is needed. Actual expenditures for research from the Alcohol, Drug Abuse, and Mental Health Administration (incorporating the former National Institute of Mental Health) amounted to $141,300,000 in 1976. The trend in appropriations for mental health research is shown in Fig. 8-3. About 30% of the current mental health research budget is devoted to alcoholism and drug abuse, and the remainder is diluted by pressures on the government to devote these resources to major social problems, including rape and other forms of violence as well as the problems of

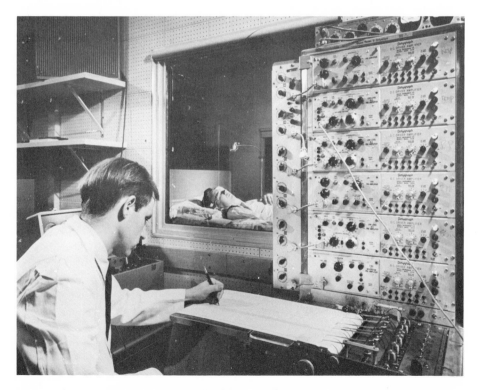

Fig. 8-2. Sleep studies. Today mental health research is far-reaching and uses sophisticated instruments. Using the electroencephalograph, it is possible to get recordings of brainwave changes during different phases of sleep, all of which can aid investigators in understanding brain function. (Courtesy National Institutes of Health)

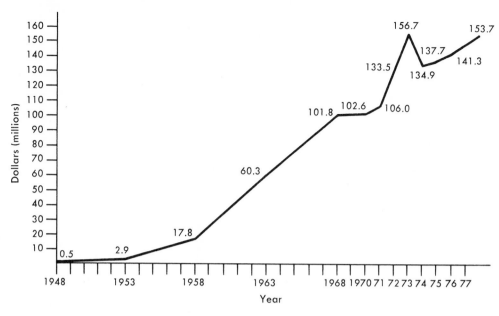

Fig. 8-3. Appropriations for mental health research, 1948 to 1977. (From Forward Plan for Health, FY 1978-82, DHEW Publication No. [OS]76-50046)

minorities and women. These are all important problems, but they are so complex as to diffuse scarce mental health resources for service as well as research.

As formidable as $150 million appears to be, it represents but a small fraction of the funds invested in research in other areas of health. The many recognized problems in mental illness that cry out for solution indicate that, as a nation, we ought to double or triple our efforts in mental health research.

The most fruitful area of research would be in the preventive aspect of mental illness (Harper and Balch, 1975). The use of alkaloids has enabled many individuals to remain at home who otherwise would have been sent to a psychiatric hospital for treatment. As important as preventive medication procedures are in dealing with mental illness, functional or psychological measures for the prevention of mental illness may be an equally productive field of research, but one in which very little organized research has been completed.

Investigations into the cause, prevention,

treatment, and cure of mental illness could be intensified if more resources were devoted to the pursuit. Research is also needed in the mental health of the normal individual. America's advances in the health and medical fields in the past quarter-century have included only modest progress in our understanding of the mental health of the normal individual. Research in the motivation of human conduct, the genesis of emotional disturbance, the nature of mild deviations, procedures for improving and fortifying personality attributes, and the measures by which an individual of normal health may cope with stress (Green and associates, 1976) are all in need of intensive study. Perhaps new methods of research need to be developed and more behavioral scientists prepared to do research in the mental health of the normal individual as well as in the problems of the mentally ill. Research on methods of mental health education will become more urgent as other research findings accumulate. Community leaders, particularly those in the health professions, must take the lead in emphasizing the need for intensive research in the field of mental health.

QUESTIONS AND EXERCISES

1. With what phases of mental health should the community mental health program concern itself?
2. Why is social health properly regarded as a phase of mental health?
3. Describe some adult in your community who has excellent mental health and analyze the attributes he or she possesses.
4. Why is public health education fundamental to a community mental health program?
5. Give several examples of conduct by an adult that indicate emotional immaturity.
6. What can a community mental health program do to assist people in improving their social personalities?
7. Why do citizens with marked aggressions represent a special community mental health problem?
8. State the case for and against having the staffs of the state's mental hospitals in charge of the total state mental health program.
9. Why has a mental health program been slow in developing in your community?
10. Appraise the mental health program of the official mental hygiene agency of your own state.
11. What statewide voluntary mental health agencies function in your state and what are their programs?
12. Survey the mental health needs of your community.
13. Propose a program to meet the mental health needs of your community.
14. Based on the available data, make a prediction of the future epidemiology of mental illness in America.
15. Show how personality maladjustment can be the true cause of a divorce.
16. If you had good reason to believe that one member of a family of your close acquaintance was in need of psychiatric service, what measures would you take to bring this about?
17. If you had good reason to believe that one member of a family you did not know was in need of psychiatric service, what measures would you take to bring this about?
18. To what extent is it correct to say that every person has his mental measles and emotional chicken pox?
19. Evaluate this statement: "Research in the field of mental disorder will create the problem of preparing professional specialists in the field of rehabilitation."
20. What research is needed in the area of normal mental health?

REFERENCES

American Medical Association: Distribution of physicians in the United States, 1973, Chicago, 1974, A.M.A. Center for Health Services Research and Development.

Autor, S. B., and Zide, E. D.: Master's level profes-sional training in clinical psychology and community mental health, Professional Psychology **5:**115, 1974.

Bellak, L., and Barten, H. H., editors: Progress in community mental health, vol. 1, New York, 1969, Grune & Stratton, Inc.

Boris, H. N.: Cultures in conflict, mental health and the hard-to-reach, Mental Hygiene **51:**351, 1967.

Broskowski, A., and Baker, F.: Professional, organizational, and social barriers to primary prevention, American Journal of Orthopsychiatry **44:**707, 1974.

Butler, R. N., and Lewis, M. I.: Aging and mental health: positive psychosocial approaches, St. Louis, 1977, The C. V. Mosby Co.

Clinebell, H. J., editor: Community mental health, Nashville, 1970, Abingdon Press.

Craft, M. J.: Psychopathic disorders, New York, 1966, Pergamon Press, Inc.

Cromwell, P. E., editor: Women and mental health: selected annotated references, 1970-1973, Health, DHEW Publication No. (ADM) 75-54.

Curran, W. J.: Community mental health and commitment laws: a radical new approach is needed, American Journal of Public Health **57:**1565, 1967.

David, H. P.: International trends in mental health, vol. 1, Community and school, New York, 1966, McGraw-Hill Book Co.

Dohrenwend, B. P.: Sociocultural and social-psychological factors in the genesis of mental disorders, Journal of Health and Social Behavior **16:**365, 1975.

Faberow, N. L.: Bibliography on suicide and suicide prevention, Rockville, Md., 1972, National Institute of Mental Health, DHEW Publication No. (HSM) 72-9080.

Fairweather, G. W., and associates: Community life for the mentally ill: an alternative to institutional care, Chicago, 1969, Aldine Publishing Co.

Felix, R. H.: Mental illness: progress and prospects, New York, 1967, Columbia University Press.

Fish, J. J.: Clinical psychiatry for the layman, Baltimore, 1964, The Williams & Wilkins Co.

Freeman, H., and Farndale, J.: New aspects of mental health services, New York, 1968, Pergamon Press, Inc.

Green, L. W., and associates: Coping and self-care patterns of normal adults in response to mild symptoms of stress, Paper presented at American Public Health Association, Miami, October 18, 1976.

Grob, G. N.: State and the mentally ill, Chapel Hill, 1966, University of North Carolina Press.

Grunebaum, H.: Practice of community mental health, Boston, 1970, Little, Brown and Co.

Hall, B. H., editor: Menninger, W. C., psychiatrist for a troubled world, New York, 1967, The Viking Press, Inc.

Halpern, W. I., and Kissel, S.: Human resources for troubled children, New York, 1976, John Wiley & Sons, Inc.

Hanlon, J. J.: Public health: administration and practice, ed. 6, St. Louis, 1974, The C. V. Mosby Co.

Harper, R., and Balch, P.: Some economic arguments in favor of primary prevention, Professional Psychology **6:**17, 1975.

Huessy, H. R.: Community psychiatry and community mental health, New York, 1966, Grune & Stratton, Inc.

Huessy, H. R.: Mental health with limited resources: Yankee ingenuity in low-cost programs, New York, 1966, Grune & Stratton, Inc.

Jones, F. H.: A 4-year follow-up of vulnerable adolescents: the prediction of outcomes in early adulthood from measures of social competence, coping style, and overall level of psychopathology, Journal of Nervous and Mental Disease **159:**20, 1974.

Kaplan, L.: Education and mental health, rev. ed., New York, 1971, Harper & Row, Publishers, Inc.

Katz, J., and associates: Psychoanalysis, psychiatry and law, New York, 1967, The Macmillan Co.

Keezer, W. S.: Mental health and human behavior, ed. 3, Dubuque, Iowa, 1971, William C. Brown Co., Publishers.

Kline, J., and King, M.: Treatment dropouts from a community mental health center, Community Mental Health Journal **9:**354, 1973.

Kocher, G. P., editor: Children's rights and the mental health professions, New York, 1976, John Wiley & Sons, Inc.

Lawrence, M. M.: Mental health team in the school, New York, 1971, Behavioral Publications, Inc.

Leonard, C. V.: Understanding and preventing suicide, Springfield, Ill., 1965, Charles C Thomas, Publisher.

Marmor, J.: Psychiatrists and their patients: a national study of private practice, Washington, 1975, American Psychiatric Association.

Matthews, A. R.: Mental illness and the criminal law: is community mental health the answer? American Journal of Public Health **57:**1571, 1967.

McLean, A.: Mental health and the business community, New York, 1967, The Macmillan Co.

Menninger, K. A.: The human mind, ed. 3, New York, 1953, Alfred A. Knopf, Inc.

Murred, S. A.: Community psychology and social systems: a conceptual framework and intervention guide, New York, 1973, Behavioral Publications, Inc.

Nash, K. B.: Supervision and the emerging professional, American Journal of Orthopsychiatry **5:**93, 1975.

National Center for Health Statistics: Health resources statistics, 1974, DHEW Publication No. (HRA) 75-1509.

National Center for Health Statistics: Parent ratings of behavioral patterns of youths 12-17 years, United States, Vital and Health Statistics, Data from the National Health Survey, Series #11, No. 137, DHEW Publication No. HRA 74-1619, 1974.

National Institute of Mental Health: The comprehensive community mental health center, Rockville, Md., 1970, PHS Publication No. 2136.

National Institute of Mental Health, Alcohol, Drug Abuse, and Mental Health Administration: Serving mental health needs of the aged through volunteer services, Rockville, Md., 1974, DHEW Publication No. NIH 74-669.

Panzetta, A. F.: Community mental health, myth and reality, Philadelphia, 1971, Lea & Febiger.

Resnick, H. L. P., and Hawthorne, V. C., editors: Suicide prevention in the 70's, Rockville, Md., 1973, National Institute of Mental Health, DHEW Publication No. (HSA) 72-9054.

Riess, B. F., editor: New directions in mental health, 2 vols., New York, 1968, Grune & Stratton, Inc.

Rosenzweig, S.: Compulsory hospitalization of the mentally ill, American Journal of Public Health **61:**121, 1971.

Ross, D. M.: Hyperactivity: research, theory and action, New York, 1976, John Wiley & Sons, Inc.

Ruiz, P., and Behrens, M.: Community control in mental health: how far can it go? Psychiatric Quarterly **47:**317, 1973.

Samuels, H.: Mental health, Dubuque, Iowa, 1970, William C. Brown Co., Publishers.

Shapiro, D. S., and associates: Mental health counselor in the community, Springfield, Ill., 1968, Charles C Thomas, Publisher.

Shochet, B. R.: The role of the mental health counselor in the psychiatric liaison service of the general hospital, International Journal of Psychiatry in Medicine **5:**1, 1974.

Sutherland, J. D., editor: Towards community mental health, New York, 1971, Barnes & Noble, Inc.

Szaz, T.: The myth of mental illness, New York, 1961, Harper & Row, Publishers, Inc.

Task Force on Community Mental Health: Issues in community psychology and preventive mental health, New York, 1971, Behavioral Publications, Inc.

Wax, D. E.: A collaborative-interactive model for mental health consultation, Child Psychiatry and Human Development **5:**78, 1974.

Welu, T. C.: Broadening the focus of suicide prevention activities utilizing the public health model, American Journal of Public Health **62:**1625, 1972.

Williams, C. L., Henderson, A. S., and Mills, J. M.: An epidemiological study of serious traffic offenders, Social Psychiatry **9:**99, 1974.

9 ▪ COMMUNITY RECREATION AND FITNESS

Regular, vigorous physical activity provides a pleasant and relaxing way of filling leisure hours. But more than this, it enhances health, improves mental and physical performance, and even helps to prolong life.

Gerald R. Ford

Recreation serves many purposes, but perhaps none is more important than the contribution it makes to health. The primary values of recreation include health promotion, prevention of certain disorders, and treatment of certain disabilities. Recreation personnel generally regard recreation as a parahealth profession.

Many individuals can provide for their own recreational needs. A large portion of the citizens in the community, however, are unable to fulfill an adequate portion of their needs without the benefit of an organized community recreational and fitness program.

THE PROBLEM

According to the President's Council on Physical Fitness and Sports, America's fitness attitudes and practices have changed positively in the following ways:

1. Physicians routinely prescribe exercise as a means of maintaining and enhancing health, and exercise is accepted therapy for many heart patients and the victims of other degenerative diseases.
2. America is in the midst of a genuine participant sports boom—more bicycles than automobiles are being bought; sports fashion and athletic footwear

have become major industries; and the number of skiers and tennis players has tripled.
3. Joggers, backpackers, and bicycling commuters, once sources of amusement or amazement, are commonplace in most communities. (There are 7 million joggers, 15 million regular cyclists, and 15 million serious swimmers among America's 110 million adults.)
4. The number of young women participating in interscholastic and intercollegiate sports quadrupled between 1966 and 1976.
5. Twelve million boys and girls try out for the Presidential Physical Fitness Award each school year.
6. Ninety percent of the Americans questioned in a national survey said that we should have physical education programs in our elementary and secondary schools.

Yet despite these facts, pockets of public apathy, urban growth, and modern life-style continually threaten to neutralize physical fitness advances. Nearly half of the 110 million adult Americans never engage in physical activity for exercise, according to a national survey. Older, poorer, and less-educated Americans frequently have little understanding of the contributions that exercise can make to health, performance, or the quality of life. Millions of Americans still are willing victims of schemes that promise fitness in a few minutes a day, without sweat or strain. One-third of all American children are overweight. The continuing financial crisis of schools and the trend away from required subjects have resulted in the loss of many physical education programs. A simultaneous trend toward "elective" physical education often results in students taking courses that contribute little to fitness or development of progressive skills. Larger schools and larger cities often diminish opportunities for participation in sports and other active forms of recreation.

Community recreation mushroomed in the decade from 1950 to 1960, perhaps as a phase of the do-it-yourself trend inherent in the modern era of suburbia. The 1920s and 1930s were characterized by the development of spectator sports and box-office attractions. These were decades that created glamorous films and professional athletics. At present the trend of the public is toward participation in physical activities, and the community finds it necessary to serve citizens who desire to occupy their leisure hours in stimulating pursuits.

The most pervasive impact on our physical and recreational patterns has been television, which has substituted passive entertainment for creative recreation and sedentary recreation for physical activity. By the time a child reaches school age, he or she is watching an average of 23.5 hours of television per week, while adults are watching 44 hours in the same week, according to Arthur C. Nielsons' ratings. Newsweek (February 21, 1977) estimates that a 17-year-old has logged at least 15,000 hours of television time, more than any other activity except sleep. This will include 350,000 commercial advertisements (70% of which on Saturday mornings are for junk foods).

A community is obliged to develop a recreational and fitness program providing for a wide diversity of participation. Recreation is no longer regarded simply as play or games but includes creative and esthetic interests as well as those of a predominantly physical nature. A community doubtless can exist without formal recreational and fitness programs, but the community is better for having an organized recreational program that provides for many of the social, creative, esthetic, communicative, learning, and physical activities of its people. Funds put into a community recreational and fitness program can be an investment in a higher level of well-being for the people of the community. The program can provide not only more enjoyable living, but more effective living for a large segment of the population.

RECREATION AS HEALTH PROMOTION

More effective and enjoyable living through recreation can contribute to mental, social, and physical health. By breaking from the dull, commonplace routine of existence, recreation contributes to a greater realization of the individual's potential for living. It provides a means for bringing to fuller fruition the health potential of the individual. Recreation alone cannot produce a high level of health, but combined with other factors affecting health it can elevate health for normal individuals. For some individuals the mental health contribution of recreation is the greatest value. For other individuals the physical health values or the social values are most important. Whatever the particular health needs of an individual may be, recreation can make some contribution to that specific need. For the individual with a chronic disability or some disorder, recreation frequently proves to be of value in restoring health. The rehabilitation value of recreation is universally acknowledged.

Mental health

The normal individual seeks self-gratification and the experience of pleasant emotions that accompany gratification of the self. Every normal individual seeks self-esteem. Many individuals are able to find this self-gratification and attainment of self-esteem in their regular vocations, but in this assembly-line age of automation, where individuals find themselves a cog in a big machine, they frequently derive little gratification from the product they help to turn out or the services they give. They will seek some other avenue through which gratification can be attained. Recreation is serving as the avenue through which many individuals obtain the emotional gratification that accompanies self-fulfillment.

The normal person seeks attention, approval, and praise. Achievement, mastery, skill, and superiority bring elation and produce satisfying emotions. Through recreation, an individual can achieve a high level of personal performance, can experience mastery, and can obtain attention, approval, and praise, all of which arouse emotions of pleasure and elation. Recreation can lift the individual into an experience in which the self is of importance. Gratification, so essential to a high level of mental health, can be attained through creative, esthetic, social, communicative, and learning activities as well as through physical activities.

Aggressions can be given an outlet in competitive games. Creative urges can be satisfied through programs in crafts, painting, dramatics, music, writing, and other arts. Relaxation may be achieved through passive activities such as reading, music appreciation, art appreciation, listening to addresses, and otherwise serving somewhat the role of the spectator rather than the active participant. On the curative side is the statement of Dr. Maurice E. Linden:

The real significance of recreation as therapy lies in its capacity to promote, foster, and develop human interaction. It awakens the spirit of competitiveness and of fair play through a pleasurable system of cooperation. In this way, it serves as a sublimated outlet for aggressive drives, as a device for retraining and restoring the human capacity for mutual identification, and has a socializing influence through team participation. Few human activities offer so much for so small an expenditure [Linden, 1957].

The famous Menninger Clinic in Topeka, Kansas, which has an outstanding record for the release of patients and few returnees, prescribes specific types of recreation for each patient as part of the therapeutic procedure.

Social health

Social health is an extension of mental health. To give meaning to life, normal individuals want friendship and companionship or association with others. The interaction with fellow human beings promotes a feeling of worth, a feeling of security from group acceptance, approval, and recognition. Social drives include the desire for new experiences and adventure.

Recreation can supply the channels through which social drives may be fulfilled. It provides opportunities for participation, companionship, recognition, and security. Recreation can contribute to the social health of people of all ages. It can elevate the feeling of personal worth in the person who already enjoys a high level of social health. It can elevate the level of social health for the individual whose social adjustment has been acceptable but not satisfactory. It can be a means by which the asocial individual can become comfortable in social situations. It can be a means for preventing or correcting antisocial tendencies. Boys and girls who already are delinquents are not so attracted to physical activity (Straub and Felock, 1974). Boys and girls, nondelinquents but vulnerable to delinquency, can find both release and wholesome direction in recreational participation. Family recreation can be an aid in preventing delinquency. A Detroit study of over 2,000 court cases showed that 60% of the juveniles had little or no recreation within the family group, 32% experienced occasional family recreation, and only 8% participated regularly in family recreation.

Even highly individualistic recreation such as painting, instrumental music, crafts, and fly tying have social health values. To have an interest in common with others can provide vicarious social reinforcement to the "loner." A common recreational interest can bring a diversity of people together and promote a general understanding and appreciation of other human beings, which in turn will improve the individual's ability to adjust socially. Properly developed, recreation and fitness are means to fuller personal development, social as well as otherwise.

Physical health

A study of longevity in America has shown that regular exercise, in combination with six other health practices, can help increase life expectancy by as much as 11 years for men and 7 years for women. One of the physicians who wrote the study report declared that "the daily habits of people have a great deal more to do with what makes them sick and when they die than do all the influences of medicine" (Belloc and Breslow, 1972).

The study started with 7,000 subjects in 1965, and by 1973 there had been twice as many deaths among the men who exercised infrequently, if at all, as there were among those who exercised regularly (Belloc, 1973). The evidence is mounting that the physically fit live longer, perform better, and participate more fully in life than do those who are not fit. Regular, vigorous exercise is essential to vibrant good health, and it enhances the capacity for enjoying life (President's Council on Physical Fitness and Sports, 1976).

Most recreation requires some degree of physical exertion, and whether the activity is one requiring vigorous, moderate, or light exertion, certain physical health benefits will accrue. Physical exertion inherent in many physical activities creates organic vigor and physiological well-being and increases physiological efficiency. Physical activity develops skill, dexterity, coordination, and stamina. A recreational program is not designed to develop circus strong men or professional athletes. Recreational activities, however, do provide sufficient physical exertion to stimulate the body to a higher level of efficiency in its functioning. Physical activity is essential for an optimum of physiological functioning. By optimum is meant that level that is desirable for normal needs with sufficient additional efficiency in functioning to take care of any emergencies or special demands that may be made of a per-

son. For the person without circulatory or other serious defects, this generally means moderate exercise. The actual amount of exercise that recreation should give an individual or group should be determined by age, general condition, and the exercise the individual gets from daily vocational and other day-to-day living practices. An individual who adjusts activities to capacity and needs can gain certain established benefits. Metabolism will be improved, circulation will function more efficiently, respiration will function more effectively, muscle tone and coordination will be improved, greater flexibility may be achieved, and general body efficiency will be improved. Perhaps the greatest physical health benefits will accrue from the improved circulation. The chronically tired person will find that a recreational activity that interests him or her will have a surprising effect in eliminating the chronic feeling of fatigue. What such an individual usually needs is stimulation rather than rest (Crisp and Stonehill, 1976).

Hospitals have been slow to recognize the value of recreation, but more than one-fourth of the hospitals in the United States have organized recreational programs. Physical rehabilitation programs employ recreational activities. Actually, much of the occupational therapy in rehabilitation programs is basically a recreational program. The motivation that a particular activity can give to a rehabilitation patient is often the difference between inadequate and adequate recovery. The mental and physical stimulation that a recreational or fitness activity can give to a normal individual actually can be even greater for the individual who is recovering from extended illness or a disability.

Daily living no longer provides enough vigorous exercise to develop and maintain good muscle tone or cardiovascular and respiratory fitness. In homes and factories, and even on farms, machines have virtually eliminated the necessity for walking long distances or climbing stairs. Television holds children in captive idleness for as much as 50 hours a week. Pervasive inactivity, together with poor living habits, has resulted in a serious national fitness problem. Obesity is epidemic. Children do poorly on tests of strength and endurance. Fifty-four percent of all deaths in the United States result from diseases of the heart and blood vessels—diseases that are associated with physical inactivity (President's Council on Physical Fitness and Sports, 1976).

NATURE OF RECREATION

Specifically delineated, recreation is a diversion for the enjoyment or gratification an activity gives an individual. What may be a job to one individual can be recreation for another. Recreation usually is a leisure-time activity in which the rewards are personal rather than monetary. At least the monetary reward is a minor factor or even immaterial. Recreation can be an esthetic experience, an academic experience, a sporting experience, or any other diversion from the humdrum level of daily life.

Recreation provides relaxation needed by people who are fatigued mentally and physically. Relaxation may take many forms. For some, social gatherings are relaxing. Others require strenuous activity. Still others prefer crafts or music or some other sedentary activity. Recreation provides experiences in the enjoyment of beauty, opportunities for serving others, and sharing interests, skills, and fellowship with others. Many adults derive considerable gratification from the service they can give in helping others in the community enjoy recreation. Recreation provides opportunity for creative activities. The joy of creation is one of man's richest experiences. Recreation can be mentally challenging. Discussion groups, forums, play writing, nature study, chess, and other similar activities can afford wholesome mental stimulation. Many individuals find very little opportunity for group participation in their normal vocational pursuits but find in recreation the opportunity to satisfy their need for group participation. Recreation can promote fellowship of a sincere type and can provide adventure. The planning as well as the participation in recreational pursuits can be invigorating.

SCOPE OF RECREATION

With the changing concept of recreation, it was inevitable that the scope of recreation would expand. From the limited philosophy of recreation as a diversion in sports and allied activities, we now find recreation extended into intellectual activities, communicative interests, creative and esthetic activities, and social activities. In attempting to indicate the various activities in each of these categories, it is recognized that a specific activity may well be considered as being in all of these categories. For purposes of delineation and convenience, a particular classification will include those activities whose primary function is in that particular category even though they may serve other purposes.

Physical activities

Recreational activities whose primary purpose is to provide physical exertion, weight control, and exercise include both team and individual events.

The number of calories per minute that might be expended by an individual pursuing physical activities is dependent on many variables, such as physical build, age, skill at the activity, and adverse circumstances, for example, a strong wind while running, waves while swimming, or an awkward partner while dancing. Table 9-1 is a comparative guide to the relative benefits to expect—in terms of weight loss—based on Morehouse and Miller (1976) and Consumers Union (1974).

Intellectual activities

Many recreational activities that are primarily intellectual or learning in nature have other values, although their primary attraction is in the intellectual stimulation or the opportunity for learning that they provide.

Amateur radio	Classes
Astronomy	Coin collecting

Collecting of scientific materials
Debates
Discussion groups
Educational films
Educational television
Exhibits
First aid
Forums
Interest groups
Language study
Museums
Ornithology
Quiz programs
Reading
Scouting
Stamp collecting
Tours, motoring
Music appreciation
Musical-instrument making
Needlecraft
Orchestra membership
Painting
Photography
Pottery making
Puppet shows
Quartets
Sculpturing
Weaving
Woodworking

One could also justifiably include the activities of the 4-H Club program and Cooperative Extension Service (D'Onofrio and Wang, 1975).

Creative and esthetic activities

All creative and esthetic activities will have some aspects of learning experience and will depend on intellectual application. However, there are certain activities such as the following that particularly satisfy the creative urge of people and provide special opportunities for esthetic experiences.

Clay modeling
Dramatics
Drawing
Group singing
Instrumental music
Jewelry making
Leathercraft
Metalcraft

Social activities

Although virtually all recreation includes some social aspects, some activities such as the following are planned primarily for their social value.

Ballroom dancing
Card games
Carnivals
Church nights
Circuses
Concerts
Festivals
Hobby clubs
Holiday parties
Hosteling
Novel-theme parties

Table 9-1 ■ Calories per minute expended in various activities

Activity	Calories per minute	Activity	Calories per minute
Walking, 2 mph	2.8	Swimming/backstroke, 1 mph	8.3
Horseback riding/walk	3.0	Gardening/digging	8.6
Bicycle riding, 5.5 mph	3.2	Chopping wood	9.0
House painting	3.5	Skiing, 3 mph	9.0
Pitching horseshoes	4.0	Swimming/sidestroke, 1 mph	9.2
Walking, 3.5 mph	4.8	Figure skating	9.5
Golf	5.0	Racketball or handball	10.2
Dancing/fox-trot	5.2	Fencing	10.5
Dancing/waltz	5.7	Running, 5.7 mph (jogging)	12.0
Table tennis	5.8	Running, 7.0 mph	14.5
Swimming/breaststroke, 1 mph	6.8	Running, 11.4 mph	21.7
Bicycle riding, rapid	6.9	Swimming/crawl, 2.2 mph	26.7
Dancing/rhumba	7.0	Swimming/breaststroke, 2.2 mph	30.8
Swimming/crawl, 1 mph	7.0		
Tennis	7.1	Swimming/backstroke, 2.2 mph	33.3
Skating, 9 mph	7.8		
Horseback riding/trot	8.0		

Operettas

Pageants

Picnics

Radio broadcasts

Social teas

Square and folk
dancing

Table games (chess
and dominoes)

Variety shows

The array of recreational activities suggests that a person who could not find one particular recreational interest indeed would be destitute. With the variety of recreational outlets now available, it is not surprising to find many people with several recreational interests. These fortunate individuals are able to get physical, intellectual, creative, esthetic, and social benefits.

VALUES IN RECREATION

An information gap persists in this area. Most Americans associate fitness with good physical performance, not with good health, improved appearance, or better performance on the job and in the classroom. This is especially true among the poor, the elderly, and the less educated. Some individuals apparently live both effectively and enjoyably without a program of regular or periodic recreation. Their vocation and other interests and activities seem to be adequate to provide them with the necessary motivation and gratification in living (Warr, 1976). Whether these individuals would live more effectively and enjoyably if they would engage in some form of recreation would be difficult to determine. Many of these individuals live so effectively and enjoyably already that it would be difficult to bring about very much improvement. Perhaps community services that some of these individuals give, in effect, serve as recreation, particularly as related to their life's vocation. For some individuals in the community, recreation merely serves to fill time. If this is a value in recreation, it is of a negative type because it means only spending time. Properly regarded, recreation is a positive force in that it is a profitable investment of time. It provides many values for the individual, the family, the group, and the community.

Individual benefits

For the individual, recreation provides adventure, activity drive, a feeling of belonging, skill, release of tension, relaxation, participation, challenges, accomplishment, mastery, success, creativity, stimulation, elation, and a fullness of living. Doubtless, all of these can be acquired or experienced in pursuits other than recreation, but living in a highly organized and mechanized world, it becomes increasingly necessary for people to satisfy many personal needs through activities outside of work and normal living pursuits.

Family benefits

In an age in which there is a growing tendency to disperse the family rather than consolidate family living, recreation could serve to integrate family action through joint interests. Social changes tend to make the promotion of family recreation an increasingly difficult task. Mothers complete childbearing at an early age and thus experience an early release from maternal duties. Still young enough to accept employment, family consolidation is reduced. Well-established neighborhoods have given way to a tendency for friendships based on special interests. Groups are not often organized on a neighborhood basis. With the increasing complexity of our social structure, the resulting overorganization tends to disrupt the family. Family-centered fun is heavily inclined toward commercialized amusements. Children and parents tend not to participate in common events. The child has his or her interests in athletic groups, music, art, scouting, and similar activities. Many activities exist in which both the children and the parents have potential interest and can participate. Perhaps some degree of promotion may be necessary ("The family that plays together stays together"), but frequently an interest exists that merely needs to be activated. In other instances interest can be developed among all members of the family so that participation by all is realized. Camping seems to be the most popular family recreation, but there are other activities equally appealing and rewarding for the family unit. Music, painting, photography, crafts, picnics, hiking, motor trips, boating, swimming, fishing, skating, skiing, bowling, tennis, golf, gardening, church activities, and special family nights suggest the variety of activities that lend themselves to total family participation and consolidation (Erben and Mantek, 1973).

Benefits inherent in family recreation are apparent. To participate as a group, to enjoy common experiences, to share the gratifications of accomplishment, and to pioneer together in new ventures will promote the physical, mental, emotional, and social well-being of the individual and the members of the family. The sense of belonging that recreation cements is highly important in family integration. With each member an individual in his or her own right, free to pursue interests within the family group, joint recreational participation is a highly valuable experience in adjusting to the needs, opinions, well-being, and respect of other members of the family.

Group benefits

While social grouping as America once knew it has undergone considerable change, we still have group formation and group action. In some areas there has been a regrouping, but generally speaking, some of the primary groups of past decades still continue. For all groups, recreation can have special significance so long as man is gregarious. Recreation provides one avenue through which this gregariousness can express itself. Association with others of the same status, of the same special needs, and the same interests can be made possible through recreation. In many instances recreational activities present the best means for providing opportunities for group participation and association. Engaging in common recreational pursuits rewards members of the group with a richer experience in group participation, in group adjustment, and in an understanding of people of like interests and pursuits.

The child group, the youth group, the adult group, and the aging group have different recreational interests and different recreational needs. Age grouping, however, is not always the pattern on which group recreation is based. The physically handicapped with a great deal of time on their hands have special group recreational needs. People with impaired vision or people with impaired hearing are not like everyone else in their need for special group recreational opportunities. The mentally retarded can benefit from opportunities for group recreation.

Formal groups find recreation an ideal vehicle for the promotion of group solidarity, motivation, and attainment. Informal groups, where more individuality remains, find recreational activities that will permit individual development within group participation. Organized groups, characterized by individual sharing, and unorganized groups, characterized by a lack of cohesiveness, have equal need for recreational activities. For one, recreation provides opportunities for cooperative service to members of its group. For the other, recreation provides a community of interest that tends to hold the group together.

Whether recreation serves as a primary activity of a group or serves an ancillary role by providing a unity of interest and participation, recreation raises the general value and significance of the group to its members. In this respect recreation is a means to an end rather than an end in itself. It is a means to achieve a greater significance of the group.

Community benefits

For some well-qualified individuals, leisure time is put to good use in wholesome channels. Other citizens find their leisure time merely time on their hands. Perhaps what people do with their leisure time is the best single index of the community's cultural level. Strictly speaking, community achievement is only a composite of individual achievement. The happiness, physical health, character development, and morale of a community are but an expression of these qualities on a composite basis in its citizens. Through its social processes, a community can do much to establish the general standard or pattern of community living. People respond in terms of what is expected of them. In this highly industrial age, a community that provides opportunities for recreational activity is laying the foundation for a wholesome community atmosphere. A community that provides alternatives to the tavern or the gambling den will find its efforts reflected in greater interest in community affairs and social life. Time, effort, and funds put into community recreation and fitness are an investment in community stability, integration, and higher social values and community standards.

PROGRAMS

In affluent, urbanized communities, planned programs must provide the physical activity that everyday life no longer supplies. Regular exercise and participation in sports must become part of a way of life for young and old alike. Homes, schools, employers, and voluntary agencies must join in providing leadership and facilities.

The national physical fitness program sponsored by the President's Council on Physical Fitness and Sports has the following specific goals:

1. A population committed to physical fitness and possessed of the knowledge and skills to achieve it.
2. Acceptance by parents, schools, recreational agencies, and sports organizations of their special responsibilities for fitness.
3. Recognition by communities and employers that fitness facilities and programs should be a part of the residential and work environments.
4. Maximum utilization of all resources—human and material, public and private—for physical fitness.

The President's Council on Physical Fitness and Sports cannot compel anyone to accept its recommendations. Its task is to educate, advise, and encourage. The responsibility for action rests with parents, school administrators, teachers, coaches, recreation supervisors, civic and business leaders, and other individuals at the community level.

Classification on a basis of who controls or promotes the activity or on the basis of who participates will tend to overlap. An activity regarded as a phase of a public recreational program may be classed as commercial recreation, and in another instance, may properly be classed as private recreation. Nationwide public recreation appears to be growing faster than commercial or private recreation, but all types of programs are undergoing constant growth and development.

Commercial entertainment

Making a precise demarcation between recreation and entertainment is difficult, even impossible, but a general distinction can be made. Recreation involves actual participation, while entertainment has a connotation of the individual being a spectator or enjoying the activity vicariously. In recent years it has become fashionable in some circles to condemn entertainment of all kinds. The catchy term "spectatoritis" has been tagged to the growth of television spectators and attendance at athletic and other spectacles. If America's leisure time were devoted entirely to being entertained, there would be justification for criticism and concern. Americans are participants in a vast variety of activities, and a reasonable balance between active participation in some activities and being a spectator at other activities can have a great deal of merit (Graney, 1974). The empathy, the exhilaration, and the enjoyment that come from watching the most highly skilled perform can have educational as well as other value. Commercial entertainment in America is big business. Unfortunately, for some, commercial entertainment is a complete substitution for recreation. Rather than condemn commercial recreation as damaging to America's moral fiber, the constructive approach to the situation is to prepare people for, and provide the means for, recreational skill and interest. Commercial entertainment includes music, television, radio, professional sports, high school and collegiate athletics, theatricals, concerts, horse racing, fairs, circuses, and a number of other activities in which people derive enjoyment merely from being spectators. So long as people have time and money they will attend these various events, unless they have developed the necessary skill and motivation to get gratification through active rather than passive participation.

Commercial and semipublic recreation

Private investments have provided recreational facilities in response to recreational needs of citizens. The primary purpose in the promotion of the enterprise has been to obtain a business profit. Nevertheless, many of these enterprises provide admirable services for the community. Some of these commercial recreation enterprises actually may be semipublic in nature, but the vast majority of them are available to the general public. Semipublic recreation usually is made available through organizations that reserve their facilities for their own members, but on occasion make their facilities available to others. Athletic clubs, golf clubs, tennis clubs, and social clubs may be in this category. Billiards, bowling, roller skating, ice skating, skiing, miniature golf, golf, swimming, canoeing, and horseback riding are illustrations of commercial and semipublic recreational activities that can serve admirably as one component of a community's recreation program. In the overall evaluation of any community's recreation program, facilities available for public recreation on a commercial basis must be given full consideration.

Private recreational and fitness programs

In providing recreational opportunities in a community, sports groups and social organizations that limit their facilities and services exclusively to their own members should not be underestimated. Segregation of this type is an accepted social practice in American life, whether or not individuals in these organizations are considered privileged in other respects. Certainly from the standpoint of community recreation, these members are privileged to enjoy the kind of recreational opportunities one might hope everyone could enjoy. Even when organized primarily for recreational purposes, most of these private organizations serve more than one function. Private clubs for golf, swimming, boating, riding, hunting, skeet shooting, tennis, skiing, skating, bowling, billiards, and dancing often include creative, social, and esthetic activities.

Public recreation

Providing recreation has become an accepted public service. Providing opportunities for recreation does not mean that all recreation must be planned or in any sense formal. It would be tragic if the nation should reach a stage where the public depended solely on official agencies for all recreational and fitness activities. Indeed, it is a justifiable apprehension that, particularly among youngsters, there is too little opportunity for self-created recreational activity.

Official agencies—state, county, or city—provide various means for giving citizens an opportunity to enjoy self-directed recreation. This is classically illustrated by the 14 million hunting licenses and 19 million fishing licenses that are issued in the United States each year. Over one-half-billion man-days are invested in hunting and fishing each year. Yet, it is readily recognized that outdoor recreation is not enough. Public recreation means diversification in recreation. It must provide for the recreational needs of all ages and various groups.

Public recreation will be expanded in the years immediately ahead. For effectiveness in terms of the physical, mental, and social health of the community, it is necessary that the program be expanded in terms of more than the need for physical activity. To provide more playgrounds and more basketball courts is not enough. Provision must be made for the social, creative, esthetic, and intellectual recreational needs of people of all ages. Particular attention must be given to recreation for adults and for the senior citizens in the community (Nystrom, 1974).

Leadership

The President's Council on Physical Fitness and Sports (PCPFS), an outgrowth of the President's Council on Youth Fitness, was established in 1956. The first Council grew out of concern about the poor performance of American boys and girls on standardized physical fitness tests. Subsequently, it was recognized that the fitness problem permeates all age groups. In 1963 the Council was directed to begin promoting adult fitness. Today the PCPFS addresses its efforts to all ages, including the elderly, and its activities are part of national preventive health efforts.

Competent leadership is the key to effective community recreational and fitness programs. Paradoxically, the greatest weakness in the American recreation program is in leadership. Of the more than 17,000 communities in the United States, fewer than one-third have full-time recreational leaders. It must be pointed out that while full-time recreational leadership is essential to an effective recreation program, the employment of a full-time recreational leader does not in itself guarantee effective or even adequate leadership. Many recreational positions are political plums or are handed to a professional athlete to supplement the pay he receives for playing baseball or basketball for the city team. Some recreational leaders have drifted into the field through close association with recreation on a voluntary basis. To like children or to be interested in recreation does not in itself indicate that a person has the necessary qualifications for good recreational leadership. Many recreational positions are political plums or are handed to a professional required for other leadership. Recreation has become a professional field, and more than

150 institutions of higher learning in the United States are granting degrees. At least 143 institutions are granting bachelor degrees, eighty are granting masters degrees, and twenty-nine are granting doctorates or directorates in the field of recreation. An additional seventy junior colleges are offering courses.

The professional preparation of the recreational leader is built on a broad foundation in the liberal arts and sciences. On this foundation the college recreation major includes studies in American culture, government, city planning, public relations, social group work, counseling, speaking, social recreation, hospital recreation, club work, sports programs, recreational dramatics, recreational music, photography, graphic and plastic arts, first aid, organization and administration of recreation, and field experience.

Areas and facilities

Physical fitness and recreation are national, state, county, community, neighborhood, group, family, and individual matters. Recreation is promoted at all governmental, economic, and social levels. In 1970 the United States Department of Commerce reported that the National Park Service supervised 281 park areas with a total of 29,629,444 acres. That year, over 172 million people visited the various national park areas. The United States had 3,337 state parks with an aggregate of over 8,518,000 acres. More than 474,168,000 persons used these facilities during the year. In 1970 31,235 cities and counties reported nonschool recreational areas. This includes beaches, golf courses, picnic grounds, and camps. Throughout the United States, there are more than 300 camps for the physically handicapped and more than 100 camps for the mentally retarded. It thus is apparent that America has had the vision to see the necessity for setting aside areas for certain recreational purposes. On a national or state level, in general, lands have been made available to provide recreational facilities for the general public (Siehl, 1974).

On the local level, however, communities have been rather shortsighted. Frequently, recreational areas have had to give way to roads, housing developments, or other needs. Recreation needs more land, not less than it already has. Many communities, through zoning, require that any extended housing development set aside areas for recreation. All community planning should encompass recreational needs, long range as well as immediate. It is necessary that communities look forward to the possible recreational needs of the next quarter or even half century in anticipation of population increases. Community parks, playgrounds, swimming pools, beaches, golf courses, tennis courts, and other recreational facilities have become a recognized responsibility in community services and planning. More extended utilization of school facilities is both necessary and sensible. The school athletic fields, playgrounds, gymnasiums, and pools are part of the community's recreational facilities, and their use should be incorporated into the community recreational and fitness programs.

COMMUNITY RESOURCES

The President's Council on Physical Fitness and Sports is responsible for implementing a seven-point program including the following objectives: (1) to enlist the active support and assistance of individual citizens, civic groups, professional associations, amateur and professional sports groups, private enterprise, voluntary organizations, and others in efforts to promote and improve physical fitness and sports participation programs for all communities; (2) to stimulate, improve, and strengthen coordination of federal services and programs relating to physical fitness and sports participation; (3) to encourage state and local governments in efforts to enhance physical fitness and sports participation; (4) to seek to strengthen the physical fitness of American children, youth, and adults by encouraging the development of community-centered and other physical fitness and sports participation programs;

(5) to develop cooperative programs with medical, dental, and other similar professional societies to encourage and implement sound physical fitness practices; (6) to stimulate and encourage research in the areas of physical fitness and sports performance; and (7) to improve school health and physical education programs for all pupils, including the handicapped and the physically undeveloped, by assisting educational agencies in developing quality programs to encourage innovation, improve teacher preparation, and strengthen state and local leadership.

Many people are not aware of the many recreational opportunities and activities that exist in their community. Those who are aware of their community's recreational program generally do not recognize the many untapped recreational and fitness resources that could be utilized in their community. There are groups and organizations making no contribution to the community recreational program who could contribute measurably to both the extensiveness and effectiveness of the community's recreational program. While a comprehensive recreational program does call for the expenditure of funds, many aspects of community recreation require little or no expenditure of money. Organizations having facilities and members who are willing to contribute their services can add appreciably to the community's recreational activities. It is not just a matter of accepting those who are willing to volunteer, but of recruiting all the individuals who may have a contribution to make toward the program. By enlisting the cooperation and active participation of all the people in all the organizations and agencies in the community that might make some contribution, it is possible to have an extensive community-wide recreational program without huge expenditures.

Legal agencies

Tax-supported organizations are regarded as legal agencies. The state conservation department providing park, camping, hunting, and fishing facilities is an example of a legal agency on the state basis that serves as a valuable resource in recreation. On the county and city level, county- or city-park boards, schools, and public libraries are resource agencies. A city recreation commission, formally organized by the city council with a staff of full-time professional recreational personnel, should be the hub about which the entire community recreational program rotates. The commission's program can be financed as a part of the city's annual budget. While various recreational activities do produce some revenue, such income is merely an incidental factor in maintaining the program. Cities today accept recreation as a necessary and proper community service and appropriate the necessary funds for its promotion.

Social groups

People with common interests and needs tend either formally or informally to form groups to promote their common interests. This is notably true of recreational interests. These groups usually are limited in their numbers and usually serve only their own members but contribute appreciably to recreation in a community. Dance groups, jogging groups, bridge groups, groups of young married couples, and similar organizations are to be found in most communities. Each group in its own way meets certain recreational needs for its own members. Some social groups undertake to promote recreational activities that will be available to others than members of the group. Out of one social group, many groups may develop to enhance the overall recreational and fitness programs of the community.

Religious groups

Religious organizations provide services other than purely religious services. Recreational activities sponsored by religious groups usually are conducted on a high level, not in competition with legal agencies, but as a supplement to the program of the legal agencies. The Young Men's Christian Association, the Young Women's Christian Association,

Boys' Clubs of America, B'nai B'rith Hillel Foundations, Young Men's and Women's Hebrew Association, Diocesan Youth Councils, Boys' League, National Catholic Youth Council, Christian Endeavor, Epworth League, and Methodist Youth Fellowship are examples of religious groups that promote outstanding recreational and fitness programs. Health and fitness are integral to most religious and philosophical systems.

Youth-serving agencies

Over 250 organizations in the United States are working with children and youth under 25 years of age. The areas in which these organizations serve are so diverse that it would be difficult to imagine any recreational needs that are not provided. To name a few of these organizations would indicate the extensiveness of the list—4-H groups, Future Farmers of America, Future Homemakers of America, Boy Scouts, Girl Scouts, Camp Fire Girls, Boys State, Girls State, youth centers, settlement houses, Big Brothers of America, and American Junior Red Cross is but a partial list. Scores of boys' and girls' groups, hosteling, and other groups indicate the many agencies created to serve the youth of America. The important thing is that each community organize, support, and promote the particular youth-serving agencies necessary to provide the leisure-time activities essential for the best development of the children and youth of the community.

Service groups

Nationally known community service groups have continuing fitness and recreational programs, either competing or cooperating with another agency or sponsoring the program themselves. Equally important is that these service groups can be called upon to support any worthwhile recreational program in the community. This is a resource that is ever present. Rotary clubs, Lions clubs, Kiwanis, Exchange Clubs, Soroptimists, Women's groups, Grange, Parent-Teacher Associations, and other service organizations provide a diversity of services in their communities, not the least of these being the promotion of recreational and fitness programs.

Neighborhoods

Recreational activities grow out of group interests. An actual or potential neighborhood interest can serve as a catalyst in initiating and extending recreational activities. Many of these enterprises are self-starting, but others need leadership to crystallize the interest that exists and to implement the contribution of the group. Interest in having a playground developed in the neighborhood, for example, can be a starting point from which an extensive neighborhood recreational program can be developed. When a playground already exists in the neighborhood, interest may be present or can be

generated in expanding both the facilities and the activities that are carried on at the playground.

Special interest groups

In a typical community, one is likely to find a number of groups having special recreational interests, such as gardening, music, dramatics, chess, stamp collecting, and photography. Through these groups, others can be encouraged to develop new interests or to enjoy an interest they already have. There is something contagious about an intense interest in some fascinating or challenging hobby or avocation. As people become exposed to all possible recreational outlets, there is a greater likelihood that they will find those particular activities that will appeal to their particular abilities and temperament.

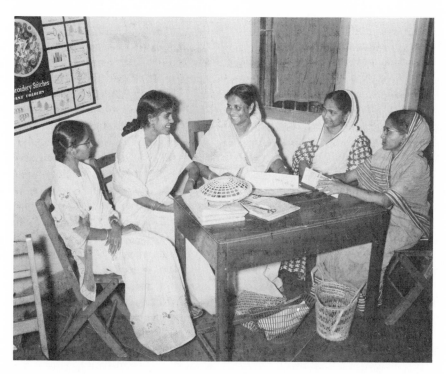

Fig. 9-1. Special interest groups are universal. In this sewing group in Dacca, Bangladesh, women discuss health and family planning concerns as well as embroidery stitches. (Courtesy Public Health Education Research Project, University of California, Berkeley)

Other community resources

As with most federal agencies, the President's Council on Physical Fitness and Sports programs falls into three major categories: public information, program development, and technical assistance and special programs.

Public information. The Council staff conducts a continuous public service advertising program designed to inform and motivate the American people; prepares articles for popular and professional publications; publishes booklets, pamphlets, a newsletter, and a research digest (free publications list available); and works with private enterprises to develop television and film materials.

Program development. The Council staff cooperates with state and local governments, voluntary organizations, professional associations, sports-governing bodies, private enterprise, and other federal agencies to promote the development of physical fitness leadership facilities and programs.

Technical assistance and special programs. Council staff members work with schools, colleges, clubs, recreational agencies, and major employers on program design and implementation. They also advise the Administration on Aging, the Community Services Administration, and other federal agencies on the conduct of fitness-related programs.

Labor unions, industrial firms, retail business houses, the Chamber of Commerce, and fraternal organizations promote and support various recreational enterprises. All of these establishments find that providing recreation is one of the finest services they can contribute to their constituents. In any community it is possible to discover public-spirited organizations that will respond to reasonable requests for support of any worthwhile community enterprise. These are the organizations that, with very little fanfare, play an extremely important role in the year-in and year-out promotion of the well-being of the community. These organizations may take an active role and actually administer a recreational or fitness program of their own, or their participation may be limited to financial or other support. Resources for the promotion of recreation are rarely more than partially tapped in most communities. To utilize all possible resources, three things are usually necessary. The first is a worthwhile program; second is qualified leadership; and the third is an informed community.

Physical fitness through recreation will increase in importance with the increase in leisure time and the extension of life expectation. Many factors enter into the extension of community fitness and recreational programs. Understanding by the public, qualified professional leadership, and adequate facilities must advance more rapidly than during the past decade if the recreational program is to serve the needs of expanding populations.

QUESTIONS AND EXERCISES

1. Appraise the statement, "How a people utilizes its leisure time is an index of its vitality and an indication of its future."
2. To what extent is recreation a vehicle for health promotion?
3. To what extent is recreation a vehicle for the treatment of disabilities?
4. Why is recreation growing as a community enterprise in America?
5. What recreational activities are available in your community for people with urges to do creative work?
6. Indicate how recreation can promote social health.
7. Why does the public place so much emphasis on recreation of a physical nature?
8. By the use of examples, indicate how an activity that is not recreational for one person may be of recreational value for another person.
9. Identify some person who does not appear to need a recreational outlet and analyze the factors that account for the absence of recreational needs.
10. Compare the recreational needs of two individuals who have widely different vocations.
11. Why is an intellectual activity recreational to one person but an unenjoyable task for another person?
12. Propose some measures to extend family recreation in your community.
13. How can group interests in your community be used to expand the community's recreational program?

14. What alternatives to the tavern and gambling den does your community offer its citizens?
15. What role does commercial entertainment play in your community?
16. To what extent does commercial recreation contribute to the total recreational program of your community?
17. What recreational activities are provided publicly in your community?
18. What areas and facilities are available in your community?
19. What additional areas and facilities should be provided?
20. What is your contribution to your community's recreational program?

REFERENCES

Belloc, N. B.: Relationships of health practices and mortality, Preventive Medicine 2:67-81, 1973.

Belloc, N. B., and Breslow, L.: Relationships of physical health status and health practices, Preventive Medicine 1:409-421, 1972.

Butler, G. D.: Introduction to community recreation, ed. 4, New York, 1967, McGraw-Hill Book Co.

Consumers Union: The medicine show, Mt. Vernon, N.Y., 1974, Consumers Union.

Crisp, A. H., and Stonehill, E.: Sleep, nutrition and mood, Somerset, N.J., 1976, John Wiley & Sons, Inc.

Danford, H. G., and Shirley, M., editors: Creative leadership in recreation, ed. 2, Boston, 1970, Allyn & Bacon, Inc.

D'Onofrio, C. N., and Wang, V. L.: Cooperative Extension and Rural Health Education, Health Education Monographs 3(1):4-119, 1975.

Dulles, F. R.: History of recreation: America learns to play, ⊙d. 2, New York, 1970, Appleton-Century-Crofts.

Erben, R., and Mantek, M.: Health, leisure and holidays, International Journal of Health Education 16:1-8, 1973.

Friedberg, P., and Berkeley, E. P.: Play and interplay: manifests for new design in urban recreation, New York, 1970, The Macmillan Co.

Graney, M. J.: Media use as a substitute activity in old age, Journal of Gerontology 29:322-324, May 1974.

Gray, D., and Pelegrino, D. A.: Readings in recreation and parks, Dubuque, Iowa, 1972, William C. Brown Co., Publishers.

Guggenheim, E. C.: Planning for parks and recreation needs, New York, 1969, Twayne Publishers, Inc.

Haun, P.: Recreation: a medical viewpoint, New York, 1968, Columbia University Press.

Heaton, I. C.: Planning for social recreation, ed. 6, Provo, Utah, 1968, Brigham Young University Press.

Hjelte, G., and Shivers, J. S.: Public administration of recreational services, Philadelphia, 1972, Lea & Febiger.

Kraus, R. G.: Recreation and leisure in modern society, New York, 1970, Appleton-Century-Crofts.

Kraus, R. G.: Recreation today, program planning and leadership, New York, 1972, Appleton-Century-Crofts.

Lee, M. P.: Grown-up activities for young people, Jericho, N.Y., 1971, Exposition Press.

Linden, M. E.: New vistas in recreation for patients, Recreation 2:259-260, 1957.

Morehouse, L. E., and Miller, A. T.: Physiology of exercise, ed. 7, St. Louis, 1976, The C. V. Mosby Co.

Nystrom, E. P.: Activity patterns and leisure concepts among the elderly, American Journal of Occupational Therapy 28:337-345, 1974.

President's Council on Physical Fitness and Sports: Organization, objectives, programs, situation report, Washington, D.C., 1976, U.S. Government Printing Office.

Rathbone, J. L., and Lucas, C.: Recreation in total rehabilitation, Springfield, Ill., 1970, Charles C Thomas, Publisher.

Rutledge, A. J.: Anatomy of a park plan: the essentials of recreation area design, New York, 1970, McGraw-Hill Book Co.

Shivers, J. S.: Principles and practices of recreational service, New York, 1967, McGraw-Hill Book Co.

Siehl, G.: Environment update, Library Journal 99:1357-1363, May 15, 1974.

Slezak, E. J.: Tips and ideas on organization and administration of recreation, Corvallis, 1970, Oregon State University Press.

Smith, F. E.: Land between lakes: experiment in recreation, Lexington, 1971, The University Press of Kentucky.

Steiner, J. F.: Americans at play: recent trends in recreation and leisure time activities, New York, 1970, Arno Press, Inc.

Straub, W. F., and Felock, T.: Attitudes toward physical activity of delinquent and nondelinquent junior high school girls, Research Quarterly: American Association for Health, Physical Education and Recreation 45:21-27, 1974.

Tillman, A. A.: Program book for recreation professionals, Palo Alto, Calif., 1971, National Press Books.

Warr, P. E.: Personal goals and work design, New York, 1976, Wiley.

PART III

Preventing disorders and disabilities

10 ▪ COMMUNICABLE DISEASE CONTROL

The prevention of preventable disease is the first purpose of a wisely governed state.

Erastus Brooks, 1882

Man has not conquered the infectious diseases to which he is heir, but through his understanding of the nature of infection he has succeeded in controlling them. Perhaps he will never eliminate infection, but it would be entirely realistic to predict that eventually he will control so effectively the organisms that cause disease that infectious diseases will be one of his minor health problems. Even today, infectious diseases as a cause of death are far less important than the degenerative diseases. Indeed, man's knowledge of and ability to control infectious diseases are far greater than his knowledge and means of controlling his own behavior.

NATURE OF COMMUNICABLE DISEASE

Disease is a harmful departure from normal. A communicable disease is one that can be transmitted from one human being to another or from lower animals to man. Communicable diseases are produced by organisms that not only are parasitic but are pathogenic, or disease-producing. Most pathogens of man are microorganisms, though some, notably the worms, are multicellular forms and can be seen with the unaided eye. Infectious disease represents a reaction of the host to the invader. The interaction may destroy the pathogen as well as produce abnormalities in the host, even to the point of causing the death of the host.

Infection and disease. Infection is the successful invasion of the body by pathogens under such conditions as will permit them to multiply and harm the host. The mere presence of organisms in the body of man does not constitute disease. A person may be harboring millions of pneumococci in his lungs without having disease. He may have billions of streptococcus organisms on his skin without having disease. Only when the organisms cause harm to the body can the condition be classed as a disease.

Disinfection consists of killing or removing organisms capable of causing infection. Disinfection mechanisms consist of destroying pathogens by dehydration or desiccation, hydrolysis or hydration, coagulation of cell proteins, oxidation, and destruction of enzymes. For practical purposes, disinfectants must possess the following desirable properties:

1. They must not damage the tissue.
2. They must not produce pain.
3. They must have a high germicidal effect or be quick-acting.
4. They must not be affected by alkalies or acids.
5. They must be low in cost.

Disinfection by the use of chemicals is the usual method. Here, the time element, concentration of the chemical, and temperature are important. The particular sensitivity of the tissue affected must always be considered in the use of a particular chemical antiseptic.

Dilute alcohol is an example of a disinfectant in everyday use. Physical disinfection includes the use of such agents as ultraviolet radiation, sound waves, and electron treatment. While all of these procedures have certain limitations, experimentation in their possibilities may lead to benefits far beyond what is now realized in their use.

Bacteriostasis is an arrest in the multiplication of pathogens and in their metabolism. Thus toxin production is reduced or ceases completely. Sulfonamides arrest bacterial action by combining with para-aminobenzoic acid (PABA), thus depriving the organism of the PABA that it must have available to carry on normal metabolic processes. This bacteriostasis enables man's phagocytes, such as neutrophils, to destroy the pathogen.

Antibiosis, such as produced by penicillin, expresses a direct antagonism to specific organisms. The antibiotics have had spectacular effects in combating certain pathogens, but they have not proved to be the panacea many in the medical sciences at first contended. Despite their magnificent contribution to man's battle against infection, the antibiotics have limitations. Bacteria develop resistant strains in response to antibiotics. This mutation, or adaptability by the bacteria, limits the use of antibiotics. Resistant strains of bacteria are found particularly in hospital-acquired infections, whereas an infection with the same organism acquired outside the hospital may be sensitive to the same antibiotics and respond well. Indiscriminate use of antibiotics, without proper indication, increases the proportion of resistant organisms. Newly developed antibiotics should only be used against organisms that have been shown to be sensitive to them and resistant to earlier antibiotics.

Contamination and decontamination. Contamination is the presence of pathogens of man or nonpathogenic organisms, such as *Escherichia coli* of man's alimentary canal, on inanimate objects. Thus articles of clothing, a door handle, a spoon, a glass, milk, or water may be contaminated. Since certain organisms, such as *E. coli*, live in the intes-

tines of man, the presence of these organisms indicates presence of human discharges. Contact with a possibly contaminated object—and thus with pathogens from the alimentary tract of man—is a present danger. The *E. coli* count is used as a standard in sanitary science and as such is a valuable index in terms of possible danger to man.

Decontamination means the killing or removing of pathogens and *E. coli* in or on inanimate objects. More drastic measures can be used here than are used in disinfection. Boiling, the use of steam, pasteurization, high levels of dry heat, long exposure to the sun, and highly concentrated chemicals are used.

INCIDENCE OF COMMUNICABLE DISEASES

Man can feel elated over the progress that has been made in the control of infectious diseases. A comparison of reported cases of selected communicable diseases in 1900 and 1976 will indicate the extent of the gain (Table 10-1). In appraising the general decline in the number of reported cases of these selected diseases, an added weight must be given to the increase in population from 1900 to 1976; the population in 1976 was 170% greater than it was in 1900.

To dispel any idea that communicable diseases no longer are a problem in America, one needs but study a table of reported cases of communicable diseases in 1976 (Table 10-2). These figures would indicate that America has not reached the point where its citizens can be complacent about communicable diseases. Communicable disease still exists in epidemic, pandemic, and endemic forms.

Epidemic (Greek—*epi* upon, *demos* people) refers to a considerable number of cases of a particular disease in a rather limited locality such as a city. What constitutes the number of cases that would classify an outbreak as an epidemic is highly flexible, depending on the particular disease and the size of the community. In a city of 12,000 people, ten cases of measles would not

Table 10-1 ■ Reported cases of selected communicable diseases, United States, 1900 and 1976 (National Center for Health Statistics)

Disease	1900	1976
Diphtheria	147,991	146
Malaria	184,165	451
Smallpox	102,128	0
Streptococcal infections and scarlet fever	161,432	433,405
Typhoid fever	35,994	384

Table 10-2 ■ Reported cases of specified notifiable diseases: United States, 1976

Disease	Reported cases
Botulism	29
Brucellosis	282
Diphtheria	146
Encephalitis, infectious	1,616
Gonorrhea	996,468
Hepatitis, infectious and serum	41,263
Malaria	451
Measles	39,585
Meningococcal infections	1,534
Pertussis	925
Poliomyelitis	9
Psittacosis	71
Rubella	12,090
Salmonellosis (excluding typhoid fever)	22,046
Streptococcal sore throat	433,405
Syphilis	23,499
Tetanus	68
Trichinosis	89
Tuberculosis	32,549
Tularemia	146
Typhoid fever	384
Typhus fever, tick-borne (Rocky Mountain spotted fever)	892

From MMWR, Morbidity and Mortality Weekly Report, Center for Disease Control, vol. 25, no. 52, January 7, 1977.

Table 10-3 ■ Deaths from infectious diseases

Cause of death	Number
Bacillary dysentery (shigellosis)	64
Botulism	6
Brucellosis	1
Chickenpox	138
Diphtheria	10
Encephalitis	350
Enteritis and other diarrheal diseases	2,322
Gonorrhea	11
Infectious hepatitis	656
Malaria	7
Measles	23
Meningococcal infections	330
Mononucleosis	25
Pertussis	5
Poliomyelitis	93
Rabies	1
Rheumatic fever	183
Rocky Mountain spotted fever	35
Salmonellosis	75
Streptococcal sore throat and scarlet fever	20
Syphilis	393
Tetanus	40
Trichinosis	1
Tuberculosis	3,875
Tularemia	4
Typhoid fever	7
Typhus fever	40

From Vital statistics of the United States, vol. 2, 1973.

be an epidemic, but in a community of 200, that number of cases of measles might be regarded as in epidemic form. Ten cases of paralytic poliomyelitis in the city of 12,000 would be regarded as an epidemic.

Pandemic (Greek—*pan* all) indicates a considerable number of cases of a wide geographical area such as a state, a section of a nation, the entire nation, a continent, or the world. Thus the outbreak of influenza in 1918-1919 was classed as a pandemic. Despite its advance in communicable disease control, the United States is not completely safe from pandemics.

Endemic (Greek—*en* in) refers to a decidedly limited number of cases in a markedly localized geographical area. The term is sometimes limited to diseases peculiar to a particular area.

Infectious diseases still account for a high death toll (Table 10-3). The table lists only a selection of the infectious and parasitic diseases that accounted for 15,669 deaths in 1973, or 0.81% of the total.

CLASSIFICATION OF INFECTIOUS DISEASES

Many bases exist for the classification of infectious diseases. Each classification has its merits, and none is without some deficiency or other. From the standpoint of practical

Table 10-4 ■ Classification of infectious diseases

Respiratory diseases	Alvine discharge diseases	Vector-borne diseases	Open lesion diseases
Cerebrospinal meningitis	Amebic dysentery	African sleeping sickness	Anthrax
Chicken pox	Bacillary dysentery	Encephalitis	Erysipelas
Coryza	(shigellosis)	Malaria	Gonorrhea
Diphtheria	Cholera	Plague	Scarlet fever
Influenza	Hookworm	Rocky Mountain spotted	Smallpox
Measles	Paratyphoid	fever	Syphilis
Pneumonia	Poliomyelitis	Tularemia	Tuberculosis
Poliomyelitis	Salmonellosis	Typhus fever	Tularemia
Rubella	Typhoid fever	Yellow fever	
Scarlet fever	Viral hepatitis		
Smallpox			
Streptococcal sore throat			
Tuberculosis			
Whooping cough			

community health promotion, the best classification would likely be one that incorporates at least a suggestion of how the disease is transmitted. The classification presented here perhaps does not do this in the strictest sense, yet it does serve the practical needs of those who are concerned with control of infectious diseases in the community (Table 10-4).

It will be noted that in Table 10-4 some diseases are listed in more than one classification. Thus tuberculosis properly can be classed both as a respiratory disease and an open lesion disease. Smallpox also can be classified both as a respiratory and an open lesion disease. In both of these infectious conditions, the avenue of spread can be from the respiratory tract or from the lesions of the body that these infections produce.

Respiratory diseases. It is not surprising that diseases of the respiratory tract rank far ahead of the other classes of diseases that plague the American citizen. In some respects, the respiratory tract is as exposed as the skin but without the defenses of the skin. Diseases of the respiratory tract are par-

ticularly prevalent in the temperate zone but exist universally. Usually acute, they pose a constant threat to the population. Only in recent years has man been reasonably effective in controlling them.

Infectious diseases of the respiratory tract follow a characteristic cycle of periods—incubation, prodrome, fastigium, defervescence, convalescence, and defection. An understanding of the typical course or cycle of a respiratory disease is helpful in controlling disease. Such knowledge points out what factors are operating at a given stage and where and what control measures should be taken.

Incubation starts with the invasion of the causative agent. Organisms multiply in the host during the incubation period, but no symptoms occur in the host. An infectious respiratory disease is normally not communicable during this period, although evidence indicates that chicken pox and measles may be transmitted to other hosts during the last 2 or 3 days of the incubation period. Length of the incubation period varies from disease to disease and from one person to another with the same disease. Generally, the more

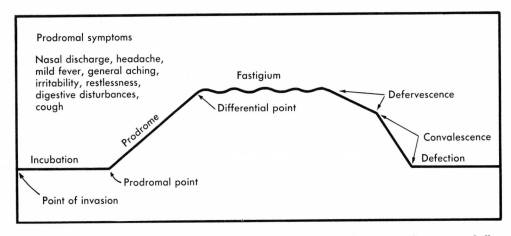

Fig. 10-1. Course of an infectious respiratory disease. The graph portrays the course of all respiratory diseases. Control of spread is most difficult during the prodrome and convalescence periods, when the infected person may be up and around. (From Anderson, C. L., and Creswell, W. H., Jr.: School health practice, ed. 6, St. Louis, 1976, The C. V. Mosby Co.)

severe diseases have a short incubation period and the less severe diseases have a longer incubation period, although exceptions to this general tendency do exist.

Prodrome period begins with the first symptoms in the host and usually lasts about 1 day. Symptoms of this period are similar for all of these respiratory infections and resemble those of the common cold. It is difficult to make a definite diagnosis at this stage because of the similarity of symptoms for all of these diseases. From a community health standpoint, there exists a great danger of disease transmission during this highly communicable stage. With the assumption that they "just have a cold," patients continue their normal routine of life and unknowingly expose a considerable number of people. Effective public education is necessary to alert people to the danger of disease transmission during the prodrome period.

Fastigium is the period during which the disease is at its height. Differential symptoms and signs appear, making accurate diagnosis possible. Although a highly communicable stage, the fastigium does not represent a serious disease control problem. Because patients are at home or in a hospital they expose only those who serve their immediate needs.

Defervescence indicates that the disease is declining in the severity of symptoms, although a relapse may occur.

Convalescence represents a recovery period. New problems in preventing disease spread arise because patients feel well enough to be up and about and expose those they come in contact with.

Defection represents the period during which the organisms are being cast off. It may run concurrently with the period of convalescence. Termination of defection is the signpost for the termination of isolation.

Alvine discharge diseases. Control of infections of the alimentary canal is essentially a problem in sanitation. Dysentery, typhoid fever, and other of the *Salmonella* infections are the principal alvine discharge diseases of consequence in the United States. *Salmonella* infections other than typhoid fever are rarely fatal, but the incidence is much higher than is generally recognized. Many cases of digestive disturbances, "intestinal flu," and "summer complaint" technically should be classed as *Salmonella* infections.

Vector-borne diseases. "Vector-borne diseases" is a better designation than "insect-borne diseases" because not all diseases in this classification are transmitted by insects. However, all of these diseases are normally transmitted to man by means of an intermediate host. These diseases pose a far greater problem in the tropics than in the United States, where only a few exist and then only in endemic form. Intensive campaigns in these affected geographical regions have brought such insect-borne diseases as malaria and Rocky Mountain spotted fever under control.

Open lesion diseases. Syphilis and gonorrhea are the open lesion type of disease of primary importance in terms of community health. Infection transfer in this class of disease normally entails direct contact with the open lesion or site of infection. In addition, only certain tissues, such as the mucous tissues, are specific for the organisms causing these diseases.

Tuberculosis and smallpox, as well as some other diseases producing skin eruptions, technically may be classed as open lesion diseases. The causative agents of these diseases leave their reservoir via the lesion of the infection.

SEXUALLY TRANSMITTED DISEASES

Though the two major venereal diseases, syphilis and gonorrhea, are spread in essentially the same way, they present very different clinical and epidemiological patterns. In addition to ensuring effective diagnostic and treatment services, control programs incorporate the similarities as well as the differences in these two diseases. The methodology for syphilis control has been developed over a long period of time and has been demonstrated to be effective in reducing the incidence of disease when rigorously applied. However, gonorrhea control methodology is still in the developmental stages and is further complicated by the following factors: (1) the short incubation period of gonorrhea, (2) its asymptomatic nature in the majority of females and some males, (3) the frequency with which patients become reinfected because of a lack of immunity, and (4) the developing resistance of the causative organism to currently available treatment.

The major thrust of gonorrhea control programs is screening by bacteriological culture of all women for asymptomatic gonococcal infection, followed by prompt treatment if they are infected.

The syphilis control program involves reporting cases, their treatment, and follow-up and interviewing patients for contact information. Named partners are traced, tested, and treated, to interrupt the transmission of disease within the community. The basic technic in syphilis control is contact investigation.

An element common to the control of both diseases is programs for venereal disease information and education. These program efforts are designed to create an awareness of the venereal disease problem and control methods and to inform the general public of the tragic consequences of these diseases. The focus is on increasing self-referrals for diagnosis and treatment and on expanding screening, contact tracing, and diagnostic and treatment programs within the community.

These two diseases represent excellent examples of the difficulty of prevention and disease control, even when the cause is known. The organisms are sensitive to drugs, yet a behavioral factor, namely promiscuity, is involved, with the resulting epidemics shown in Figs. 10-2 and 10-3.

CAUSATIVE AGENTS

Not all parasites of man are pathogenic to man, but all pathogens of man are parasites of man. Some of man's parasites—for example, *E. coli*—produce no antagonistic action in man. However, these inhabitants of man's large intestine do not live in symbiotic relationship with man because they do not return some benefit to man for the benefits they receive. Some pathogens may produce so slight a disturbance in man that the host is not aware of the disturbance. Even in a carrier condition a pathogen may produce some disturbance in the host.

A pathogen is a poor parasite because it

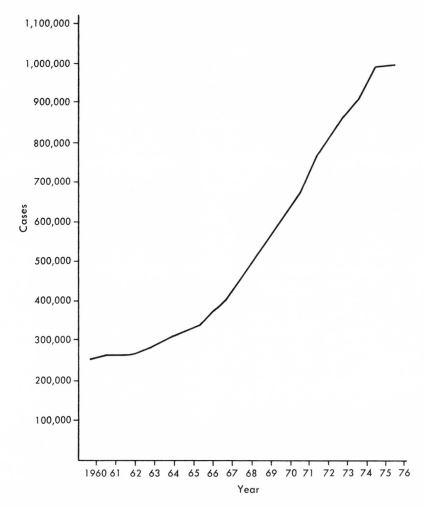

Fig. 10-2. Number of cases of gonorrhea, United States, 1960 to 1976. (Center for Disease Control, MMWR Morbidity and Mortality Weekly Report, vol. 26, no. 1, January 14, 1977)

arouses the host. It is analagous to a burglar arousing the household that he is preying upon. The response of the host is usually a defense reaction, basically of a chemical nature.

Types of infecting organisms. The vast majority of organisms pathogenic to man belong to the plant kingdom, specifically of the phylum Thallophyta. Bacteria constitute the greatest number of pathogenic organisms. Rickettsiae are small bacteria and viruses are ultramicroscopic forms. Certain true fungi, including the molds, are also pathogenic to man, although they may produce infestations

as well as infections in that they live on the body as well as in the body. In the animal kingdom certain protozoa and a few metazoa are pathogens of man. There are many classifications of pathogens of man, and all of them have a sound basis. The use of a particular classification depends on whether one criterion or particular criteria are given more weight than other criteria. For the purposes of the various people working in community health and parahealth fields, a classification that can be readily applied to existing conditions would be most logical. Of necessity, such a classification must overlook certain

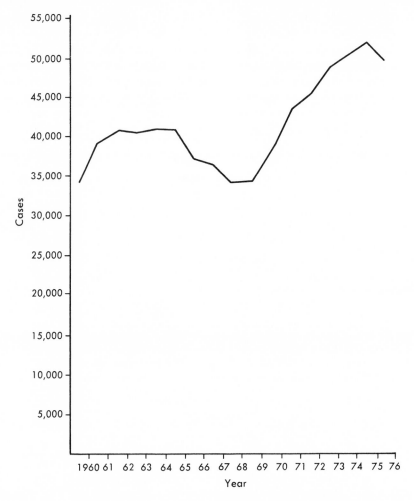

Fig. 10-3. Total number of cases of early syphilis, United States, 1960 to 1976. (Center for Disease Control, MMWR Morbidity and Mortality Weekly Report, vol. 26, no. 1, January 14, 1977)

technical criteria in the interest of functional needs.

Specificity of infecting organisms. A typhoid bacillus is derived only from a pre-existing typhoid bacillus. The virility but not the species may change from generation to generation of a particular type of organism. The severity of the reaction the organism produces in man may rise or subside with subsequent generations of the organism, but the action will always be similar in its basic nature. In addition to specific action, many organisms are harmful only to specific types of tissue. This basic tendency of all patho-

gens to be specific accounts both for the manner in which the organism functions and the reaction it produces in the host. In some respects the diphtheria bacillus may resemble the typhoid bacillus and in some respects the diphtheria bacillus may produce a somewhat similar reaction in the host, but the two different organisms have definite identities. This specificity of infecting organisms is a universal phenomenon.

Mode of action. Most pathogens of man injure human tissue by the toxins they produce. In their normal metabolic processes these pathogens produce substances that happen to be injurious to certain tissues in man. Some organisms—for example, diphtheria bacillus—produce toxins that diffuse through the permeable membrane of the bacterium and for this reason are called exotoxins. Other pathogens—for example, typhoid bacillus—produce a toxin that does not diffuse through the impermeable membrane that encloses the organism and for this reason are called endotoxins. When an organism of this type dies, its enclosing membrane undergoes changes that make it permeable to the toxins.

A small proportion of the pathogens of man invade the tissues directly. Some of the protozoa such as the malaria plasmodium and the spirochete of syphilis, as well as some viruses and rickettsiae, invade man's cells and bring about cellular change and, possibly, destruction.

RESERVOIRS OF INFECTION

Pathogens of man are relatively fragile organisms that survive only in a highly selective medium. A reported case of a new host for a particular type of organism means

Table 10-5 ■ Pathogens of man

Plants		Animals	
Organisms	Diseases	Organisms	Diseases
Bacterium (split fungi)	Diphtheria	Protozoan (one cell)	
Bacillus (rod-shaped)	Bacillary dysentery	Ameba	Dysentery
	Pertussis (whooping cough)	Plasmodium	Malaria
	Tuberculosis		
	Typhoid	Spirochete (spiral)	Syphilis
Coccus (spherical)	Furunculosis (boils)	Metazoan	
	Gonorrhea	Roundworm (e.g., ascaris)	
	Scarlet fever	Tapeworm	
	Streptococcal sore throat	Trichinella	Trichinosis
Spirillum (spiral-shaped)	Cholera		
	Rat-bite fever		
Rickettsia (small bacteria)	Rocky Mountain spotted fever		
	Typhus fever		
Virus (ultramicroscopic)	Chicken pox		
	Coryza		
	Influenza		
	Measles		
	Mumps		
	Poliomyelitis		
	Rabies		
	Smallpox		
True fungus	Mycosis		
Mold	Tinea (ringworm)		
Yeast	Blastomycosis		
	Dermatophytosis		

that the organism had been harbored in a medium favorable to the organism's survival, multiplication, and functioning. The medium in which organisms are thus harbored must possess moisture, relatively high temperature, nutrients, and an absence of light. It is rather easy to classify the reservoirs of organisms that affect man—those living hosts that provide an excellent medium and thus harbor these pathogens.

Human reservoirs. Man himself is the greatest reservoir of organisms pathogenic to man. This is the genesis of the time-tested question when a new case of disease is discovered—"Where is the other case?" Thus man himself is the source of the greatest danger of infection. *Frank cases,* or persons obviously ill with a disease, may be of great danger to an individual but not to a community. Although the individual who nurses the ill person may be greatly exposed to the disease, the community can be effectively protected by preventing transfer of infection from the known reservoir to other possible hosts, once the reservoir has been located. *Subclinical infections,* variously referred to as missed, abortive, or ambulatory cases, constitute a great community danger because the affected individuals may continue their normal daily routine. An ambulatory patient with diphtheria, scarlet fever, dysentery, or smallpox could unknowingly expose and infect a considerable number of associates before the source of the new cases of the disease is located. *Carriers* are individuals who harbor and disseminate a pathogenic organism without themselves experiencing recognizable symptoms. The longer the duration of the carrier status, the greater the danger to the community. Chronic or permanent carriers carry a long-time threat; however, once they are identified, control measures can be instituted that will minimize and almost remove the danger of communicating the disease to others. A convalescent carrier or transient carrier can be a serious danger to those in the immediate environment. Although the period of communicability may be relatively short, a sufficient

number of people can be infected by one such carrier to set off a chain reaction that may fan out and encompass a considerable number of new hosts.

Lower animals. Only a few species of lower animals harbor organisms pathogenic to man, and these are principally domestic animals. Rodents also serve as reservoirs of organisms that produce disease in man. Man has the necessary means to protect himself against diseases such as anthrax from sheep and cattle; glanders and tetanus from horses; hoof-and-mouth disease from cattle; brucellosis from cattle, swine, and goats; tuberculosis from cattle; trichinosis from swine; psittacosis from parrots and parakeets; rabies from canines and bats; and Rocky Mountain spotted fever and tularemia from rodents.

In the technical sense, the plant kingdom actually does not function as a reservoir of infection for man. However, in considering hookworm and tetanus, there is some justification for the contention that soil may serve as a reservoir for the pathogens of man.

ESCAPE OF ORGANISMS FROM RESERVOIR

The fact that a particular pathogen is harbored in a particular host is important from the standpoint of disease spread, but the organism must escape from the reservoir if other potential hosts are to be endangered. For some diseases, the mere fact that a person harbors the causative agent in itself represents no danger or a danger only under most unusual circumstances. A person with trichinosis is not endangering the health of others unless for some mystical reason they should become cannibalistic. The causative agent of trichinosis, being in the skeletal muscle of the human, has no avenue of escape. Likewise, a person who is an active case or carrier of malaria does not pose a danger to those about him under ordinary circumstances. The causative agent of malaria normally does not escape from the reservoir that harbors it. The organism can escape and endanger others only via the female

Anopheles mosquito, a blood transfusion, or perhaps the common use of a hypodermic needle among drug addicts.

It is a common observation that most of the pathogens of man can escape from the human body. The avenue of escape depends on the site of infection. The respiratory tract represents the most common and most dangerous avenue of escape. While an individual harbors an infection of the respiratory tract, it is realistic to assume that the escape of the organism is a continuous process. The escape may utilize such vehicles as droplets from coughs and sneezes, eating utensils, or the human hands. Escape via the intestinal tract would be through discharges of the colon and via the urinary tract through the urine. Open lesions provide an easy means of escape. With tubercle bacilli this is true whether it is a lesion of lung tissue or of the surface of the body. Likewise, the open lesions of syphilis, gonorrhea, and common furunculosis (boils) provide ready means of escape for the pathogens that produce the lesion. Mechanical escape of organisms from the human body is possible by biting or sucking insects, but here the organism must be aided by a specific vector or intermediate host.

Preventing the organism from escaping from the reservoir obviously provides one means of communicable disease control. Efforts must be based on a knowledge of the nature of the organism and the specific avenue through which it must escape.

TRANSFER OF INFECTION

Once the organism has escaped from the reservoir it still must be transferred to a new host if a new case of the disease is to occur. The normal pathogens of man do not walk or run or swim or fly. They must be transported by some vehicle. This transfer can be effected from person to person either directly or indirectly.

Direct transmission. Organisms can be transmitted directly from one person to another without an intermediate object. This requires intimate association usually, but not necessarily physical contact. Thus coughing and sneezing can be a direct means of transmitting organisms from one person to another without physical contact being involved. This accounts for the high incidence of respiratory diseases in crowded living areas.

Indirect transmission. When an intermediate object is involved in the transmission of disease from the reservoir to a new host, the mechanism is classed as indirect transmission. Such a transfer involves no particular close relationship between the reservoir and the new host. There are, however, two basic requirements for indirect transmission. The first of these is that the organisms involved must be virile enough to survive a long time outside of a living body. Thus highly resistant organisms such as those causing typhoid, tetanus, and anthrax are most likely to be transmitted by indirect means. On the other hand, highly fragile organisms such as those causing meningitis, syphilis, and gonorrhea are less likely to be transmitted by an intermediate object except under most unusual and highly favorable survival circumstances. A second requirement for indirect transfer of infection is the existence of a favorable vehicle of transmission. It may be a specific living form of life, such as a mosquito, or a highly favorable substance, such as milk. In a high proportion of diseases that can be transmitted by indirect means, for its survival the specific organism requires a specific medium or decidedly limited media and these media must be existing under certain circumstances and must be providing certain conditions.

Vehicles of transfer

There is some presumption in using the expression "vehicles of pathogen transfer," since the objects that make the transfer from the reservoir to a new host are not truly vehicles in the accepted sense. However, to a certain degree, these objects do transport the organism from one person to another. They might also be referred to as routes of infection since they represent certain pathways by which the organisms are transferred. Vehicles of transfer may be animate or inanimate.

Vectors. Animate vehicles are spoken of as vectors. These are intermediate hosts of the organism and represent the connecting link between one case of a disease and a susceptible new host. Transfer by vectors can be either biological or mechanical. In a biological transfer, the organism spends part of its life cycle in the body of the intermediate host. Biological vectors are specific for specific diseases. Malaria is transmitted only by the female *Anopheles* mosquito, yellow fever by the *Aedes aegypti* mosquito, typhus fever by the louse, plague by the flea, and Rocky Mountain spotted fever by the tick. When a vector makes possible the mechanical transfer of organisms, such specific action does not prevail. In this instance the vector comes in contact with infectious agents that mechanically become attached to the vector's body, legs, or other parts and thus are transmitted.

In unusual cases a vector that normally produces a biological transfer may also effect a mechanical transfer. Normally, the *Anopheles* mosquito harbors the plasmodium of malaria for about 14 days while the pathogen goes through a life cycle. The resulting young forms are then introduced into a host. This is true biological transfer. However, the *Anopheles* mosquito can get some blood from feeding on a human being with malaria, leave this reservoir, and immediately attach to a new host, where the organisms from the original reservoir can be mechanically introduced. This would be a mechanical transfer.

From the standpoint of knowledge of how to block the transfer of infection via vectors, man is well equipped. Theoretically, it would be possible to eliminate all disease transfer via vectors, but it is not possible to apply this knowledge because of the practical problem of extensiveness involved. Man knows how these vectors operate and how they can be destroyed, but, with the almost limitless number of vectors, man has to content himself with concentrating on the destruction and other control of vectors in specific areas

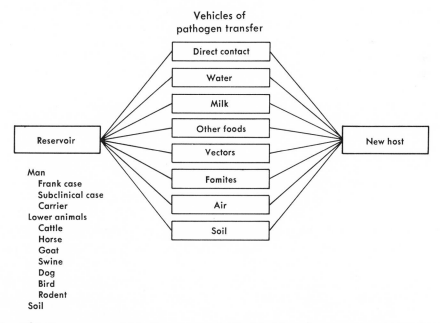

Fig. 10-4. Routes over which diseases travel. The blocking of routes over which infectious diseases travel prevents pathogens from reaching potential susceptible new hosts.

Table 10-6 ■ Means of pathogen transmission

Indirect contact			Direct contact
Airborne	**Water- and food-borne**	**Vector-borne**	
Anthrax†	Botulism†	Glanders†§	Anthrax†
Cerebrospinal meningitis*‖	Brucellosis†	Jaundice, infective*	Brucellosis†
Chicken pox*	Cholera*	Malaria*	Gonorrhea*
Encephalomyelitis, equine†	Diphtheria*	Plague*	Smallpox*
	Dysentery, bacillary*	Relapsing fever*	Syphilis*
Influenza*	Hoof and mouth disease‡§	Rocky Mountain spotted fever*§	Tetanus*
Measles*	Poliomyelitis*‖		Tularemia*
Mumps*	Streptococcus*	Tularemia*	
Pneumonia†	Tuberculosis†	Typhus fever*§	
Psittacosis†	Tularemia*	Yellow fever*§	
Tuberculosis†	Typhoid fever*		
Typhus fever*‡			

*Infects man only.
†Infects man and animals useful to man.
‡Infects animals or birds only.
§Artificially transmissible by air in laboratory.
‖Means of transmission unknown.

where the incidence of vector-borne diseases is pronounced.

Inanimate vehicles of disease transfer pose a special problem as society becomes more complex and people congregate in ever greater numbers in restricted areas. If an inanimate object is to serve as a vehicle of pathogen transfer it must have certain characteristics; otherwise, the organism will not survive the interval between the time it comes into contact with the object and the time it is transmitted to the new host. If the organism is to survive and remain sufficiently virile to set up a new infection, the time interval during which the organism is carried by the medium must be relatively short. The medium must be moist, bland, warm (near 100° F), and exist in relative darkness. Water, milk, other foods, air, fomites, and soil are the recognized inanimate vehicles of disease transfer.

Water. Water serves as a medium for the transfer of organisms from the human alimentary tract. Typhoid, paratyphoid, cholera, and bacillary dysentery are transmitted via water. Organisms normally do not multiply in water, yet an organism such as the typhoid bacillus can live for 2 or 3 weeks in relatively cool water. Man has developed the necessary measures to protect himself against disease transmission via water. Filtration and chlorination of community water supplies have been effective in controlling water-borne diseases.

Milk. Milk is an excellent medium for several organisms pathogenic to man. Contamination of milk can come from three sources. The first is infection within the udder from a disease with which the cow suffers, such as brucellosis and bovine tuberculosis. The second is infection within the udder by organisms accidentally introduced into the udder by a human being. Septic sore throat and scarlet fever are typical of this type of contamination. The third is direct contamination of the milk by a human being after it has left the cow. Thus a milk handler harboring diphtheria, typhoid, or dysentery bacilli may introduce the organism into the milk in the course of milk processing. Through herd testing, dairy sanitation, and pasteurization, man has been able to prevent the spread of infectious disease via the vehicle of milk.

Other foods. Other foods can be a means of transmitting pathogens but are not offenders as often as the lay public believes. For solid foods to serve as a vehicle of disease transfer, they must be moist, nonacid, not cooked, and handled a great deal. If a clerk in a bake shop, through handling, should leave typhoid bacilli on baked goods, the likelihood is rather remote that these few organisms would survive over the considerable length of time that would intervene before the pastry is eaten. This does not suggest that a typhoid carrier should be working in a public bake shop, but it does indicate that disease transfer by this means is not as frequent as is commonly thought. There are three common sources of contamination by food. The first of these is food handlers conveying organisms to the food by coughing or by their hands. The second is contamination during growth, such as shellfish developing in a body of water contaminated with typhoid bacilli. The third is from infected animals, such as the transmission of trichinosis and the tapeworm. Here, however, proper cooking would destroy pathogens. This is the key to protection against transfer via the common foods. Boiling or heating to the boiling point will destroy the usual pathogens of man that may be transferred via the food he eats.

Air. Air as a vehicle of disease transfer is not ideal. The dryness, low temperature, and light of the air are highly unfavorable to pathogenic organisms. Droplets from sneezing and coughing may give pathogens a moist vehicle that will help them survive long enough to set up an infection if they are inhaled into the respiratory passage of a new host. Measles and chicken pox appear to be more readily transmitted by this means than any of the other known respiratory diseases of man. A cubic foot of air may contain a considerable number of pathogens, but they would be so attenuated before being inhaled into the respiratory tract of a person that the likelihood that they would set up an infection in the new host is somewhat limited.

Fomites. Fomites are inanimate objects—other than water, milk, food, and air—that might be vehicles of disease transfer. The term embraces such things as clothing, bed linen, books, toys, handrailings, and similar objects. Fomites are no longer regarded seriously as vehicles of disease transfer because they do not provide a good medium for pathogens. However, it is possible that a patient, by handling an object, may leave a considerable number of organisms on the fomite and, if another person immediately handles the same object and gets his hands up to his mouth, the fomite may serve as a vehicle of spread. Increasing use of disposable items in the health care field minimizes this route.

Soil. Soil may harbor the organisms that cause hookworm, tetanus, anthrax, and botulism. Each of these presents a particular type of control procedure, but by the use of immunization, boiling, wearing of clothing, and other procedures, man has various effective means for preventing soil from being an actual vehicle of disease transfer.

In any situation where an intermediate object is the vehicle for the transmission of disease from a reservoir to a new host, it should be possible to block that route and thus prevent disease spread. In practice, however, man does not utilize the knowledge available to him, primarily because of a lack of understanding or because of carelessness or indifference. Through proper education of the public and the exercise of community control, it is possible to reduce the transfer of disease via animate and inanimate objects. In practice, public health officials find that the control of the social contact route is a much more difficult task than the control of disease spread routes involving vectors or inanimate objects.

ENTRY OF ORGANISMS
INTO NEW HOST

Arrival and entry are not synonymous. When the organism arrives at the place of the new host, it still has to find its proper port of entry and must overcome certain body barriers. Pathogens producing respiratory diseases must arrive at the mouth or nasal entry to the respiratory tract. Likewise, the organism causing an infection of the alimentary canal must find its way to the mouth. However, even when such an organism finds its way into the alimentary canal, acid in the stomach may destroy the organism. Direct infection of mucous membranes such as occurs in gonococcus infection requires that the organism come in contact with mucous membranes. While the hookworm can go through the unbroken skin and mosquitoes can penetrate the skin sufficiently to introduce pathogenic organisms, nevertheless percutaneous infections generally require a cut or an abrasion of the skin if the organism is to enter the body and create an infection.

DEFENSES OF THE HOST

After leaving the reservoir, being transferred to the new host, and by chance reaching the right port of entry, the pathogen still encounters a series of defenses the new host possesses. Indeed, virile organisms in a large number must enter the new host if all of the defenses of the new host are to be overcome and infection produced.

Resistance. The nature of resistance is expressed in the ability of the host to ward off pathogens. General resistance against infection is nonspecific in that the various resistance factors that the human possesses serve as barriers or are antagonistic to all pathogens of man. The skin serves as a mechanical barrier, and its natural acid state provides a further defense against pathogens that usually require a neutral or alkaline medium. The secretion of mucous tissue serves as a defense against most, and in a sense, all pathogens. The ciliated epithelium tissues of certain passages such as the respiratory tract provide an added defense, as the cilia tend to propel organisms to the exterior of the passageway. Acidity of such structures as the stomach, bladder, urethra, and vagina provides additional resistance to infection. Leukocytes with their phagocytic action destroy foreign organisms and perhaps represent man's most salient defense against infection. Lymph nodes filter out infectious organisms and are capable of destroying them. A highly important defense, not generally recognized as such, is the ability of the body to produce an elevated temperature or fever. The optimum temperature for pathogens of man is about 100° F, which is the approximate normal temperature of the body of man. In elevating the temperature by only 2 degrees, the body is able to inactivate the pathogens so that they are unable to multiply and carry on normal metabolism involving toxin production. During this stasis, the phagocytes of the body are able to engulf and destroy the pathogens.

It is apparent that from time to time small numbers of pathogens enter the human body without setting up infections. Man's general resistance is normally able to provide the necessary defenses to prevent infection.

Immunity and susceptibility. This concept distinguishes the status of the host regarding defense against specific diseases. The host with no specific resistance is termed susceptible and may be converted to immunity status by a variety of mechanisms. Complete resistance is termed "immunity" and is specific for a particular disease. Immunity is dependent on the presence of specific substances in the body that are most easily identified in the bloodstream but are present in all tissues. These chemical substances are called antibodies and may be in the form of antitoxin, which neutralizes a particular toxin, agglutinin, which causes organisms to clump together, or precipitins, which produce a precipitation.

Active immunity exists when an individual's own body produces the necessary antibodies. This occurs either through the actual attack of the disease or by artificial introduction of the necessary antigenic substance into the body. An antigen is a substance (for example, toxin) that, when introduced into the body, causes the formation of antibodies.

Passive immunity is "borrowed" immunity and exists when antibodies produced in some other individual or animal are introduced into a person. The duration of passive immunity is relatively short because the protective substances tend to disappear, not to be replaced by the individual's own body action. Passive immunity is employed when a susceptible person has been exposed to a disease and there is insufficient time to produce active immunity. The injection of convalescent serum into a susceptible child exposed to measles would give the child temporary immunity or at least measles with very mild symptoms. The infantile immunity that a child experiences during the first 6 months of life is an example of natural passive immunity in that antibodies from the mother's bloodstream diffuse through the membranes of the placenta into the bloodstream of the fetus. The immunity exists only while the mother's antibodies survive in the child. No stimulation of the child's tissues to form antibodies occurs.

Natural immunity expresses the concept that a species has a genetic immunity to a particular disease to which some other species is susceptible. Mammals are immune to many of the microorganisms that cause infection in birds. Domestic animals are susceptible to some diseases, such as distemper, to which man is immune. Likewise, domestic animals are immune to diphtheria, smallpox, typhoid fever, and other infectious diseases to which man is heir. These are examples of natural immunity in species. Fortunately, the human species possesses an immunity to a vast number of microorganisms that conceivably could be disease-producing except for man's distinctive biochemistry. However, man, by chance or by design, is able to add to this general protection or defense by acquiring artificial immunity to those diseases to which he could be susceptible.

Acquired immunity comes from having an attack of a disease or from artificially inducing a body reaction to produce the necessary protective antibodies. In man, second attacks are common in such diseases as influenza, pneumonia, gonorrhea, streptococcal sore throat, and the common cold but are relatively rare in such diseases as chicken pox, diphtheria, measles, poliomyelitis, scarlet fever, smallpox, typhoid fever, and yellow fever. Artificial active immunity is available for diphtheria, tetanus, pertussis, smallpox, poliomyelitis, typhoid fever, cholera, Rocky Mountain spotted fever, measles, German measles, mumps, and influenza. Various immunization schedules are in use.

Because no cases of smallpox have been reported in the United States since 1949, the Surgeon General of the United States Public Health Service has recommended that smallpox vaccination be discontinued. His reasoning is that there is a greater threat to human life in possible complication from vaccination than in not being immunized. The spread of an epidemic through a population is determined by the immune/susceptible ratio. When the supply of susceptibles is exhausted, the epidemic ceases.

AGENT-HOST-ENVIRONMENT

The outcome of disease in the individual is determined by the interaction of these three factors. The agent may be of high virulence or present in high dosage. The host defenses may be compromised by age or concomitant disease, or the immune system may be affected by drugs given for chronic disease.

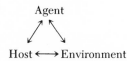

The environment may be hostile in respect to climate, such as air pollution. In intervention, action may be applied at any of the three points. Resistance of the host may be enhanced by nutrition or by vaccination, for example. The agent may be directly attacked by antibiotics, and the environment may be altered by sanitation.

This model may also be used to consider other conditions in addition to infectious diseases, such as automobile accidents, where the agent is the automobile, the host is the driver, and the highway is the environment.

EPIDEMIOLOGY

Epidemiology is the study of the distribution and determinants of disease in the population. The unit of study is not the individual, as in clinical medicine, but the community. Epidemiology compares and contrasts, studying both sick and well groups. Variables such as age, sex, race, and occupation are analyzed in an attempt to determine which are found frequently in the sick yet are found rarely in the well. The validity of the conclusions reached is subject to statistical tests. Epidemiological methods may be used to study chronic as well as infectious diseases, and disease in the community is first categorized under time, place, and person. By studying the time of onset in an epidemic, a shared event, such as a meal, may be identified. It can then be determined if this particular meal was attended by many of the sick persons but by few of a comparison group of well people. Food histories may then be assembled and a suspect vehicle identified. The place of the epidemic may help to identify the offending vehicle, such as the density of cases in an area sharing a common water supply, or cases predominantly on the route of a mobile food vendor. The persons involved in an epidemic may point to its cause, for example, they might share a common exposure to toxic inhalants in an industrial plant or to asbestos fibers in construction work.

Legal controls. Communicable diseases are controlled through the exercise of police power, which is the authority or power of

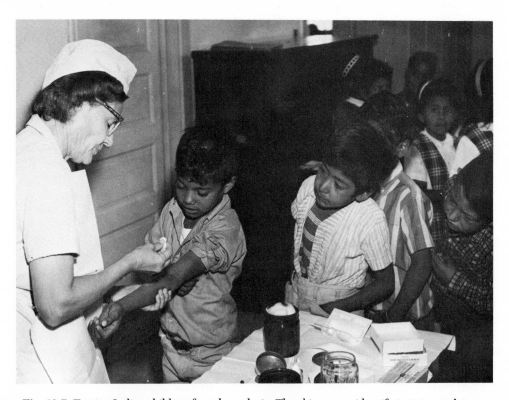

Fig. 10-5. Testing Indian children for tuberculosis. The skin test to identify incipient tuberculosis is a valuable screening procedure in the tuberculosis control program. (Courtesy Public Health Service)

the people to do whatever is necessary for the protection and general well-being of the public. Basically, sovereignty or ultimate authority rests with the people, who vest it in the state to exercise for them. The state may in turn delegate police power to counties to exercise within their geographical boundaries. Cities may be granted a charter that gives broad authority, including police power, to do whatever is necessary for the well-being of the people within the political limits of the city. It is clear that city authorities have the power to take the necessary measures to control communicable diseases within the city limits. Likewise, counties have the authority to exercise control measures outside of corporate municipalities.

The state reserves its power to take necessary action on a statewide or an area basis for the protection of the public against the spread of communicable diseases. In practice, the state enters into communicable disease control practice in a broad advisory capacity to the community governmental units and by direct action when communicable diseases spread beyond a single county and become a threat to a considerable portion of the state's population. It is apparent that the state does not usually step in and take action unless local authorities are unable to cope with the situation or unless the state is requested by local authorities to assist in the problem of disease control.

In the exercise of police power, the one governing principle recognized by the courts is that whatever action is taken must be reasonable. Thus it may be reasonable for health authorities to isolate an individual in his home for a period of 5 days when he suffers from a diagnosed case of a certain communicable disease, but a court may rule that it would not be reasonable to require that patient to be removed to a hospital and isolated there for 2 weeks. Actually, the science of epidemiology has advanced to a point where the action taken is usually reasonable because it is based on sound principles of microbiology and medical science. Further, citizens today are saved from a great deal of

inconvenience suffered by their grandparents because modern public health science has displaced much of the empiricism applied in disease control less than half a century ago.

In exercising police power, health authorities cannot ignore the personal and religious rights of the individual as guaranteed by the Constitution of the United States. However, courts have been very reluctant to censure public health official action exercised reasonably in the interest of the general population. Courts have ruled that while official health boards cannot require a person to be immunized in opposition to religious beliefs, action of health officials in imposing quarantine on some nonimmunized people when an epidemic threatens the community is just and reasonable. In the present era, however, control measures are so highly effective that if a relatively small percent of the population is not immunized against a disease, the fact that 85% of the people are immune virtually limits the spread of the particular disease by means of immunity level. From the standpoint of public health administration, communicable disease control is a much less difficult task than it was half a century ago. The present scientific approach to epidemiology encompasses certain well-established, effective measures of action.

Segregation of reservoir. An effective program of communicable disease control must direct itself to preventing the spread of disease and increasing the resistance of the new potential host. Logically, preventing the spread of disease is the most desirable and the most profitable in results in terms of the extended effort. Theoretically, perfect prevention of spread would mean perfect control of communicable diseases. It is possible to establish certain barriers around a reservoir of infection and thus block the spread of the disease.

Isolation, the oldest communicable disease control measure, is the segregation of an infected person or lower animal until danger of conveying infection has passed. Isolation can be a highly effective control measure, but in practice isolation will occasionally fail resulting from variability in the duration of the communicable state and from human failures in observing regulations.

When bacteriological methods are used to determine the interval of isolation, the termination of the communicable state can be made with precision. Laboratory examination of the secretions of a patient with tuberculosis will establish the presence or absence of the tubercle bacillus and thus determine the continuance or termination of isolation. Likewise, examination of secretions from the nose and throat in a patient with diphtheria will provide an accurate bacteriological determination of whether isolation should be terminated. If two smears from the nose, taken 24 hours apart, and two smears from the throat, taken 24 hours apart, are all found to be negative, isolation can be terminated with assurance that the patient is in a noncommunicable state.

Laboratory examination of respiratory secretions will also indicate whether viable streptococci are present and will thus serve as a marker for the continuance or termination of isolation. Laboratory examinations of the excretions of patients with typhoid fever and dysentery likewise can give a reliable indication of whether isolation should be continued or terminated. However, typhoid in particular poses a special problem because a typhoid carrier tends to discharge the bacilli intermittently. In some cases, positive fecal specimens may be a month apart. The use of laboratory methods to terminate isolation requires that a good laboratory and a qualified technician be available and that the tests be practical.

An arbitrary period of time for isolation is far more common than the use of laboratory methods for determining the period of isolation. The arbitrary time designated by law or by board of health regulations is usually based on practical experience through observation. To designate too short a period of isolation would mean exposing others and thus defeat the true purpose of isolation. The longer the period of isolation the greater the safety but the greater the injustice be-

cause many patients reach a noncommunicable state long before the maximum isolation period is reached. No definite rule applies; for this reason, great variation is found from state to state and even from community to community. To set an inflexible isolation period would make no provision for individual variation. For this reason, the usual practice is to set a minimum time that experience has demonstrated will be ample in perhaps 80% to 90% of the cases, and then leave to the discretion of the attending physician the need for extending the isolation in individual cases. An arbitrary period of isolation can be quite satisfactory for diseases such as measles and chicken pox where no convalescent carriers occur, but unsatisfactory for a disease such as scarlet fever where convalescent carriers are always a possibility.

Isolation has certain limitations. Hidden cases—those never reported by parents—are not technically under isolation. Missed, subclinical, or ambulatory cases—those so mild that no medical services are obtained—are not subjected to isolation measures. Carriers of a disease do not usually have overt symptoms and thus are not identified as potential hazards. In addition, during the early or prodrome stage of a respiratory disease, individuals may not be ill enough to remain home; yet they are in a highly communicable state and capable of communicating the disease to others. In all of these cases isolation will not be applied.

Quarantine is the detention of susceptible individuals who have been exposed to a communicable disease. These individuals are often spoken of as "contacts." Nonsusceptible people are not included as contacts. Quarantine is infrequently used in disease control at present because the individual is rarely in a communicable state during the incubation period of a disease. As a consequence, not until first symptoms appear does the individual represent a danger, and, at this point, isolation can be imposed. Measles and chicken pox are exceptions in that they may be communicable during the last 2 or 3 days of the incubation period. However, even in the case of these two diseases, quarantine is of questionable control value.

When quarantine is imposed, the period of time is based on laboratory findings, the maximum incubation period, or both. Thus if several laboratory specimens are negative the person is released from quarantine, or if the usual incubation period for the disease in question is 7 days, then after the seventh day following exposure to the disease the subject is released from quarantine if no disease symptoms are exhibited.

Reducing communicability. Treatment of a patient represents an important procedure in communicable disease control. Medical treatment of patients can be highly effective in reducing communicability of certain diseases. Through the use of chemotherapy and antibiotics, syphilis can be rendered noncommunicable.

Reservoir eradication. Logically, the most permanent and thus the most desirable measure of communicable disease control would be the complete elimination of the reservoir. This is possible when the lower animals serve as reservoirs of organisms pathogenic to man. Bovine tuberculosis has been eliminated in the United States by an orderly widespread program of testing cattle and then slaughtering those that are reactors. A similar program now under way seeks to eliminate all lower animals harboring *Brucella* organisms and thereby prevent undulant fever in man.

Paradoxically, the principle of reservoir eradication can be applied to the human. However, not the entire individual but the particular organ harboring infectious organisms is eliminated. This procedure is directed to the carriers of disease. The major obstacle in the promotion of this program lies in the unwillingness of carriers to submit to the necessary surgery. A high percentage of typhoid carriers are rendered a noncarrier by the removal of the gallbladder. Health officials and the family physician can explain to the carrier that there is a strong likelihood that, by having the gallbladder removed, the carrier may no longer have to be bound by restrictions imposed by health regula-

tions. However, no absolute guarantee can be made that the surgery will eliminate the source of typhoid bacilli in the carrier.

Sanitation. Environmental control measures are directed toward the vehicles of disease transfer and are effective in limiting the spread of such diseases of the intestinal tract as hepatitis, typhoid, paratyphoid, dysentery, salmonellosis, staphylococcus infection, and cholera. In the control of these diseases, the application of the principles of sanitation of water supplies, milk, and other foods and to sewage disposal has played an important role in the reduction of the incidence of alvine discharge diseases during the past half-century. Sanitation has also been effective as a measure in controlling vector-borne diseases such as malaria and yellow fever. By destroying the breeding places of the vectors and by the use of effective insecticides, programs in sanitation can effectively control the spread of insect-borne diseases.

Sanitation is ineffective and of little value in the control of such respiratory diseases as measles, chicken pox, scarlet fever, streptococcus sore throat, diphtheria, smallpox, and whooping cough. Decontamination measures may possibly be of some value in preventing spread of the respiratory diseases, although their actual effectiveness has never been scientifically determined. Concurrent decontamination and terminal decontamination are still practiced on the assumption that contaminated fomites may, under certain circumstances, be a mode of respiratory disease transmission.

Increasing resistance of new host. Even though organisms of sufficient number and virility to establish infection should invade a new host, measures still may be taken to protect the host and prevent further spread of the disease. Passive immunization can give transient emergency protection. Before this procedure is employed, it must be ascertained that the person actually was exposed and is susceptible to the disease. Because passive immunization lasts but a few weeks, it provides only a stopgap for a particular situation when no other measures are feasible. Passive immunization has one marked disadvantage in that the serum usually used may sensitize the individual so as to set up the future danger of an anaphylaxis—extreme reaction to a second exposure to the foreign serum. For this reason, passive immunization is not regarded as a good community project to be used on a widespread basis. In practice, it is used only for selected cases.

Modification of the severity of a disease should be regarded as a control measure. Diseases such as diphtheria and scarlet fever can be modified by treatment, and by this procedure communicability can be reduced.

From the practical standpoint, the obvious approach is to immunize all prospective new hosts. This means artificial immunization of all adults against diseases such as poliomyelitis and all children against such diseases as diphtheria, pertussis, and poliomyelitis. The need for immunization against typhoid fever and Rocky Mountain spotted fever should be determined by the prevalence in a specific area or of special danger to particular individuals such as nurses, public health workers, or foresters.

Community education. Fundamental to the effectiveness of any measures designed to control communicable disease is an effective continuous program of community education. Government authority is necessary but not sufficient for a high level of effective disease control. The public must be informed far in advance of any outbreaks. A community health education program that week after week is keeping its citizens informed about the nature, the spread, and the control of communicable diseases will have ready a highly potent means to check the spread of any infectious disease that may break out. Knowledge not only helps in the prevention of disease but in proper control when disease does occur. In addition a well-informed public will not be stampeded by scare rumors or fantastic reports such as fatal reactions to immunization. Further, a good community health education program will assist in obtaining funds for the promotion of immunization and other control measures. Community health education means utilizing all resources available. The printed word, the spoken word, visual aids, and demonstrations must be employed. The need is not an appeal to the emotions but an appeal to reason through understanding and an appreciation of the obligation to one's community, neighbors, family, and oneself.

No communicable disease control program will be perfect. The application of present knowledge, methods, and techniques can yield a near-perfect result. Any communicable disease control program requires constant effort and analysis. What has proved to be effective will be continued. What can be improved will be changed. The decline in the incidence and death rates of the various infectious diseases is mute evidence that man has devised successful, though not perfect, means for preventing disease spread. Effective though present measures may be, there is still room for improvement, although public health workers do not expect to see the millenium when no infectious disease plagues man.

DISEASE CONTROL MEASURES

Many individuals and agencies serve in one capacity or another in the control of communicable diseases. Legal authority for the control of communicable diseases rests with the official health agencies, yet the medical profession, the hospitals, clinics, voluntary health agencies, and the schools all play important roles in disease control. In practice, official health agencies welcome the cooperation and assistance of individuals and agencies competent to assist in the general problem of disease control. Health education of the public is fundamental to effective communicable disease control measures, and official health agencies recognize that the supplementary health education contributed by other agencies is highly valuable in the general control program. Indeed, health education of the public represents the primary approach of the official health agencies in controlling diseases. In the philosophy of modern community health, a department of health that must continually rely on its legal authority for an effective program would be regarded as an outdated and ineffective agency.

Official health agencies. Legal responsibility and authority for the control of communicable diseases rests with the tax-supported agencies on the national, state, and community level. The United States Public Health Service has responsibility for the prevention of disease coming from outside the nation. This encompasses international quarantine of harbors and air fields. In addition the Service has responsibility and authority for the prevention of spread of disease between states. In this capacity the Service has jurisdiction over travel of infected persons as well as the shipment of infected animals and contaminated articles such as meat. In addition the United States Public Health Service has supervision over the shipment of biologics via interstate carriers. The United States Public Health Service also grants assistance to states in dealing with severe epidemics or special disease problems. This is more a professional service courtesy than a legal obligation.

State health departments provide communicable disease control measures within their states through their divisions of communicable diseases, laboratory services, and sanitation. State sanitary codes set up provisions for isolation and quarantine, vaccination, reporting of communicable diseases, examination of school children, exclusions from school, hospitalization standards, treatment of syphilis, protection of water supplies, disposal of human wastes, and protection of foods for sale. The state health department laboratory serves the medical profession and other qualified individuals in the diagnosis of disease and in the termination of isolation when laboratory tests are of value. In addition routine laboratory services such as water and milk analysis are valuable in disease control. The state health department gives assistance to local health

agencies when severe epidemics occur or when special disease problems exist. Under most circumstances the state health department has authority to step into a local situation only on invitation from the local health authorities.

Local health agencies—district, county, and city—touch the individual citizen and, because of their close relationship with the people, represent the most important and most effective agency for disease control. Community health agencies may set up their own communicable disease regulations or codes to exercise within their own boundaries. These regulations may not be in conflict with the state regulations nor establish lower standards than those of the state regulations, but the local standards may be higher than those of the state. Essential to an effective program of local control, the health department must have an informed public and must work cooperatively with the medical profession, the schools, and all other agencies and individuals having a role in the control of communicable diseases.

Physicians' reporting of communicable disease cases is made as easy and effective as possible. As a practical measure, physicians use the telephone in reporting diseases, particularly the more serious diseases. Official isolation of a patient is done through the attending physician, who also is contacted concerning the release of the patient from isolation. A health department representative informs the family of official isolation requirements and usually places responsibility on the family for the observance of these requirements.

The most difficult disease control problems arise when no physician has been called. However, health department staff members, through their contacts in the community, will usually have information channeled to them about families having illness. Public health nurses particularly will get such information and will visit the reported family. In addition to the information they may give the family on the care of the illness, they will also likely refer the matter to one of the medical physicians on the health staff, who will make the necessary diagnosis for official control purposes.

Communicable disease control measures on the local level must be carried every day of the year. Educating the community in the prevention and control of disease is a never-ending task. It goes on when there is not a single known case of infectious disease in the community as well as when an epidemic exists. It involves the promotion of immunization, particularly of infants and preschool children. It involves constant attention to the community water supply, sewage disposal, food handling, and vector control. It involves special programs at different times of the year when particular communicable diseases are most prevalent. Communicable disease control is but one phase of the total official community health program, but it commands the best efforts of the local health department.

Schools. Within their own premises, schools have the legal authority and the responsibility to take reasonable measures for the prevention and control of communicable diseases. In cooperation with the local health department, the medical profession, and the parents, the school can contribute to the control of communicable disease by the promotion of immunization, the early recognition of signs of infectious disease, and the effective control of exclusions from school and readmissions to school. This requires school personnel versed in the fundamentals of communicable disease control and an appreciation of the schools' obligation to the students, the family, and the community in controlling infectious disease.

In general, immunization as a requirement for admission to school is regarded as a local measure and is left to the discretion of local school boards. Courts have upheld the right of a local board of education to require immunization as a condition for school admission when exceptions are made on religious grounds. As a general practice, the local board of education requires immunization against diphtheria and smallpox as a requisite for school entrance. In a growing number of school districts, poliomyelitis and measles immunizations are being added to the required list. Paradoxically, at the same time there is a growing tendency to displace compulsory immunization with voluntary immunization. As more parents understand and appreciate the necessity for immunization there becomes less need for compulsory measures.

Through inspections, reviews, and observations of children, teachers are able to detect early indications of possible communicable disease. Early detection of disease will result in early exclusion of the pupil with greater protection to other youngsters in the school. The child with indications of communicable disease should be segregated immediately. An emergency rest room should be available where the child can lie comfortably on a cot. Parents are usually informed by telephone that their youngster is not feeling well and it is suggested to them that the youngster be brought home. Informing the parents and enlisting their confidence and cooperation in the exclusion of the child is a desirable courtesy. However, the school has a responsibility to exclude any youngster who appears to have a communicable disease. This principle is clearly stated in the case of *Stone v. Probst*, in which the court said: "Pupils who are suffering or appear to be suffering from a communicable disease may menace the well-being of all pupils and therefore should be denied the privilege of school attendance."* After the child has been taken home by a member of the school staff or other designated person, responsibility for futher isolation of the youngster legally rests with the local health department. Consequently, the school keeps the local health department informed on all matters relating to the illness of children who have been excluded from school. A high degree of cooperation between

---

*Supreme Court of the State of Minnesota, 165 Minn., 1925, 361,206 NW 642; appeal from the District Court, Hennepin County.

school and health department is necessary if the interests of the community are to be served best by both agencies.

In the event of an epidemic, the school works cooperatively with the community health department and is governed by the regulations and recommendations of the health department staff. In practice both health and school officials are reluctant to close the schools during an epidemic. Usually, with the schools in session, it is easier to control the spread of disease through morning and noon inspections of the children and constant observation throughout the day. Likewise, the opening of school in the fall is not delayed because of an epidemic. Experience has demonstrated that opening the schools and applying control measures that include the school are as effective as any other means for limiting the spread of disease. Occasionally, for efficiency reasons, a school may be closed when such a high percentage of youngsters is absent that the schoolwork will have to be repeated for the benefit of those who were absent. As an illustration, more than 70% of the students in a high school were absent because of influenza on a Wednesday. After consultation with the health department, school officials closed the school until the following Monday. This, however, was an education or economic measure rather than a communicable disease control measure.

Voluntary health agencies. All nontax-supported voluntary health agencies that receive their financial support from private sources have neither a legal responsibility nor, strictly speaking, an official status except as they may be incorporated under the laws of a state or otherwise recognized. Yet the voluntary health agencies serve an important role in communicable disease control. Normally, a voluntary health agency is organized to deal with one specific health problem or a disease such as tuberculosis or poliomyelitis. From its founding, the National Tuberculosis and Respiratory Disease Association has devoted itself to public health education by keeping the public informed

and urging the public to take certain measures. As a supplement to this basic public health education program, the Association has sponsored testing programs and research. On the local level, the state associations in many instances have branched out into the broader field of health education, encompassing fields other than tuberculosis. Through the years, the efforts of this voluntary agency have contributed measurably to the battle against tuberculosis, even though it has never undertaken to contribute financially or otherwise to the treatment of patients.

On the other hand, the National Foundation for Infantile Paralysis, almost from its outset, gave direct financial assistance to families having a member afflicted with poliomyelitis. The Foundation has also promoted research and an extensive public health education program. Several other national and local voluntary health agencies also contribute to community communicable disease control programs. In the main their contribution has been that of educating the public and supporting the official and other health agencies engaged in matters of health that include disease control.

Medical profession. The keystone in the entire communicable disease control program is the practicing physician who diagnoses and supervises the disease case. In the treatment and supervision of the patient and in instructions to the patient's family, the physician represents the first line of defense against the spread of communicable disease. Further, through advocacy of immunization and by immunizing as a routine part of medical service to the family, the practicing physician daily makes an invaluable contribution to communicable disease control in the community.

Clinics and hospitals. A special arm in the community communicable disease control program is represented by the clinical and hospital services that exist in the community. Clinics, whether of the broad service type or of a specialized nature, serve as an immunizing and diagnostic service for special tests or other highly specialized techniques. The availability of such a medical center lends confidence and assurance to the public and community health service alike that the highest level of medical skill is available when a crisis or other unusual situation arises. Special immunization clinics may be set up when an epidemic threatens. An outbreak of typhoid fever may justify setting up immunization clinics. This is particularly true during disasters such as floods.

Hospitals may not be an indispensable agency in communicable disease control because most patients with a communicable disease remain at home. However, circumstances may arise that make it not only highly desirable but imperative that a patient be hospitalized.

That man has made progress in the battle against infectious diseases is apparent. To be lulled into the complacent frame of mind that the battle has been won would be foolhardy and even tragic. The battle against infectious diseases goes on, day in and out. Research must find answers to many problems and questions as yet unsolved. In the meantime, communities employ the knowledge, methods, and techniques now available and thus hold the incidence of infectious diseases to a practical minimum. Doubtless, much effort in this field seems to be wasted, but to paraphrase a common expression: "Eternal vigilance is the price of freedom from communicable disease."

QUESTIONS AND EXERCISES

1. What distinction can be made between infectious disease and communicable disease?
2. What significance do you attach to the fact that the number of reported cases of streptococcal infection was greater in 1976 than in 1900?
3. Evaluate this statement: "If effective methods of immunization were developed for all of the communicable diseases, mankind would eliminate the communicable diseases with which he is now plagued."
4. Recall three recent outbreaks of communicable diseases you observed or otherwise were acquainted with. Do you class these outbreaks as endemic, epidemic, or pandemic?
5. What communicable respiratory diseases are most likely to appear in epidemic form in your community?
6. What disease do you predict will cause the next worldwide pandemic?
7. To what extent is there justification for saying that an epidemic is evidence of an inadequate public health education program?
8. Is pasteurization of the community milk supply less necessary today than it was 25 years ago?
9. Enumerate the various services your state department of health provides in its communicable disease control program.
10. What are the various organizations or agencies in your community contributing to communicable disease control?
11. What steps should an ordinary citizen take when he has evidence that a case of communicable disease may exist in a household where no physician has been called and no precautions are being taken to prevent possible spread of the disease?
12. What is being done and what further should be done in your community to prevent the spread of communicable diseases via foods other than milk or water?
13. From the standpoint of public health education, how would you change this prevailing attitude: "It's just a cold"?
14. Why should passive immunization be rejected as a community-wide procedure?
15. An individual diagnosed, with laboratory confirmation, as having syphilis refused free treatment and was isolated in the county jail. Evaluate the action taken by the county health department.
16. What disadvantages in respect to communicable disease control does a democracy have that a dictatorship does not have?
17. Why does undulant fever exist in the United States, when slaughtering all brucella-infected cattle, swine, and goats would prevent the disease in man?
18. Is there any evidence that new infectious diseases are appearing?
19. Design an experiment or study to show whether nonfatal infections shorten life expectancy.
20. Make a general comparison of the incidence of communicable disease cases and deaths in the United States in 1975 and predicted in 2000.

REFERENCES

American Public Health Association: Control of communicable diseases in man, ed. 11, New York, 1970, The Association.

Chelsky, M.: A method of interpreting infectious disease incidence, American Journal of Public Health **59:**1661, 1969.

Ellis, R. W., and Mitchell, R. G.: Diseases in infancy and childhood, ed. 6, Baltimore, 1968, The Williams & Wilkens Co.

Gallagher, R.: Diseases that plague modern man, Dobbs Ferry, N.Y., 1969, Oceana Publications, Inc.

Hanlon, J. J.: Public health: administration and practice, ed. 6, St. Louis, 1974, The C. V. Mosby Co.

Henschen, F.: The history and geography of diseases, translated by Joan Tate, New York, 1966, The Delacorte Press.

Krugman, S., Ward, R., and Katz, S. L.: Infectious diseases of children, ed. 6, St. Louis, 1977, The C. V. Mosby Co.

Rouché, B.: Annals of epidemiology, Boston, 1967, Little, Brown and Co.

Smith, I. M.: Infectious disease, Baltimore, 1967, The Williams & Wilkins Co.

Top, F. H., and Wehrle, P. F., editors: Communicable and infectious diseases, ed. 8, St. Louis, 1976, The C. V. Mosby Co.

11 ■ SAFETY IN THE COMMUNITY HEALTH PROGRAM

Carelessness does more harm than a want of knowledge.

Benjamin Franklin

Safety is a state of mind. Many agencies in a community concern themselves with safety, often with a special interest in one aspect such as home, occupational, recreational, motor vehicle, school, or fire safety. These agencies make their most effective contribution to community safety when there is a well-organized, well-integrated community safety program. This is a role and a service the official community health department can provide.

EPIDEMIOLOGY OF INJURIES

As a despoiler of expected years of life, a producer of human misery, a waster of national financial and other economic resources, and a degrader of the quality of human existence, accidents probably rank first among all health problems of American people.

Norvin Kiefer, M.D.
Equitable Life Insurance Company, New York

Accidents are the fourth leading cause of death in the United States; however, among patients aged 1 to 37 years, they are the leading cause of death. One in four Americans will be involved in an accident each year. Of the 115,821 accidental deaths in 1973, the ranking was:

Automobile	55,111
Home	Approximately 30,000
Work	Approximately 15,000
Miscellaneous	Approximately 15,000

The ranking for frequency of all accidents was home, work, automobile, and miscellaneous.

AUTOMOBILE ACCIDENTS
Factors influencing occurrence

Age and sex. Male motor vehicle occupants in the 15- to 24-year age group have an exceptionally high death-to-injury ratio. Age difference in resistance to injury and in the ability to survive a given injury influence the age distribution of injuries and death. As a result, decreased ability to survive crashes is a major factor that causes older persons to be overrepresented among fatally injured drivers. It is important to separate the effect of age on the initiation of an event from the effect of age in the outcome of the event.

Table 11-1 reveals that half of all deaths of white males aged 20 to 24 years are caused by injuries and that over one-third of all deaths in this age group are caused by automobile accidents alone. The influence of age is demonstrated by comparing the distribution in the 50- to 54-year age group, where only 2.4% of deaths are the result of automobile accidents.

Alcohol. The most important human factor known to be causally related to all types of accidents and a factor in over half of all fatal injuries is alcohol. It is a factor that increases the severity of the outcome and makes it harder for a passenger to escape from a burning or submerging car. It makes emergency treatment difficult and obscures the diagnosis.

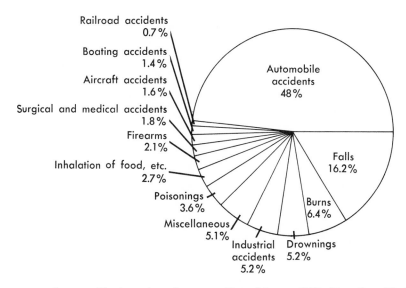

Fig. 11-1. Distribution of fatal accidents by cause, United States, 1971. (Data from Vital statistics of the United States, vol. 2, 1973)

Table 11-1 ■ Proportionate mortality for white males, ages 20 to 24 and 50 to 54 years in the United States, 1970

Ages 20 to 24 years		Ages 50 to 54 years	
Cause	**Percent**	**Cause**	**Percent**
Automobile accidents	36.8	Arteriosclerotic heart disease	40.2
Suicide	7.8	Cancer of the lung	6.0
Homicide	4.0	Vascular lesions affecting central	5.0
Drowning	2.5	nervous system	
Aircraft accidents	2.5	Cirrhosis of liver	3.4
Lymphosarcoma and	2.5	Suicide	2.4
Hodgkin's disease		Automobile accidents	2.4
Firearm accidents	2.0	Cancer of the rectum and bowel	2.0
Water transport accidents	2.0	Pneumonia	2.0
Nephritis and Nephrosis	2.0	Chronic rheumatic heart disease	2.0
Pneumonia	2.0	Cancer of the stomach and esophagus	2.0
Arteriosclerotic heart disease	2.0	Hypertensive heart disease	2.0
Other	33.9	Other	30.6

From Robbins, L. C., and Hall, J. H.: How to practice prospective medicine, Indianapolis, 1970, Slaymaker Enterprises.

Age, sex, and alcohol are significant variables in accidents. While psychological factors may also play a role, they are very difficult to separate from cultural and social components of behavior.

Intervention to reduce injury caused by accidents

Intervention may be directed at the agent, host, or environment. Most effort is directed at the host, for the urge to reform and alter other people's behavior is very strong. Investigation frequently reveals the cause of accidents to be human error. Unfortunately, this approach is the least rewarding of the three available. Consideration of automobile-related injuries illustrates this point. Three classes of people—young males, alcoholic persons, and elderly people—are most likely to be involved in automobile accidents, and these three groups are particularly resistant to education programs. For the amount of effort expended, the results of education programs for the general population are disappointing. Seat belts are used by less than half of the people who have them, despite their recognized efficacy in reducing injury.

Much more rewarding is intervention at the agent level, modifying it so that the potential harm is lessened and the product made safer. This has been done to a limited extent in the automobile. In the area of medication containers have been designed so that children cannot open them and poison themselves. Children's pajamas are made of flameproof fabric. Safety is now built into the design of many products. The doctrine of manufacturers' liability for harm resulting from faulty design or operation has done much to accelerate this trend. Legal accountability for products used by the public has forced companies to incorporate safety features. Ralph Nader is to be thanked for his early crusading efforts on behalf of the consumer.

The most effective site of intervention is the environment. The environment should be modified so that it is safe and is designed so that accidents will rarely happen, and that when they do little harm will result. The most obvious and familiar example is the highway. By using a wide median strip featuring a sturdy guardrail, fatal accidents can be immediately and permanently reduced. Safe access and exit ramps, clear signs, lighted junctions, and rest areas contribute to safe driving. Other safety features well known to highway engineers and now available, such as frequently struck highway structures being covered with compressible materials such as a collection of oil drums, also reduce accidents. This principle can be applied to housing and pedestrian areas, which may be made safe by nonslip surfaces, grading, and lighting. The environment in industrial areas may be modified to increase safety by reduction of air and noise pollution and the use of guardrails. The environmental changes necessary for safety frequently involve enforcement of existing regulations (for example, the 55 mph limit) or enactment of new legislation, for example, gun control and prohibition of all firearms. Such radical changes need to be preceded by campaigns to influence public opinion as to the benefit of the change proposed. However, once a measure has been successfully enacted, the people appreciate the benefit to the public health that ensues, and such laws are not rescinded. The battle only has to be won once.

In summary experience has shown that priority in injury control should be given to measures that require little or no human action or cooperation.

SAFETY PROGRAM
Home safety

"Safe at home" is one of those cliches that is something of a mockery in the United States. Each year about 30,000 people in America lose their lives as the result of an accident in the home and about 4,500,000 more suffer disabling injuries. The health implications are starkly apparent.

At home the most dangerous area for accidents is the bedroom, because it is most often the site of falls, chiefly among older

Situations:

1. Driver performance with failure

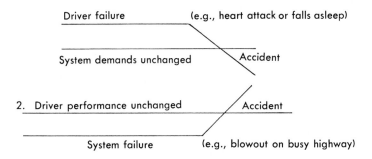

2. Driver performance unchanged

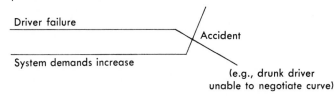

3. Driver performance decreased

Driver failure

System demands increase

Accident

(e.g., drunk driver
unable to negotiate curve)

Fig. 11-2. Automobile/highway conditions and driver performance. (Adapted from Blumenthal, 1968)

Table 11-2 ■ Basic matrix for classifying highway crashes and countermeasures

	Human	**Vehicle and equipment**	**Modification of environment**
Precrash	Alcoholism control programs	Improved braking ability for heavy trucks	One-way street
Crash	Safety belt usage	Bumpers that reduce crash forces	Removal of unyielding structures from the roadside
Postcrash	Emergency medical care	Extrication	Emergency systems

Adapted from Haddon, W.: A logical framework for categorizing highway safety phenomena and activity, Journal of Trauma **12**(3):193-207, 1972.

---

people. The second most dangerous area is the kitchen.

Community home safety programs. Year after year more people are injured in accidents in the home than in motor vehicle accidents, yet few communities have an organized continuing program of home safety promotion. In addition to the prevention of injuries, home safety programs could make inroads on the nearly 30,000 deaths a year that occur as a result of accidents in the home.

Some communities have an established fire prevention program that is laudable even

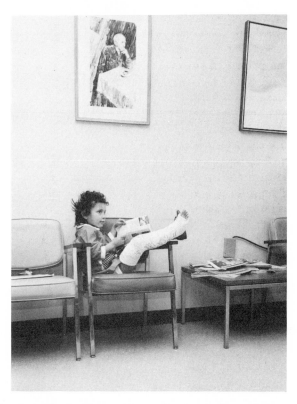

Fig. 11-3. Childhood accidents. Home safety and safety and community injury control programs tend to be too broadly oriented to multiple problems. More focus on the specific groups experiencing specific types of accidents is needed. (Courtesy Johns Hopkins Medical Institutions)

though limited to one phase of home safety. For more than 15 years, Cincinnati has had a "Target System" of fire inspections supported by a Tactical Inspection and Educational Unit. Inspections are made of structures by assigned members of each fire company. Frequency of inspections is determined by the "Target" or category of the structure, and the five categories are determined by the inspectors based on the nature of the occupancy and the past inspection record. In the poorest category, inspections are made as frequently as every 2 weeks. When persuasion does not result in getting hazards corrected, court action may be taken against noncompliance with fire department orders.

In some communities the fire department encourages citizens to request fire inspection by the department staff. This is often associated with Fire Prevention Week. These programs are not to be discouraged, but obviously such piecemeal home safety programs are not adequate. A community-wide home safety program spanning all aspects of home accident prevention is the urgent need.

Because education is a basic ingredient of home safety promotion, the health education division of the community health department can provide the leadership and responsibility for a community program to prevent accidents in the home. With the health department spearheading the program, safety activities and contributions of various organizations (for example, the fire department) and individuals can be correlated with the efforts of the health department. A community-wide home safety council can serve as a sounding board and an entree to the public and their homes.

Like other accidents, home accidents are caused by improper practices and unsafe conditions. Safety promotion in homes must be directed toward the correction of practices and conditions. An extensive and intensive program of education of the public must precede any action directed to specific circumstances. This means the use of all possible media of communication and the promotion of special measures for alerting the public to the need for safety in the home.

Once the interest of the public has been aroused, the next step will be home safety surveys by householders themselves. Participation by the individual citizen is the key to effective home accident prevention. A *home safety survey* form should be delivered to all households and to other structures in the community. Such a survey should be a simple form based on conditions and practices of importance in safety.

Basement and laundry

1. Are all flues, stovepipes, and chimneys clean and tight?
2. Are combustible surfaces near stoves, furnaces, and vents insulated?
3. Is kindling wood stored at a safe distance from the furnace?
4. Are furnace fires started without the use of gasoline, kerosene, or other explosive materials?
5. Are ashes always placed in metal containers?
6. Are old newspapers and other inflammable materials removed promptly from the basement?
7. If the laundry floor tends to be damp, is a rubber mat provided?
8. Are cords that are exposed to water coated with rubber?
9. Are soap powder and other detergents kept off the floor to prevent slipping?
10. When not in use, are electrical appliances disconnected from the wall socket?
11. Are the basement and laundry room adequately lighted?

12. Are all gas connections checked twice a year to detect leaks or defects?
13. Are noninflammable cleaning fluids used and only out of doors?
14. Is a regular place provided for tools?
15. Is an inspection made once a month to check any special hazards peculiar to a particular basement or laundry?

Kitchen

1. Is the floor clean and free from hazards such as upturned linoleum edges?
2. Are matches in metal containers and out of children's reach?
3. Is a short, sturdy stepladder used for reaching high places?
4. Are electrical appliances disconnected from the wall when not in use?
5. Is the electric iron rested on a proper stand when not in use?
6. Are the handles of pots and pans on the range turned out of the reach of children?
7. Are receptacles with water emptied immediately after using?
8. Are all gas connections checked twice a year to detect leaks or defects?
9. Is care taken to prevent gas flames from being extinguished by liquids boiling over or by drafts?
10. Are knives and other sharp instruments kept out of the reach of children?
11. In using a knife, do you always cut away from the body?

Living room and dining room

1. Are small rugs anchored so that they do not slip on polished floors?
2. Are the edges of rugs prevented from curling?
3. Is there a storage place for toys, and are they kept there when not in use?
4. Is nonskid wax used on floors?
5. Are chairs and other furniture in good repair?
6. Are scissors kept out of reach of small children?
7. Are pins and razor blades wrapped and disposed of properly?

8. Are extension cords placed where they will not be tripped over?
9. Are open wall sockets plugged?
10. Are all electric fixtures of an approved type and in good condition?
11. Is a sturdy stepladder used in reaching high places?
12. Are cigarette stubs extinguished and placed in convenient noninflammable containers?
13. Is a screen placed in front of a fireplace?

Stairs

1. Are stairs well lighted and unobstructed?
2. Do light switches operate from top and bottom of the stairs?
3. Is carpeting fastened securely to the floor and in good repair?
4. Is there a strong handrail on at least one side of the stair?
5. Are there secure gates at the bottom and top of stairs to protect young children?
6. Are all members of the household careful not to carry heavy loads on stairs?
7. Do the aged live entirely on the first floor and avoid the use of stairs?
8. Is the bottom step on the basement stairs painted a luminous white?

Bathroom

1. Is a rubber mat placed in the tub and a handhold installed on the wall?
2. Are electric fixtures made of porcelain or other insulating material?
3. Are portable appliances and cabinets moved to an out-of-the-way place when not in use?
4. Are medicines and poisonous substances placed in a locked cabinet or other place inaccessible to children?
5. Are all poisons kept in clearly marked containers?
6. Is a pin stuck in the cork of every bottle containing poison, and are labels double checked under clear light before the poison is used?
7. Are little children never left alone in the bathroom?

Bedroom

1. Is the passageway from the bed to the door unobstructed?
2. Are dresser drawers and closet doors always closed when not in use?
3. Are window screens securely installed?
4. Are electric heaters disconnected at the wall before the occupant goes to sleep or leaves the room?
5. Is there a convenient light switch for emergency night use?
6. Is it a practice never to smoke in bed?
7. Are safeguards provided to prevent children from falling out of cribs or beds?

Garage, yard, and porch

1. Are garage doors open while the car motor is running?
2. Is there a safe place to store garden equipment?
3. Is rubbish burned in a metal container on windless days and are children kept away?
4. Is the ladder of sound construction and properly anchored when used?
5. Are snow and slush promptly removed from porch and walks?
6. Is ice covered with sand, ashes, or other gritty materials?
7. Do the porch steps have a strong handrail?
8. Are the porch steps and walks unobstructed?

A survey is a means to an end, not an end in itself. A follow-up to correct unsafe conditions and practices is the logical corollary to the survey. Through the various media of communication, continuous emphasis must be placed on the importance of corrections if this approach is to yield tangible results.

Objective data may be obtained on injuries and how they occur in the home by providing all households with a form for reporting the time, place, factors involved, and the nature of the injury. These collective data can be highly meaningful in pinpointing where emphasis should be placed in the home safety program. It also will yield some comic relief in the way of oddities associated with accidents in the home.

In a novel approach to the study of accidents in the home, the Kalamazoo, Michigan, health department distributed a safety packet, including a home safety calendar, to more than 7,000 households. Residents were asked to record all home accidents and report them to the health department each month for 4 months. From the collected calendars the health department obtained data on home accidents.

FARM SAFETY

Safety on the farm is a complexity of occupational, home, motor vehicle, and recreational safety. From the standpoint of occupation, 23% of all industrial accident deaths occur in farming. The number of accidental deaths in farming, which is higher than in any other industry, is partially explained by the large number of persons engaged in farming. On a basis of deaths per 100,000 workers, farming ranks third, exceeded only by mining and construction.

State departments of agriculture and federal extension services carry on programs for promoting farm safety. Farm organizations such as the Farmers Union and the Grange also have continuing and special farm safety programs. These programs of action are usually supported by a variety of statewide safety education programs that include farm safety education. The state department of education usually promotes statewide safety education in the schools of the state, and farm safety is included in the program, particularly in the farm areas.

Farm accidents. In 1970 farm residents in the United States suffered 6,700 accidental deaths. Of these, 3,400 were caused by motor vehicle accidents, 2,000 by work accidents, and 1,300 by home accidents. The same year there were 580,000 disabling injuries to farm residents. Of these, 120,000 were caused by motor vehicle accidents, 200,000 by home accidents, 190,000 by work accidents, and 70,000 were listed as public.

Farm life places the agricultural family in a variety of situations with unique problems in safety. Machinery poses a special hazard. U.S. Department of Agriculture studies provide interesting data on farm accidents (Table 11-3). These data can be equated with comparable data for nonfarm people presented by the National Safety Council. These data give an indication of respects in which fatal accidents on farms differ from fatal accidents not on farms and point up where the greatest emphasis should be placed in safety promotion on the farm. The U.S. Bureau of Agricultural Economics presents further information on the location of accidents causing injury to farm residents. It is thus apparent

Table 11-3 ■ Fatalities on farm and comparable nonfarm fatalities*

Cause	Farm (%)	Nonfarm (%)	Cause	Farm (%)	Nonfarm (%)
Machinery	34.1	5.6	Electric current	3.4	3.4
Drowning	15.0	22.3	Lightning	2.5	0.4
Firearms	12.0	3.8	Poisoning	1.7	1.1
Falls	9.1	35.6	Suffocation	1.4	1.0
Blows	5.7	4.7	Other	5.0	17.0
Animals	4.9	0.1	Total	100.0	100.0

*Data for farm accidents are from U.S. Department of Agriculture; nonfarm data are estimates by the National Safety Council.

that accidents pose a special problem for the farm population, calling for more effective action than thus far has been expended.

Home	16%
Barn	22%
Elsewhere on farm	34%
Road or street	11%
Elsewhere or unknown	17%

Prevention of farm accidents. Preventing farm accidents includes the prevention of home accidents as well as the prevention of accidents elsewhere on the farm. A program of prevention must be vested in the farm families through self-direction as an outgrowth of an intensive and extensive program of farm safety education. Correlated with safety education should be a *farm safety survey* that farm families themselves can use profitably.

Farmyard
1. Do farmyard driveways provide a clear vision for automobile drivers and pedestrians who may use them?
2. Are automobiles driven slowly in the farmyard?
3. Is the parking place provided for automobiles one that will promote safety in backing out or in driving away?
4. Are unused lumber and materials piled or properly put away?
5. Are bins, racks, gates, and fences in good repair?
6. Are postholes and other holes properly covered or barricaded?
7. Are highly inflammable materials, sharp objects, and rubbish disposed of properly?

Buildings
1. Are all buildings in good repair?
2. Are stairs and ladders in good condition and free from obstruction?
3. Are all loose boards nailed down?
4. Are slippery floors covered with sand, straw, or other materials to prevent slipping?
5. Do only qualified people climb the silo, windmill, barn, or other high places?
6. Are hayloft and other openings properly covered or barricaded?

7. Is smoking in the hay barn prohibited?
8. Is the hayloft properly ventilated to help prevent combustion?

Equipment, machinery, tools, and supplies
1. Are dangerous tools locked up away from the grasp of children?
2. Are insecticides and other poisons properly locked up?
3. Is gasoline stored separately in a proper tank?
4. Is a definite place assigned for all tools and equipment?
5. Are handles on tools secure?
6. Are children not allowed on farm machinery while the motor is running or while the team is hitched to it?
7. Is the motor shut off when the operator is not in the seat?
8. Are all machines and motors stopped before repairs are attempted?
9. Are all pulleys, hoisting equipment, and parts required to hold heavy loads inspected carefully before being used?
10. Is machinery properly stored and kept in good repair?

Animals
1. Do only qualified people handle livestock?
2. Are dangerous animals properly penned?
3. Is a lead staff always used in handling bulls?
4. Are animals always approached by speaking to them to avoid frightening them?
5. Are children properly instructed in necessary safety measures to avoid being injured by animals?

Combined with the home safety survey, this farm safety survey can be used as the basis for an evaluation of hazards and safety in farm life. All farm families should take the time necessary for safety surveys and should have the wisdom to follow up the survey by correcting the hazardous conditions and practices revealed by safety surveys.

A local committee of key leaders in agriculture leads and coordinates efforts in farm safety. In some communities a farm safety committee under the community safety council coordinates the efforts of organizations and invididuals in farm promotion. More than twenty organizations participate in farm safety on the local level. Agriculture Extension Service, Grange, Farmers Union, Farm Bureau, Future Farmers of America, 4-H clubs, and Future Homemakers are but a few of these. Meetings, campaigns, contests, demonstrations, and studies are the channels through which these organizations operate in safety promotion.

Most states have full- or part-time farm safety specialists. With a professional safety expert working with a farm safety council, statewide programs serve to bolster local efforts as well as to promote special safety programs.

OCCUPATIONAL SAFETY

Industrial safety refers to accident prevention in a branch of trade or production on a wide geographical stage, such as in the steel industry or auto industry. Occupational safety refers to accident prevention within the confines of a single operational unit. It is an intramural program, such as the safety program in a chemical plant. Industrial safety is of value because of the pooling of experience and know-how among the various units within an industry. Yet it is on the local operational level where accidents must be prevented and where a safety program will yield the greatest results.

Of the major safety programs, occupational safety appears to have made the greatest progress in accident prevention. While the enactment of Workman's Compensation Laws beginning in 1912 made safety economically profitable, management has more than a business interest in safety promotion. Management is interested in protecting the lives and health of employees. The effectiveness of safety programs is attested in the drop in the accident frequency rate for companies reporting to the National Safety Council. The lost-time disabling injuries per 1 million man hours of work dropped from 31.87 in 1926 to 5.90 in 1970. This is a remarkable accomplishment, but the record is not yet at a level safety experts regard as acceptable.

Congress passed the 1970 Occupational Safety and Health Act, which makes mandatory the reporting of occupational injuries and illnesses by employers. A new system of uniform reporting and recording will be used. This should result in more complete reporting.

Occupational accidents. Generally speaking, industries with the highest accident frequency rates (disabling injuries per 100,000 work hours) also have the highest severity rates (days lost per 1 million work hours). By their very nature, certain industries such as mining, marine transportation, quarrying, and construction tend to be hazardous. Other industries have a minor degree of hazard. While data for a total industry are of value in a local operation, each plant or place of employment must deal with the hazards it has in its own operation.

In any consideration of occupational accidents it must be pointed out that workers suffer more accidental deaths and injuries off the job than they do on the job. Further, the probability of an injury incurred at work being fatal is only half that for injuries incurred away from work. This is shown in the National Safety Council report for 1970 (Table 11-4). These data speak loudly for the effectiveness of occupational safety programs, but they also raise the question of carry-over from the safety education in industry into the off-job activities of daily living.

Table 11-4 ■ All deaths and injuries of workers, 1970

Place	Deaths	Injuries
At work	14,200	2,200,000
Away from work	42,500	3,200,000
Motor vehicle	26,100	950,000
Public non- motor vehicle	8,600	1,100,000
Home	7,800	1,150,000
Total	56,700	5,400,000

Prevention of occupational accidents. Organization, a planned program, expert direction, and the enlistment of all personnel are the ingredients of an effective accident prevention program in occupations. Usually the program consists of the following eight aspects:

1. Leadership of management
2. Assignment of responsibility
3. Safe working conditions
4. Safety training of all personnel
5. Accident records
6. Analysis of accidents and research in safety measures
7. Employee acceptance of responsibility safety
8. First aid and medical services

Industry has recognized and developed safety experts who are usually designated as safety engineers. This concept could well be applied to other provinces of human activity where accidents play an even more important role than in industry.

SCHOOL SAFETY

For school-age youngsters, accidents loom as a greater threat to life and limb than do diseases. In the age group 5 to 19 years, accidents are the leading cause of death. In a year more than 10,000 American school children lose their lives in accidents.

School accidents. About 43% of accidental deaths among school children are connected with school life. Of these accidents about 6% occur when children are on their way to or from school, about 20% in school buildings, and about 17% on school grounds. Approximately 2 million school youngsters are injured in a year. Reports of the National Safety Council indicate that 20% of these injuries occur at home, 5% when children are on their way to or from school, 28% on the school grounds, 24% in school buildings, and 23% in other places, chiefly in public places. The highest injury rate is among youngsters between the ages of 7 and 12 years. Their vigor and abandon lead to many of their injuries. However, all levels of school-age children have high accident rates.

Prevention of school accidents. Leadership, vision, organization, and teamwork are the ingredients of an effective school safety program. A designed program on paper is excellent as a working blueprint, but action is the key to a safety program. Further, the school safety program is properly regarded as one facet of the total community safety program. The school driver education-training program has long been accepted as a part of the community safety program, but it must be recognized that the overall school safety program, in the same light, is also a phase of community safety promotion.

A safety council composed of students and faculty is the guiding force of a school safety program. A school safety patrol can have subdivisions such as traffic patrol, building and grounds patrol, and a fire patrol. Student participation under teacher guidance is the working pattern.

Surveys of conditions and practices affecting safety in the school environment point up hazards and indicate preventive measures that must be taken. These surveys properly include conditions and practices going to and from home.

A system for reporting accidents is of legal significance as well as of preventive value. This is particularly true when a systematic investigation and follow-up is tied in with the reporting system.

Safety education as an integral phase of health education has been effective in the creation of safety attitudes and the establishment of safe practices. It is in the early formative years of life that safety attitudes are most readily acquired.

Schools can prevent accidental deaths and injuries among students and faculty, but a systematic, vigorous, and sustained program is necessary.

RECREATIONAL SAFETY

Safe adventure has long been the theme of recreational safety. It would be unrealistic to restrain recreation for the purpose of preventing all accidents. It would be equally unrealistic to think that recreation could be accident-free, but past experience has demonstrated that recreation can continue to expand and safety promotion can go hand in hand with this expansion.

Accidents in recreation. Each year about 22,000 Americans lose their lives in recreational activities. As there has been a yearly increase in recreational activities, the yearly death toll in recreation has tended to increase accordingly. Yet when considered in terms of the increased number of participants in recreation, the rate of fatal accidents has declined. Not all of these deaths are strictly chargeable to recreation. Flying and railway fatalities can occur in commercial travel as well as in recreational travel. However, statistical breakdown in these categories would be difficult.

Most of the people who lose their lives in accidents in recreation are in the prime of life. This is particularly true in water accidents, boating, accidents with firearms, and flying.

Prevention of accidents in recreation. In 1959 the National Safety Council created a Public Safety Department that includes sections on Recreational Boating and Water Safety, Gun Safety, and General Aviation Safety. These sections, or committees, serve in the role of program planning for national and state groups conducting public safety activities. The program includes fact finding and research, exchange of information, standards or recommendations, technical assistance, training, program aids, and measurement of performance.

On the community level we find that organized, supervised recreation is usually safe recreation. Trained personnel, definite responsibilities, established regulations, regular supervision, safety surveys, and safety education have produced results. It is in unsupervised recreation that action is most needed, and here the primary approach is safety education. However, this is not a simple matter because education in the safe use of firearms does not carry over into safe conduct in swimming or boating.

Part of the safety education in recreation is provided by such organizations as rifle clubs, boating clubs, and camping and sportsman clubs. The Red Cross, Boy Scouts, Girl Scouts, Y.M.C.A., and similar organizations have contributed greatly to the promotion of safety education for recreation. Despite these efforts, safety education for recreational needs is inadequate on all levels. Yet to conduct an organized community program of safety education in this sphere of activity is a difficult assignment. The individual efforts of all agencies and individuals promoting safety education in other activities make an indirect contribution to recreational safety.

Regulations governing recreational activities have a considerable effect on the promotion of safety. This is particularly true of regulations designed to prevent the inexperienced from participating in activities for which they are not prepared or qualified. It is the inexperienced or unskillful recreationist who is most likely to be involved in accidents. It is the reckless person who is most likely to involve others in accidents.

Each community can survey the recreational safety needs of its people and formulate a program accordingly. The cooperation of all groups sponsoring recreational activities or programs will add assurance for the success of the safety program. Recreational safety promotion should be coordinated with other safety programs in the community.

COMMUNITY SAFETY PROGRAM

The promotion of community safety poses a unique problem because safety in a community is the province of many organizations and individuals. Organizations involved in community safety include the health department, fire department, police department, recreation department, schools, industry, chamber of commerce, service clubs, civil defense, medical profession, and news media. The need is to integrate the contributions of all agencies into one unified, effective community safety program.

Organization. The community health department is the most logical agency to bring together the various forces that play upon the problem of accident prevention in the community. While the official health department can be the crystallizing catalyst in the reaction, a basic ingredient is a community safety council with representation from the various groups that have a contribution to make to safety and that have a dynamic interest in safety. This voluntary, nonofficial body is at one and the same time a sounding board, a source of information, an expression of community thinking, and a supporter of the various safety programs operating within the community.

Community safety promotion. Each agency will continue its ongoing program, expanding as conditions and the council indicate. Unnecessary duplication can be eliminated, but it should be recognized that certain duplication is highly desirable. Unmet needs will be recognized, and an underst•nding will be reached on which agency will deal with a recognized need.

A *poison control center* is a valuable segment of the community safety program. It is the place where people can call for help in case of poisoning—accidental or intentional. Properly a center is open 24 hours of the day and is manned by a person who knows how to use the standard references on poisons and recommended countermeasures. He needs to know both the physiology and pathology involved. In small communities a hospital is the logical location for such a center. In larger communities a poison control center may be located elsewhere.

Surveys of safety are sponsored by safety councils or may be initiated by member organizations. The essential factor is to discover where hazards exist in the community. Once hazards are located, measures can be initiated to reduce or even eliminate them.

Safety education is a province of all agencies concerned with safety in the community, but safety education must be coordinated and integrated to be extensive enough to be fully effective. Safety consciousness in a community can be developed but it takes a lot of

doing. This is a continuous job, as are all aspects of community safety promotion.

QUESTIONS AND EXERCISES

1. Evaluate this statement: "Even if all accidental deaths could be eliminated, the promotion of safety would be essential to the health of the nation."
2. If you were to study the epidemiology of accidents in your community, what factors would receive your attention?
3. A certain community (M) has a much better safety program than another community (N), yet community M has a higher accident rate, a higher accidental death rate, and a higher injury rate per 100,000 population. What factors would account for this paradox?
4. The accidental death rate in the United States has declined since the turn of the century, yet accidents as a cause of death now rank fourth. In 1900, accidents ranked seventh. How do you explain this apparent contradiction?
5. How is your state highway safety program organized and administered?
6. Make proposals to improve your state highway safety program.
7. Why is the state industrial safety program generally more effective than the state traffic safety program?
8. On the state level, who has responsibility for the promotion of home safety in your state?
9. What agencies in your state promote farm safety on a statewide basis?
10. Why have the people of the United States failed to go all out in halting the slaughter on our highways?
11. Make some proposal for eliminating the unsafe driver.
12. If a car travelling 55 miles per hour crashes into a fixed concrete abutment, with how much force will a person of 160 pounds be thrown forward? Use the equation $MV = Ft$, in which M = mass, V = velocity, F = force, and t = time (1 second).
13. Set up an organizational chart for a model motor vehicle safety program for some community.
14. Design a model community home safety program.
15. Who in your county is engaged in the promotion of farm safety?
16. Evaluate the safety record and safety program of one of the industrial firms in your community or in some other community.
17. How effectively have the schools of your community taken advantage of their opportunity to promote safety, particularly safety education?
18. What are some obstacles to the promotion of recreational safety?
19. If you were to set up a safety council for your community, who would be on the council and what

would be the specific provinces of the council's program?

20. What is the greatest safety need in your community?

REFERENCES

American Public Health Association: Accident control in environmental health programs, New York, 1966, The Association.

Bergner, L.: Falls from heights: a childhood epidemic in an urban area, American Journal of Public Health **61**:90, 1971.

Blumenthal, M.: Traffic safety research review, National Safety Council **12**(1):1968.

Chisholm, J. J.: Lead poisoning, Scientific American **224**:15, February, 1971.

Collins, J. C., and Morris, J. L.: Highway collision analysis, Springfield, Ill., 1967, Charles C Thomas, Publisher.

Florio, A. E., and Stafford, G. T.: Safety education, ed. 3, New York, 1969, McGraw-Hill Book Co.

Greenshields, B. D., and associates: Development of a method of predicting high accident and high viola-tion drivers, Journal of Applied Psychology **51**:205, 1967.

Haddon, W.: A logical framework for categorizing highway safety phenomena and activity, Journal of Trauma **12**(3):193-207, 1972.

Hirschfeld, A. H., and associates: The accident process: an overview, Journal of Rehabilitation **33**:27, 1967.

Iskraut, A. P.: The epidemiological approach to accident causation, American Journal of Public Health **57**:1708, 1967.

Kraus, H.: Prevention of low back pain, Journal of Occupational Medicine **9**:578, 1967.

Luchterhand, E., and Sydiaha, D.: Choice in human affairs: an application to aging-accident-illness problems, New Haven, Conn., 1967, College & University Press.

National Safety Council: Accident facts, Chicago, annual, The Council.

Seaton, D. C., and associates: Administration and supervision of safety, New York, 1968, The Macmillan Co.

Stack, H. L., and Elkow, J. D.: Education for safe living, ed. 4, Englewood Cliffs, N.J., 1966, Prentice-Hall, Inc.

12 ▪ COMPULSIVE BEHAVIORS

*Today's American citizen lives in
a drug using culture.*

Anonymous

Four habits will be considered in this chapter—alcoholism, cigarette smoking, obesity, and drug addiction. All share a compulsive and dependent component in behavior and result in major increases in mortality, morbidity, and social pathology in the community.

ALCOHOLISM

Alcohol is the second most important known cause of mortality and morbidity in this country, second only to tobacco. Epidemiological, clinical, and laboratory evidence have made it clear that cirrhosis of the liver in the United States is caused primarily by alcohol consumption. However, cirrhosis is only one in the impressive list of diseases associated with alcohol. These include acute and chronic intoxication; toxic psychoses; gastritis; pancreatitis; cardiomyopathy; peripheral neuropathy; automobile, home, and occupational accidents; suicide; homicide; injuries; and cancer of the mouth, pharynx, larynx, esophagus, and liver. Alcohol contributes to ill health, crime, poverty, broken homes, divorce, social conflicts, loss of earning power, social degradation, and other social pathology.

Alcohol is undoubtedly the most abused drug in the United States today. Four to 6 million Americans have been diagnosed as alcoholics, and another 5 million are believed to have a serious drinking problem. The Science News Letter in 1971 estimated that 50% of traffic fatalities were alcohol related. Employees suffering from alcoholism are estimated to cost the nation 10 billion dollars in lost productivity costs.

Cirrhosis of the liver was the seventh leading cause of death in the United States in 1974 with 33,319 deaths, compared with 32,132 for breast cancer. Cirrhosis is very prevalent in both sexes and all races, but the rates are higher in males and blacks.

Low socioeconomic groups have a higher prevalence of cirrhosis than do high socioeconomic groups. There is a relationship to occupation—those involved in handling alcohol show increased rates of hepatic cirrhosis. Mortality from hepatic disease drops suddenly if alcohol is removed from the community.

Prevention of alcoholism may again be considered under intervention at agent, host, and environment levels. Alcohol is an anesthetic and is toxic in overdose. The healthy adult liver can oxidize about ¼ ounce of absolute alcohol per hour. The alcohol content is half the proofage, so ¼ ounce is equal to 0.6 ounce of 86% proof alcohol. The absorption of alcohol into the bloodstream is delayed by food in the stomach, thus peak blood levels are not reached so quickly after eating. It is alleged that there is a safe level of drinking in terms of dosage and that 45 ml/day of absolute alcohol may not harm the liver if the alcohol is taken diluted and is spread throughout the day. This is equivalent to 3½ ounces of 86% proof alcohol daily. The effects of alcohol are strictly dose related, regardless of the form (whisky, wine,

Table 12-1 ■ Hepatitic cirrhosis mortality rates

Higher	Lower
Males	Females
Blacks	Whites
Low socioeconomic status	High socioeconomic status
Occupation, handling alcohol	All other occupations
Residents in areas where alcohol is available	Residents in "dry" areas or "dry" times

beer, etc.) in which the alcohol is taken. It does not seem possible to detoxify alcohol, and dosage must be regulated.

Altering behavior of the host is the most popular way of intervening, and exhortation, coupled with deprivation, is usually tried. Group therapy using behavioral modification technics is most likely to succeed, and Alcoholics Anonymous is the leading exponent of this approach. Counselors are frequently former alcoholics, who are better able to appreciate the difficulties of abstinence than are those who have never overcome such a problem. A nonjudgmental, supportive, understanding relationship must be established. Medical treatment employing aversion therapy using disulfiram (Antabuse) is most effective. However, this therapy must be restricted to the motivated alcoholic and used in conjunction with the supportive group therapy described.

Most medical treatment merely results in rendering the alcoholic fit enough to resume drinking. Survivorship in cirrhosis depends on cessation of alcohol consumption. If, in the alcoholic, consumption persists, all medical and surgical measures are to no avail.

It is essential that the alcoholic, during a period of remission, understand that if he or she resumes drinking death will result. All social networks to help alcoholics, such as Alcoholics Anonymous and the support of family and friends, should be employed.

Altering the environment is the most effective way of reducing alcoholism in the community. Education should be used to inform people of the dangers of alcohol, and all negative education, for example, advertising of alcohol, should be banned in all media. Social ambience must be altered so that alcohol is not regarded as a reward, as a status symbol, or as something that is glamorous. The cost of alcohol should be greatly increased by taxation, so that a significant part of discretionary income must be expended to buy alcohol, and competing needs considered. There is an excellent correlation between a low relative price, high consumption, and high cirrhotic mortality in international comparisons (Popham, Schmidt, and Lint). France has the highest cirrhotic death rate, over twelve times that in Britain. Alcohol costs 3.6 times as much in Britain, and only 31% as much is consumed in Britain as in France. The level of acceptance of drinking in a society also positively correlates with cirrhotic death rates. Community values are thus reflected in community health.

CIGARETTE SMOKING

Cigarette smoking is the greatest community health hazard, a self-imposed risk. Mortality and morbidity is greatly increased in smokers versus nonsmokers, especially in respiratory and cardiovascular diseases.

Although cigarette smokers suffer the highest relative risk with respect to the cancers listed in Fig. 12-2, the community impact of smoking is greatest in cardiovascular disease because the latter is so prevalent.

Cigarette smoking accounts for 19% of

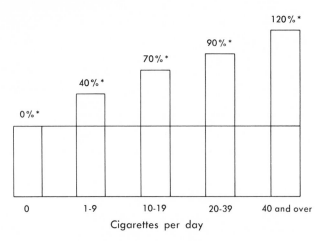

Fig. 12-1. Daily cigarette consumption and death rates. Asterisk indicates percent increase in death rates from all causes. Note dose/response effect. (From *Progress against cancer* 1970, a report by the National Advisory Cancer Council, p. 40)

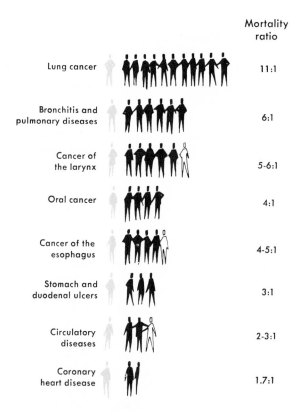

Fig. 12-2. Mortality ratio of smokers to nonsmokers for several diseases. A mortality ratio of 11:1 means that the death rate for smokers is eleven times that for nonsmokers. (From *Progress against cancer* 1970, a report by the National Advisory Cancer Council, p. 41)

cancers among all persons and 32% among males. Selected sites, where the attributable risk (AR) caused by smoking is high, are listed in descending order of incidence in Table 12-2.

Attributable risk is the percentage of total cases that can be ascribed to the particular risk factor, in this case cigarette smoking. It is computed by using the relative risk of smokers and the prevalence of smoking in the community.

Although the trend in smoking has been upward in the past 25 years, from 1965 to 1971 there was a sharp decline, presumably resulting from the impact of education anti-smoking campaigns. In 1965 43% of the total adult population was smoking, whereas in 1975 this had fallen to 34%, 39% among males and 29% among females (Adult Use of Tobacco 1975, Department of Health, Education and Welfare).

Cigarette smoking is a social class habit. It is also a city dwellers' habit. Cigarette smoking began and first spread in cities. The cities have remained ahead of the rest of the country both in the numbers of smokers and in the average number of cigarettes smoked each day. Studies in this country have shown that the prevalence of cigarette smoking increases as the socioeconomic

status (SES) decreases. The habit starts at an earlier age the lower the socioeconomic status.

Although women used to feel safe from lung cancer because their death rate was low compared with that for men, this picture is beginning to change alarmingly. The female lung cancer death rate has doubled in the past 10 years. Female death rates from lung cancer are now 25% of the death rate for men and are increasing more rapidly.

The recent upsurge in the lung cancer death rate for women can be attributed to the fact that women began to smoke in much greater numbers about 30 years ago and the trend has increased since then, possibly as a result of advertising.

Smoking habits are established in the teens, and in the great majority of cases, teenage female smokers will become adult female smokers. Teenage girls, who never smoked to the extent that teen-age boys did, have now caught up. In 1968 only about half as many teen-age girls smoked as boys. But, by 1974 15.3% of girls between ages 12 and 18 years were smoking, only slightly less than the boys' 15.8%. This means that in about another 10 years there should be as many adult female smokers as there are adult

Table 12-2 ■ Sites of high attributable risk of cancer from cigarette smoking

Site	Attributable risk (smoking)	Number of cases* (incidence)	Number of deaths* (mortality)
Lung	85%	98,000	89,000
Bladder	52%	29,900	9,800
Pancreas	48%	21,800	11,800
Buccal cavity	67%	17,300	4,650
Larynx	82%	9,200	3,350
Esophagus	76%	7,600	6,900
Pharynx	86%	6,600	3,800

From American Cancer Society: CA—A Cancer Journal for Clinicians **27**(1):34-35, January/February, 1977.

*Estimates for 1977—American Cancer Society.

male smokers, with a commensurate increase in lung cancer deaths for women.

Smoking parents set the example for children. Studies show that youngsters whose parents smoke are more likely to adopt the habit than are children of nonsmoking parents.

Women seem to find smoking more difficult to give up. Of women smoking in 1966, 25% had quit by 1970. Men, in the same period, had a quitting rate of 39%. One woman in nine who was an exsmoker in 1966 had returned to the habit by 1970.

The rise in the number of women smokers has not been lost to the attention of cigarette manufacturers, who have stepped up advertising campaigns for new brands of cigarettes designed expressly for women.

Prevention of smoking. Reducing the toxicity of the agent is possible. Most American adults who continue to smoke are smoking cigarettes with lower tar and nicotine levels. In 1975 only 20% of smokers said they used cigarettes with 20 mg or more of tar, down from 55% in 1970. The proportion of persons smoking cigarettes with nicotine levels of 1.4 mg and above declined from 45% to 18% (Adult Use of Tobacco 1975, Department of Health, Education and Welfare). Dosage can be reduced by smoking fewer cigarettes, inhaling less, leaving a longer stub, taking fewer puffs from each cigarette, and taking the cigarette out of the mouth between puffs.

Education. Communities can mount antismoking campaigns, and local groups can reinforce national leadership on this issue. People must be made aware of the hazards of cigarette smoking. This awareness results in (1) individuals being motivated to quit smoking, and (2) smoking becoming less socially acceptable. This is very important in the young. Advertising presently directed at youth establishes that smoking is socially acceptable and desirable.

In the young, it is also necessary to negate peer influence. Risk taking is part of peer group culture. During the socialization process, nonsmoking must be instilled. Role models—persons teenagers admire—may prove effective. The difficulty is that not smoking is a "nonaction" and not a dynamic force, thus associations cannot be made with hero figures. Smoking may also be a symbol of independence and rebellion to teenagers against the norms of the family or group to which they belong.

OBESITY

Obesity is very common in the United States, where it is estimated that 25 million persons are overweight and 7 million are 20% above optimal weight.

Overweight infants become obese adults (Charney and associates, 1976); and during adolescence they are obese children. Prevention must begin early, before learned patterns of overeating are established. Obesity is associated with increased rates of coronary heart disease, diabetes, hypertension, stroke, and accidents, and the combined toll on community health is very large.

Obese people can change their learned habitual patterns of overeating in response to a behavioral approach to weight management. This involves unlearning or modifying old behaviors and substituting them with new. People must value the outcome (that is, weight loss) that they believe will result from these new behaviors. The popular image of the ideal figure must stress being slim. Exercise is most important in weight control and good health, and communities can provide exercise programs and facilities.

"HARD" DRUGS AND PILLS

In the United States as recently as the close of World War II, the term "problem drugs" generally meant only morphine or its derivative, heroin. This limited concept of problem drugs has now been expanded to a point where morphine represents one of the lesser drug problems. As more and more people become dependent on drugs, there has arisen an alarming abuse of stimulants, depressants, hallucinogens, and narcotics, cutting across all social strata.

To say that we are a "pill happy" society

is not an exaggeration, and reliance on pills is the genesis of much drug abuse.

Drugs can be variously classified, but four classes are recognized: narcotics, stimulants, hallucinogens, and depressants. These are based on the effects produced.

Drug abuse is a complex social and health problem. Its solution must come through education and social change, not punishment. Perhaps there is a place for a "crash" program based on education, but the problem of drug abuse calls for a long-term, continuing program of education and social change.

Addiction and habituation

Drug addiction is a psychosomatic entity in which a derangement of cellular metabolism occurs causing a physiological alteration and having psychological effects. The altered state of the body tissue produces a physical dependence that becomes known only after discontinuation of the drug. This dependence is masked while the drug is being taken.

Physical effects of dependence exhibited on withdrawal include body aches, hot flashes, fever, perspiration, nausea, nasal discharge, muscle cramps, body jerks, tremors, and irritability. All of these effects produce anxiety, restlessness, and insecurity. The drug is sought to obtain relief from the distress. Thus a drug can be a danger to the individual and to the community if it produces drug dependence that can result in impaired judgment, physical damage, and psychotic reactions. Morphine, heroin, and alcohol produce physical and psychological dependence.

The National Commission on Marihuana and Drug Abuse has divided the entire spectrum of drug-using behavior into the following five patterns:

1. Experimental. The most common type of drug-using behavior—a short, non-patterned trial of one or more drugs, motivated primarily by curiosity or desire to experience an altered mood state

2. Recreational. Voluntary or patterned use of a drug, usually in social settings; behavior is not sustained by virtue of the dependence of the user on the drug

3. Circumstantial. Behavior generally motivated by the user's perceived need or desire to achieve a new and anticipated effect in order to cope with a specific problem or situation (for example, students preparing for examinations; long-distance truckers)

4. Intensified drug-using behavior. Drug use that occurs at least daily and is motivated by an individual's problem or stressful situation or a desire to maintain a certain self-prescribed level of performance (for example, housewives who regularly consume barbiturates or other sedatives, business executives who regularly consume tranquilizers, youths who have turned to drugs as sources of excitement or meaning); the salient feature of this group is that the individual still remains integrated within the larger social and economic structure

5. Compulsive use. Patterned behavior at a high frequency and high level of interest, characterized by a high degree of psychological dependence and perhaps physical dependence as well. This category encompasses the smallest number of drug users. The distinguishing feature of this behavior is that drug use dominates the individual's existence, and preoccupation with drug-taking precludes other social functioning (for example, chronic alcoholics, heroin-dependent persons)

Personality and its relation to drug misuse and abuse is difficult to categorize because one can identify a wide spectrum of personalities misusing and abusing alcohol and, to some degree, morphine and heroin. The misuse of marijuana and LSD involves unique social behavior; perhaps some degree of personality identity is discernible.

While a vast range of personality structure may be found among drug addicts, it

Table 12-3 ■ List of drugs—medical uses, symptoms produced, and their dependency

Name	Slang name	Chemical or trade name	Classification	Medical use
Heroin	H, horse, scat, junk, smack, scag, stuff, Harry	Diacetyl-morphine	Narcotic	Pain relief
Morphine	White stuff, M	Morphine sulfate	Narcotic	Pain relief
Codeine	Schoolboy	Methylmorphine	Narcotic	Ease pain and coughing
Methadone	Dolly	Dolophine Amidon	Narcotic	Pain relief
Cocaine	Corrine, gold dust, coke, Bernice, flake, star dust, snow	Methylester of benzoyl ecgonine	Stimulant, local anesthesic	Local anesthesic
Marijuana	Pot, grass, tea, gage, reefers	*Cannabis sativa*	Relaxant, euphoriant in high doses, hallucinogen	None in U.S.
Barbiturates	Barbs, blue devils, yellow jackets, phennies, peanuts, blue heavens	Phenobarbital, Nembutal, Seconal, Amytal	Sedative-hypnotic	Sedative, relieve high blood pressure, epilepsy, hyperthyroidism
Amphetamines	Bennies, dexies, speed, wake-ups, lid poppers, hearts, pep pills	Benzedrine, Dexedrine, Desoxyn, Methamphetamine, Methedrine	Sympathomimetic	Relieve mild depression, control appetite and narcolepsy
LSD	Acid, sugar, big D, cubes, trips	d-Lysergic acid diethylamide	Hallucinogen	Experimental study of mental function, alcoholism
DMT	AMT, businessman's high	N,N-Dimethyl-tryptamine	Hallucinogen	None
Mescaline	Mesc	3,4,5-Trimeth-oxyphenethylamine	Hallucinogen	None
Psilocybin		3-[2-(dimethylamino) ethyl]indol-4-ol dihydrogen phosphate	Hallucinogen	None
Alcohol	Booze, juice, etc.	Ethanol, ethyl alcohol	Sedative-hypnotic	Solvent, antiseptic
Tobacco	Fag, coffin nail, etc.	*Nicotinia tabacum*	Stimulant-sedative	Sedative, emetic (nicotine)

From Ray, O. S.: Drugs, society, and human behavior, St. Louis, 1974, The C. V. Mosby Co. Adapted from Natio
*Question marks indicate conflicts of opinion.

How taken	Usual dose	Effects sought	Long-term symptoms	Physical dependence potential	Mental dependence potential
Injected or sniffed	Varies	Euphoria, prevent withdrawal discomfort (4 hr)	Addiction, constipation, loss of appetite	Yes	Yes
Swallowed or injected	15 milligrams	Euphoria, prevent withdrawal discomfort (6 hr)	Addiction, constipation, loss of appetite	Yes	Yes
Swallowed	30 milligrams	Euphoria, prevent withdrawal discomfort (4 hr)	Addiction, constipation, loss of appetite	Yes	Yes
Swallowed or injected	10 milligrams	Prevent withdrawal discomfort (4 to 6 hr)	Addiction, constipation, loss of appetite	Yes	Yes
Sniffed, injected, or swallowed	Varies	Excitation, talkativeness (varies, short)	Depression, convulsions	No	Yes
Smoked, swallowed, or sniffed	1 to 2 cigarettes	Relaxation, increased euphoria, perceptions, sociability (4 hr)	Usually none	No	Yes?
Swallowed or injected	50 to 100 milligrams	Anxiety reduction, euphoria (4 hr)	Addiction with severe withdrawal symptoms, possible convulsions, toxic psychosis	Yes	Yes
Swallowed or injected	2.5 to 5 milligrams	Alertness, activeness (4 hr)	Loss of appetite, delusions, hallucinations, toxic psychosis	Yes?	Yes
Swallowed	100 to 500 micrograms	Insightful experiences, exhilaration, distortion of senses (10 hr)	May intensify existing psychosis, panic reactions	No	No?
Injected	60 to 70 milligrams	Insightful experiences, exhilaration, distortion of senses (less than 1 hr)	?	No	No?
Swallowed	350 milligrams	Insightful experiences, exhilaration, disortion of senses (12 hr)	?	No	No?
Swallowed	25 milligrams	Insightful experiences, exhilaration, distortion of senses (6 to 8 hr)	?	No	No?
Swallowed	Varies	Sense alteration, anxiety reduction, sociability (1 to 4 hr)	Cirrhosis, toxic psychosis, neurologic damage, addiction	Yes	Yes
Smoked, sniffed, chewed	Varies	Calmness, sociability (time varies)	Emphysema, lung cancer, mouth and throat cancer, cardiovascular damage, loss of appetite	Yes?	Yes

stitute of Mental Health: Resource book for drug abuse education, October, 1969, pp. 34-35.

is possible to identify certain personality traits that indicate persons more likely than others to resort to drugs. For example, the psychopathic personality type of individual uses drugs to gain a certain mental state or emotional thrill, while the neurotic person turns to drugs to relieve tensions and anxieties. A person who is psychopathic will seek to suppress delusions or relieve depression through drugs. Morphine users seek to escape from or avoid situations that they find distressing. Alcoholic persons may have been depressed, hostile, dependent, or otherwise socially inadequate, to their own way of thinking.

In any consideration of the relationship of personality to drug use is the social environment in which persons find themselves. Social conditioning is extremely important, especially when chance, accessibility, and curiosity combine with a social background weak in personal responsibility and community standards of self-esteem.

Habituation has the connotation of the customary use of a practice of one kind or another that a person finds pleasurable, either as relaxation or activation. Habituation to a drug means that the drug has not produced a physical or psychological dependence because the individual can easily terminate the use of the drug without discernible side effects. Habituation to coffee, tea, and cola drinks is widespread in the United States, but no evidence exists that addiction occurs.

Heroin addiction and social pathology

In the United States the heroin addiction problem is actually not as great as that of several other drug problems such as alcoholism and the use of hallucinogens and depressants. The Bureau of Narcotics and Dangerous Drugs estimates 515,000 heroin users in the United States. This figure is extrapolated from the number of reported deaths from heroin overdoses. More than half of known addicts live in four cities— New York City, Washington, D.C., Chicago, and Los Angeles. By states, the concentra-

tion is heavy in three states—New York, 48.3%; Illinois, 14.6%; and California, 14%.

That addiction to heroin or morphine is a phenomenon predominantly of early adulthood is revealed by the age distribution of known addicts.

Age (years)	Percentage
17 and under	0.2
18 to 20	3.1
21 to 30	47.4
31 to 40	38.1
Over 40	11.2

While studies show that young adults constitute a disproportionate part of the addict population, it has been difficult to identify a particular personality vulnerability or pattern. While some addicts are dullards, many are above normal in intelligence. Some are loafers, some are hard workers.

People who become addicted generally tend to be noncompetitive people who prefer to avoid difficulties rather than face them. They tend to be people who will look for the easiest, least painful solution to their problems. It is true that most people who become addicted had personality problems, but most people with the same problems do not turn to narcotics as a solution.

It takes three things to produce an addict —a poorly adjusted person, an available drug, and the means for bringing the person and drug together. Usually bringing the person and drug together is neither premeditated nor planned but sheerly accidental. Associates usually introduce the drug to the person.

Blighted areas in the large cities are the breeding grounds for narcotics addiction. Where social and economic deprivation exists, drug addiction flourishes. Before World War II a high proportion of addicts was among the foreign-born and first generation of Americans with parents of European ancestry. Today, blacks have replaced the foreign-born and account for a disproportionately high percentage of drug addiction.

Boys and girls with a delinquent orientation toward life are most likely to experiment with drugs. Juveniles are prime targets for addiction when they come from homes in which there exists hostility, divorce, separation, personality clashes, low ambitions, distrust, or little opportunity for identity. Association with a delinquent group can then lead the way to drug addiction.

The mere fact of narcotics addiction does not turn addicts into criminals unless they find it necessary to commit crime to obtain drugs. Addicts are usually arrested for possession or selling drugs, not for using drugs.

An infectious disease model of drug abuse

If drug abuse is seen as a practice that is transmitted from one person to another, it may be considered for operational purposes as a contagious illness. This approach makes it possible to apply to its study the methods and terminology used in the epidemiology of infectious disease.

In the epidemiological model the infectious agent is heroin, the host and reservoir are both man, and the vector is the drug-using peer. The conventional notion of the "pusher" as the vector is effectively dispelled by a careful review of those studies in which an effort was made to trace the spread of heroin use from person to person. In these studies it is clear that, in the vast majority of instances, an addict was introduced to the use of heroin by a well-meaning friend, usually in the setting of previously established peer group activity. Beginners must learn advanced intravenous injection techniques from other addicts.

The disease presents all the well-known characteristics of epidemics, including rapid spread, clear geographic bounds, and certain age groups and strata of the population being more affected than others.

Treatment of addiction. The physician may not legally dispense heroin to an addict without attempting to cure the addict. This usually means treating the addict in a hospital or referring him or her to a facility where effective treatment can be received. The Public Health Service hospitals for narcotics addicts at Lexington, Kentucky, and Fort Worth, Texas, have accommodations for 1,800 patients. Voluntary patients compose about half the hospital population and pay a nominal fee if they are financially able. While treatment has been excellent, there have been difficulties in providing posthospital care and rehabilitation service. As a replacement for the federal hospitals, subsidies would support state and community centers that can provide local posthospital care and rehabilitation service.

State and community centers have been established to provide care for narcotics. New York City and Los Angeles have such centers, through which highly effective programs have been developed. Physicians, psychologists, nurses, social workers, and other personnel work out effective treatment and posthospital programs to fit the needs and situation of each specific patient. This can be duplicated in the moderate sized communities of the nation. Certainly, every state should provide a complete narcotics control and treatment program.

Drugs are now available to help the narcotics addict through the withdrawal phase. The drugs used temporarily replace heroin and can be withdrawn gradually without the physiological distress created by withdrawing heroin. However, successful treatment requires further psychological, sociological, and personal supervision in the hospital, the home, and the community. A guidance center is not adequate. Posthospital care must go with patients, especially if they go back to their old environment.

The methadone maintenance approach is the most widely used treatment for heroin addiction. Methadone, a synthetic substitute for heroin, can be made available legally. It is administered in a fluid, and heroin addicts stop at the treatment center only long enough to take the drink containing methadone. It appears that methadone induces a cross-tolerance to heroin so there is no craving for heroin. Because methadone treatment in fact substitutes methadone addiction for heroin addiction the treatment leaves something to be desired, but until something better is developed methadone programs are valuable, being used on an ambulatory basis is a community.

In California any addicted person may voluntarily seek treatment in the California Rehabilitation Center, a hospital to which an addict may also be committed by a court. All admissions must stay at least 6 months. On release some patients may be transferred to a halfway house to prepare for entrance to the outside world. Patients are released on parole from the hospital and remain on parole until they have remained drug-free for at least 3 consecutive years.

To deal in the community with the narcotics addict, Great Britain decrees that a physician may administer drugs to an addict if withdrawal would be harmful to the patient or if he or she would not be capable of continuing a normal, useful life without the drug. This removes the profit incentive from illicit drug sales. Responsibility for the control of the addicts rests with their physicians, and the plan has been highly successful. This program might well be tried in America, but it must be recognized that conditions in the United States differ from conditions in Britain, and modifications of the plan would doubtless be necessary.

Prevention of heroin addiction. Legal control of heroin traffic is essential at all times. The federal Harrison Narcotic Act and its enforcement by the Bureau of Narcotics has been effective in control, although the law does have some deficiencies. On the local level, communities generally have

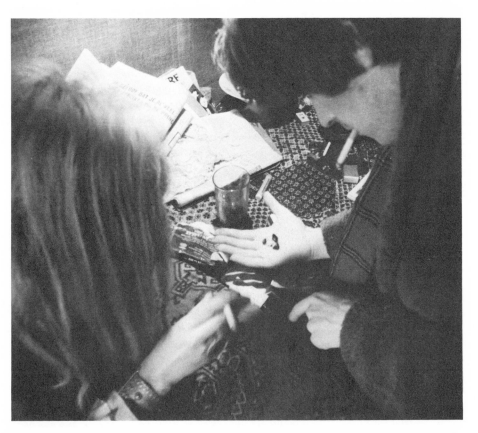

Fig. 12-3. Drug addiction (Netherlands). Hippies in a drug tryst. Some take drugs for the mind-altering effects, others to symbolize their membership in a special group. (Courtesy World Health Organization)

not carried their end of the program to control narcotics.

Upgrading of social conditions that spawn drug addiction is the great preventive. Better housing, better neighborhoods, better recreation and jobs, participation in community affairs, better health promotion, and respect for every human being are the foundations on which rests the prevention of narcotics addiction. Education to supplement and complement social and economic development completes the foundation of any community program to prevent heroin addiction.

Abuse of other drugs

The mounting menace of drug abuse is alarming. More and more Americans are becoming dependent on drugs, either for thrills, to relieve tensions, or for escape. Americans take pills for all conceivable purposes. There exists a general instability as an aftermath of a series of major wars, yet most people living in the world do not resort to drugs.

Rebellion, boredom, curiosity, seeking new experiences, fun, kicks, pressures, feelings of being trapped, rejection of society, the impersonal nature of our complex society, peer group conformity, revolt against the older population that has created the present state of the world, depression, escape, quest for identity—the possible reasons why people take drugs are almost endless. Heavy users of drugs are frequently people with inner conflicts who rarely look to external experiences or what is happening about them. They seek change in their inner thoughts to relieve pain they feel or to obtain a more pleasing mental state. Many are psychotics, and a greater number are neurotics.

Marijuana. Marijuana, a hallucinogen, is obtained from the dried flowering tops of the pistillate (female) plant *Cannabis sativa.* The plant grows in all of the fifty states. In America the dried, crushed leaves and flowering top are smoked as a cigarette. Some smokers develop a certain psychological dependency on marijuana, but there is no hangover.

Marijuana is neither as good nor as bad as has been claimed. The federal marijuana law is far too severe in terms of the drug's danger. State laws against use generally are also too severe. The sale of marijuana should be the focus of the law, and penalties imposed for trafficking in the drug should receive more attention.

Lysergic acid diethylamide (LSD). More than a quarter of a million people in the United States have taken LSD. In its pure form the drug cannot be distinguished from water, being tasteless and odorless. It can be transported via sugar cubes, liquor, gum, and virtually any food.

LSD is dangerous. It produces hallucinations, delusions, distortions, anxieties, and even psychoses. Under the influence of LSD, some users take their own lives, and some take the lives of others. The drug can produce damage to the brain, to bone marrow, and to chromosomes. The consequences of chromosome damage can be awesome in terms of genetic and other effects that are the concern of the community and its present and future welfare.

Many who experiment with LSD could be classed as normal individuals. Fortunately for these people, one "trip" may not cause permanent damage, although the danger is always present. Repeat trips insidiously produce long-term deleterious effects.

Prevention of LSD use must be directed toward education of the public and the prevention and correction of conditions that lead a person to turn to LSD as an escape from the present environment.

Barbiturates. Americans consume more than 3 billion sleeping pills in a year. Most of these are barbiturates in some form and are used for producing sleep or for purposes of sedation. Barbiturates have been beneficial to man when properly used. It is in the indiscriminate misuse of barbiturates that the problem lies, and the extent of barbiturate addiction may be exceeded only by alcohol addiction.

The person intoxicated with barbiturates is drowsy, confused, depressed, morose, irritable, and quarrelsome. Withdrawal results in severe physiological disturbances and may be fatal. The drug should be withdrawn only under medical supervision.

While some people deliberately take an overdose of barbiturates, some deaths regarded as suicides resulting from an overdose of sleeping pills are accidental. Barbiturates produce a twilight zone in some people, causing individuals to forget that they have taken a pill, so they take one pill after another.

In the United States the growing specter of barbiturate addiction and death poses a most difficult problem. Barbiturates have a role in medical practice, but the abuse of the drug is becoming widespread.

Education of the public has been woefully inadequate in preventing and controlling barbiturate addiction. Public health officials may well consider the seriousness of the barbiturate problem and take necessary preventive measures. Treatment facilities on the local level are necessary. This is desirable on several counts, but particularly because the public health service hospitals do not accept barbiturate addicts unless they are also addicted to morphine or heroin. Barbiturates constitute a community health problem of much greater importance than the public recognizes and public health officials acknowledge.

Amphetamines. Pep pills such as benzedrine and dexedrine are prescription drugs, yet their misuse appears to be on the increase. Amphetamines are used to reduce the appetite in obesity. Any success will depend on social conditioning. These drugs reduce the feeling of fatigue and are used as rejuvenators by people who burn both ends of the candle and by those who seek to "get high" on occasion.

APPRAISAL OF COMMUNITY RESPONSIBILITY

Misuse of drugs is an intertwined social and health problem. Any program to deal with the problem must encompass the social, economical, psychological, and physiological factors encompassed by the phenomenon of drug misuse. Laymen and health officials alike recognize the importance of the problem, yet only sporadic attempts have been made to deal with the problem.

Too much reliance is made on the federal government to deal with the matter. Limitations of the federal program are apparent in the 1966 Drug Abuse Control Law, which is not aimed at the user but at the trafficker. The program of the federal agencies has been important and should be expanded, but the solution to the problem must come on the community level with support from a state program. Health officials must concern themselves with mental health, safety, communicable disease, environmental health, and all other factors affecting the well-being of people. The focus of the program must be the person who uses drugs as well as the person who misuses drugs.

The old legal approach to drug abuse must be replaced by a broad, constructive program of prevention and control. While the legal approach to possession and sale of drugs must be continued, the use of drugs must be placed in the category of health, and the individual concerned must be regarded as a person with a health problem. An effective community program for the prevention and control of drug abuse should include the following five aspects:

1. Improvement of conditions in the deprived neighborhoods, where addiction is most common
2. Promotion of mental health programs for the normal individual and clinical and other services for disturbed persons
3. Public health education on the use and misuse of drugs
4. Increased measures to reduce the availability of drugs
5. Providing treatment for people with addictions, including the necessary follow-up and guidance in rehabilitation

Responsibilities and programs of health departments change as the relative importance of different problems changes. Drug abuse is not new but it has attained an importance in our society, and immediate, tangible action is long overdue. Just as some people misuse the automobile, so some people misuse drugs. Motor vehicles and drugs both serve mankind, but, when misused, both produce physical, mental, and social pathology. It is a relatively small percentage of the population that misuses drugs, but the best interests of this segment and of society as a whole require greater attention and a more effective program than exists at present.

QUESTIONS AND EXERCISES

1. Distinguish between addiction and habituation.
2. Why is there no justification for the popular view that drug addicts fit into a common personality pattern?
3. Design an alcoholism control and treatment program for your community.
4. What should the schools teach in alcohol education?
5. Distinguish between stimulant and hallucinogen.
6. Why has there been no recent increase in heroin addiction?
7. Not all poorly adjusted people are drug addicts. Why?
8. What provisions does your state make for the treatment and care of heroin addicts?
9. What are the merits and demerits of the British program for dealing with heroin addicts if the program were to be considered for your state?
10. To what extent does the tension of the present world enter into the mounting menace of drugs?
11. For a person with personality problems, what does your community have to offer as an alternative to drugs?
12. Why not legalize the use of marijuana in your state?
13. Why would you expect a marijuana smoker to be a person who most likely would try LSD?
14. Why do today's youth tend to be attracted to LSD?
15. Under what circumstances should a user of LSD, marijuana, or barbiturates be classed as psychotic?
16. As a part of a community drug control program, what purpose, would a suicide prevention center serve?
17. Survey the drug addiction prevention, control, and treatment facilities of your community and recommend an effective program.

REFERENCES

Adult Use of Tobacco 1975, Department of Health, Education and Welfare.

Alpert, R., and associates: LSD, New York, 1967, The New American Library, Inc.

Blachley, P. H.: Drug abuse: data and debate, Springfield, Ill., Charles C Thomas, Publisher.

Block, M. A.: Alcohol and alcoholism, Belmont, Calif., 1970, Wadsworth Publishing Co., Inc.

Calahan, D., and associates: American drinking practices, New Brunswick, N.J., 1969, Rutgers University Press.

Carney, R. E., editor: Risk-taking behavior: concepts, Springfield, Ill., 1971, Charles C Thomas, Publisher.

Charney, E., Goodman, H. C., McBride, M., Lyon, B., and Pratt, R.: Childhood antecedents of adult obesity: do chubby infants become obese adults? New England Journal of Medicine 295(1):6-9, July, 1976.

Claridge, G.: Drugs and human behavior, New York, 1970, Praeger Publishers, Inc.

Cohen, S.: The drug dilemma, New York, 1969, McGraw-Hill Book Co.

Gellman, J. P.: The sober alcoholic: an organizational analysis of Alcoholics Anonymous, New Haven, Conn., 1967, College & University Press.

Harris, R. T., and associates: Drug dependence, Austin, 1971, University of Texas Press.

Hoffer, A., and Osmond, H.: The hallucinogens, New York, 1967, The Macmillan Co.

Ketcham, F. S.: Alcoholics and the community, Journal of the American Medical Association 202:980, 1967.

Love, H. D.: Youth and the drug problems, Springfield, Ill., 1971, Charles C Thomas, Publisher.

Lucas, B. G.: ABC of drug addiction, Baltimore, 1970, The Williams & Wilkins Co.

McCarthy, R. G., editor: Drinking and intoxication: selected readings in social attitudes, New Haven, Conn., 1967, College & University Press.

Maddox, G. L., and McCall, B. C.: Drinking among teenagers, New Haven, Conn., 1967, College & University Press.

Moscow, A.: The merchants of heroin, New York, 1967, The Dial Press.

Pittman, D. J., and Snyder, C. R.: Society, culture and drinking patterns, Urbana, 1968, University of Illinois Press.

Popham, R. E., Schmidt, W., and Lint, de J.: Law and drinking behavior (Ewing, J. A., and Rouse, B. A., editors), Chicago, Nelson-Hall Publishers.

Terris, M.: Drinking: our no. 2 killer, Medical Opinion, pp. 23-29, February, 1975.

Treatment of alcoholism: A study of programs and problems, Joint Information Services of the American Psychiatric Association and the National Association for Mental Health, Washington, D.C., 1967, American Psychiatric Association.

PART IV

Environmental health

13 ▪ COMMUNITY WATER SUPPLIES

All water has been through living systems
and must be used over and over again,
so man is required to regenerate the environment.

Anonymous

Environment in the modern complex community projects itself into more and more factors in an increasing variety of threats to health and life. Water, air, land, waste, shelter, and food represent what is regarded as the inanimate environment; but other people—individually, in the family, in groups, and in masses—represent an important and formidable aspect of the environment in which one operates. From the earliest times man has been striving to control the environment, but man himself makes the environment a greater and greater threat to his own health and life. Hence he has compounded the problem of environmental control. Greater congestion of people in metropolitan areas, the concentration of industry, population mobility, and sheer increase in numbers have made control of the environment more imperative and equally more challenging.

WATER CONSUMPTION

Communities need water for recreation, irrigation, industry, and domestic use. The population increases, industry expands, and other water uses multiply, yet the quantity of water remains fixed. Water must be reused in most places in the world. Man's ingenuity is economically and technically challenged by the task of retaining the quality of water.

Water is the most important commodity man consumes, and the consumption of water goes steadily up, so that today in the United States the average daily use for domestic purposes is 130 gallons per person. Communities with industries requiring vast amounts of water may have a total use that reaches 1,600 gallons per person per day. No nation in the world approaches America in demand for water, and no nation wastes more water. Community leaders tend to be too conservative in estimating future water requirements. Many areas in America will experience an increasing shortage for the rest of this century unless low-cost desalinization is employed or the harnessing of runoff from glaciers is successful.

The price of water to the consumer is reasonable but, with the supply becoming inadequate, new costly procedures such as desalinization of sea water will double and even triple the cost of water for the nation.

WATER-BORNE DISEASES

Pathogens of man do not normally multiply in water, yet they can survive in water and remain virile enough to set up an infection in a new host. Water serves as a vehicle of transfer of diseases of the alimentary canal and of transfer of certain worms, notably the schistosomes. No evidence exists that the respiratory diseases of man are conveyed via water.

Evidence is conclusive that four infectious diseases—typhoid, paratyphoid, cholera, and bacillary dysentery—are transmitted by water. The contention that viral hepatitis, amebic dysentery, and poliomyelitis are transmitted by water is not substantiated.

189

CHARACTERISTICS OF WATER

For community purposes water must be in sufficient supply and free from contamination, pollution, and turbidity. Water that may be suitable for household purposes may not be satisfactory for individual use if it is high in mineral content.

The ultimate source of water is rainfall, whether it is surface water impounded in a lake, pond, river, or reservoir created by a dam, or whether it is groundwater that has percolated through the ground to a stratum of gravel. In nature there is no pure water. It contains dissolved gases, minerals, and organic matter from the decay of such forms as algae and fungi.

Hardness of water is caused by the presence of calcium and magnesium salts. Hardness of 100 parts per million (ppm) or less, expressed as calcium carbonate, is soft enough for household use. Softening can be done at the time of filtration by adding lime and soda, and the calcium carbonate formed will precipitate out and leave a residual hardness of less than 100 ppm. To reduce alkalinity, the effluent from the softening process may be carbonated with carbon dioxide.

Drinking water containing too much sulfate (2,000 ppm), chloride (1,000 ppm), or calcium carbonate (300 ppm) will cause digestive disturbances in most people. Osmotic balance in the human colon can be upset by water high in mineral content, and severe diarrhea can result.

GROUNDWATER SUPPLIES

Groundwater is usually the preferred source for communities under 50,000 population. Rarely will a larger city locate sufficient groundwater for its needs, although San Antonio, Texas, with more than a half million people, has a groundwater supply. Groundwater has certain merits. It is free from contamination, pollution, turbidity, and color. However, it is scanty and highly mineralized.

As a community supply, groundwater is usually safe, and the low capital funds and operating costs make ground water an economical source. The first requirement is to locate an adequate supply. This means locating a gravel bed that serves as a natural reservoir. Test wells are drilled to outline the reservoir. The object is to locate a yard-thick gravel bed below an impervious layer 60 feet or more beneath the surface. At least one more gravel stratum should be located to assure an uninterrupted flow of water by having a second and even a third source. The rate of underground flow can be measured by putting dye into one hole and timing the interval required for the dye to get to another hole that is being pumped. An electrical conductor can also be used for this purpose. When the conductor put down into one hole reaches the next hole, the electrical circuit is completed and is recorded on a dial.

Producing wells are cased with pipe that is 6 to 24 inches in diameter and that has a brass intake screen where the pipe is embedded in the gravel. Spacing of wells depends on the underground flow and community needs. Electrically operated centrifugal pumps raise the water into a receiving reservoir of concrete construction. A second set of pumps forces the water up into a large storage or pressure tank.

Bacteria attach to sand grains and secrete a sticky covering that causes other bacteria to stick to this biological film. As water percolates into the ground, bacteria are filtered out by the sticky film. Groundwater may be contaminated by seepage along the well casing, by limestone, by other previous material above the groundwater supply that does not intercept bacteria, and by direct surface contamination into the groundwater stratum.

Well water is normally free from turbidity and can be chlorinated without filtration. Frequently it is unnecessary to chlorinate groundwater, although it may be done as an extra precaution. Many communities do not chlorinate their groundwater but have a chlorination unit standing by in the event the water should become contaminated.

SURFACE WATER SUPPLIES

New York City requires about a billion gallons of water a day. Multiply this by 365 and one gets some concept of the task that city has supplying its citizens with water. Consider what would happen if the city were without water for 48 hours. New York gets 10% of its water from wells. The remainder comes from surface water and necessitates a number of protected storage reservoirs and flumes. Cities like Chicago and Milwaukee are fortunate in having Lake Michigan as an excellent water source. The Mississippi River serves as both a water source and a sewage disposal receptacle for a long string of cities, including Minneapolis, St. Louis, and New Orleans. Surface water has certain merits. It is more abundant, more easily measured, and softer than ground water. However, it is frequently polluted by shore wash, transportation waste, and human waste. It is usually contaminated, is highly colored, and is often turbid.

With the increasing population and the high mobility of people today, virtually all surface water must be treated before it is safe for human consumption. Some lakes and streams have clear water, so no filtration is necessary, however, chlorination may be required. Most surface water is so turbid, polluted, and contaminated that both filtration and chlorination are necessary.

Rapid sand filtration was developed in America and is designed to filter out particles and bacteria. If the water contains considerable sediment, a preliminary settling chamber may be used to precede the treatment process. Otherwise, the water is pumped directly from the intake in the river or lake into the series of tanks comprising the treatment plant. These tanks are usually of concrete construction and, frequently, more than a sufficient number of tanks will be constructed so that some tanks may be shut off and cleaned or repaired while the rest of the tanks carry on the treatment process.

The treatment usually consists of five steps: flash mix, flocculation, sedimentation, filtration, and chlorination as shown in Fig. 13-1.

Flash mix is done in a relatively small tank.

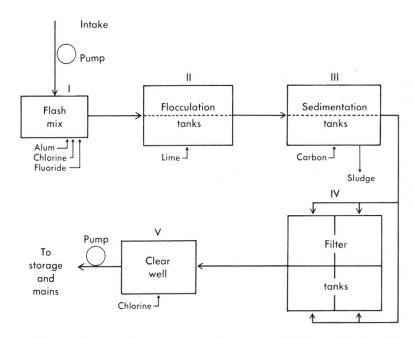

Fig. 13-1. Schematic diagram of water treatment, beginning with the introduction of floc material, then through flocculation, sedimentation, and filter tanks. After this process, the water is clear and ready for final chlorination to assure potability of the water.

Aluminum sulfate is fed into the incoming water and forms a flaky hydrate or floc. At the same time, chlorine is added and, if the water is being fluoridated, the fluoride is also added in the flash mix.

Flocculation consists of trapping particles of turbidity by the mechanical process of absorption of suspended solids. Because flocculation causes an increase in the density and size of coagulated particles, floc particles settle at a fast rate. Flocculation tanks are fitted with slowly rotating wooden paddles to ensure an even and continuous water-chemical mixture. In some plants, lime is added to assist the alum in forming floc and also for pH control. It takes about 30 minutes for the water to go through the flocculation tanks.

Sedimentation is the settling of the flocculation and is carried out in sedimentation tanks connected directly to the flocculation tanks. Water is retained here for about 2 hours to allow the floc to settle to the bottom of the tanks. From the bottom of the tanks floc will be scraped into troughs. Other troughs around the top of the tanks collect the upper layer of water, which is relatively free of floc.

If the water has an odor, activated carbon may be added to the water in the sedimentation tank, although the carbon may be added at some other stage of treatment. The activated carbon is effective in removing odor and objectionable taste.

Filtration is necessary to remove whatever turbidity may remain after the flocculation and settling. At the bottom of a filtration tank is a layer of gravel, topped by either sand or anthracite coal. Water percolates through this medium and goes out via drains at the bottom of the tank. To clean floc that accumulates on the anthracite coal or sand, the water level is lowered to the top of the troughs just above the coal level. The water flow is then reversed so that the accumulated floc is flushed into the troughs and carried off as waste. In some plants the water goes from the filtration tank to a temporary storage tank called a clear well, but this is not always essential.

Chlorination, the final step, decontaminates the water and is a simple, effective method for destroying bacteria. Postchlorination is designed to bring the residual chlorine to a level between 0.25 and 0.7 ppm. The chlorine residual properly is determined on water in the distribution system as well as at the plant of origin. Two samples a day at the plant and one from the system are recommended. A chlorine residual between 0.2 and 0.3 ppm will destroy all pathogens of man and, at this concentration, the chlorine cannot be detected by either taste or smell. In emergencies a chlorine residual of 0.7 ppm may be maintained. Although chlorine can be detected at this concentration, it is not harmful to humans.

The slow sand (European) method of filtration is similar to the rapid sand method except that instead of an artificial gelatinous layer, a film produced by bacteria is the interceptive medium. The method is too slow and the intercepting layer is not reliable. The rapid sand method is forty times faster and more reliable. Thus the rapid sand method is preferred in the United States.

Addition of fluorides

Based on available knowledge, the most effective, inexpensive, and simple method of preventing dental caries is the fluoridation of the public water supply. Beginning with studies of local areas where people had a low incidence of dental caries, scientists discovered that these areas had water that naturally contained about 1 ppm of fluorides. Where the fluoride content of water was much lower than this, the incidence of caries was high.

On the recommendation of dentists, physicians, and scientists, municipalities began adding fluorides to water supplies as a preventive measure against dental caries. Most water supplies contain a small amount of fluorides and the need is simply that of adding enough fluorides to bring the concentration up to 1 ppm. Northern cities raise the fluoride content slightly above this level and southern cities hold the fluoride content just

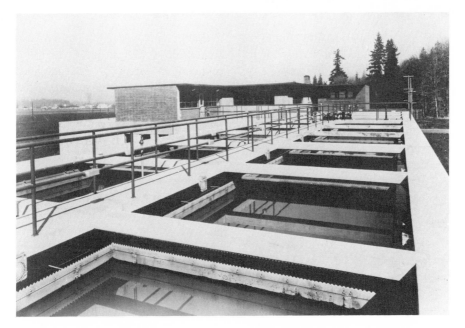

Fig. 13-2. Flocculation tanks in a series. The advantage of this arrangement is that not all tanks need to be in use at the same time, thus providing a favorable situation for cleaning or otherwise servicing the tanks. (Courtesy CH₂M-Hill, Corvallis, Oregon)

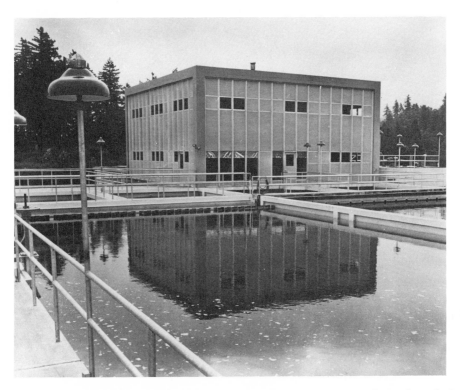

Fig. 13-3. Large flocculation tanks. In large cities where community water demands are high, the large tanks may be most effective. (Courtesy CH₂M-Hill, Corvallis, Oregon)

a little below 1 ppm. This is an adjustment to the difference in water consumption.

In 1976, more than 9,500,000 people in the United States were drinking water with a natural fluoride concentration between 0.7 and 3.0 ppm. Another 83 million people were drinking water to which fluoride had been added. People in more than 7,500 communities had public water supplies containing a caries preventive concentration of fluorides. It has been the history of public health that the small communities are the last to adopt new health measures, and this has held true for fluoridation. New York City, San Francisco, Baltimore, Chicago, Philadelphia, Pittsburgh, Milwaukee, St. Louis, and Washington, D.C. have fluoridated water supplies. Only about 40% of cities with populations between 2,500 and 10,000 have adopted fluoridation, and less than 20% of communities under 2,500 now fluoridate. Sweden, Netherlands, West Germany, Japan, and many other nations are making fluoridation available to their people.

Public health people are not surprised by the opposition to fluoridation, because health innovations have always been opposed. Vaccination, pasteurization of milk, chlorination of water supplies, and even indoor plumbing were, in turn, opposed by the easily frightened, those who resist change, the uninformed, people with aggressions, and others. Fortunately, fluoridation is gradually gaining acceptance, and this is repeating public health history. Unless effective means are used to reduce dental caries in the United States there will not be enough dentists to provide the necessary dental service for the more than 210 million people. Courts have ruled fluoridation is a reasonable legal exercise of the local police power in the interest of the public health and not a violation of individual rights. One state after another is requiring fluoridation of community water supplies.

Some communities have water supplies with a high natural fluoride content of 8 ppm. This concentration prevents caries but causes mottling of the teeth, although no other harm

to the human body has been detected. These communities add phosphate to the water to reduce fluorides to a level of 1 ppm. In communities having a water supply with a natural fluoride content of 2 ppm, people have health histories showing no deviation from that of the population at large.

TESTING OF WATER

Quality of community water is always a first consideration, and health considerations are of primary importance. Thus, bacteriological examination of a municipal water supply is of primary consideration. Physical and chemical properties of water can be of great importance to industry and of significant importance to the general public as well. Radiological examination of water is of more recent vintage and not generally a concern, but in specific instances the possibility of radioactive contaminants in water can be significant. Bioassays are necessary to evaluate toxicity in fish, and biological examinations are used to determine the extent of plankton and other life forms.

Bacteriological examination of water is necessary to ascertain possible contamination. Samples are collected at representative locations throughout the community water system. Frequency of collection is adjusted to the likelihood of contamination. A groundwater supply may be so safe that a sample once a month may be adequate. The size of a community, as well as possible contamination, may require more frequent sample collections. For routine purposes, the usual minimum is as follows:

Population	Minimum samples per month
Under 2,500	1
25,000	25
100,000	100
1,000,000	300

Pathogens are not routinely isolated in the water. The coliform group of bacteria has been used as the index of contamination. United States Public Health Service standards require that, of the 10 ml samples examined each month, not more than 10% shall show the presence of the coliform group. These standards set a maximum monthly density of coliform organisms at 1 per 100 ml of water tested.

A sample is collected under sterile conditions so that any contamination discovered would have to be in the water. A milliliter is spread over an agar medium and incubated at 37° C. A colony will form from each of the *E. coli* in the sample and thus a bacteria count can be made.

Water may have *E. coli* and be safe. The contamination may come from lower animals. Citizens do not relish the idea of drinking water from the discharges of either lower animals or man. The test is merely an indicator of contamination. Investigation is necessary to determine the source of contamination before the discharges of a typhoid carrier or of a patient with cholera get into the water. Every precaution should be taken to prevent the community water supply from being a vehicle of disease transmission.

Chemical examination of water varies, depending on the specific chemical one wishes to detect. Tests for hardness are most frequent. A test for chlorine residual is used to determine the decontamination effect of chlorination. Nitrite and nitrate determinations indicate recent and old pollution of water. Iodine, iron, phosphate, and sulfate content are of interest. Dissolved oxygen and carbon dioxide indicate water quality before treatment. Most community water supplies are tested routinely for chlorine residual and this may constitute the only chemical examination unless some special problem arises.

REGULATION OF PUBLIC WATER SUPPLIES

Providing water to a community is a recognized function of local government. The city government usually constructs and operates the water system as a corporate function. This is not a responsibility of the health department, but a special water department or the department of public works usually operates the water system. A few communities grant a franchise to a private corporation to sell water as a commodity to the public.

Providing water to the community is a local government function, but the regulation of public water supplies is the responsibility of the state, which usually delegates this authority to the state department of health. A public water system is one that provides piped water for human consumption that has at least fifteen service connections or that regularly serves at least twenty-five people. If a city wishes to erect a water plant, the plans must be approved by engineers from the state department of health. In practice these engineers actually serve as advisors for the city in developing the plans. This advisory service is without cost to the city. Even though the city pays to have plans drawn and the water system constructed, it is the state that passes on the adequacy of the plans and the construction.

Once the plant is in operation, the state continues its supervisory authority. Plant operators must be certified by the state. Regular reports on water analysis must be submitted to the state as the state department of health decrees. However, there is usually an amiable relationship between the representatives of the state and community officials. Both groups are interested in safe water for the people of the community. Cooperation extends to the level where the state representative serves as a consultant if the community should encounter a problem in the operation of its water system. This consulting service is given without cost to the community. It is an expression of the dedication in service to the public that is characteristic of truly professional public health personnel.

Safe Drinking Water Act of 1974

Drinking water supplied to most American homes is usually recognized as being safe. Yet the National Community Water Supply Study of 1970 reveals that the quality of household water is declining. Part of this decline is attributed to the careless use of various chemical substances and other toxic wastes. As an outgrowth of this study by the U.S. Environment Protection Agency (EPA), Congress enacted the Safe Drinking Water Act of 1974.

This Act provides for the establishment of water standards. Congress also authorized the EPA to support state and local community drinking water programs by providing financial and technical assistance. It is recognized that the federal government—through the EPA—has the authority and responsibility for enforcing standards and otherwise supervising public water systems.

The major provisions of this Act provide for an extended list of guidelines and responsibilities such as the following:

1. Establishment of primary regulations for the protection of the public health
2. Establishment of secondary regulations relating to the taste, odor, and appearance of drinking water
3. Measures to protect underground drinking water sources
4. Research and studies regarding health, economical, and technological problems of drinking water supplies; specifically required are studies of viruses in drinking water and contamination by cancer-causing chemicals
5. A survey of the quality and availability of rural water supplies
6. Aid to the states to improve drinking water programs through technical assistance, training of personnel, and grant support; a loan guarantee is provided to assist small water systems in meeting regulations if other means of financing cannot reasonably be found
7. Citizen suits against any party believed to be in violation of the Act
8. Record-keeping, inspections, issuance of regulations, and judicial reviews
9. A fifteen-member National Drinking Water Advisory Council to advise the EPA Administrator on scientific and other responsibilities under this Act
10. A requirement that the Secretary of Health, Education and Welfare ensure that the standards for bottled drinking water conform to the primary regulations established under the Act or publish reasons for not doing so
11. Authorization of appropriations totaling $156 million for fiscal years 1975, 1976, and 1977

Thus, we see that a vigorous, organized program is underway to assure the people of the nation of safe drinking water. Standards ultimately will include maximum contaminant levels and general criteria for operation, maintenance, and intake water quality. Interim primary regulations established by the EPA on March 14, 1975, became effective in 2 years. Secondary standards have also been prescribed relating only to taste, odor, and appearance of drinking water. These standards will be enforced only when the individual states want to enforce them.

A state can continue to enforce its own laws and regulations governing drinking water supplies if they meet certain requirements such as the following:

1. Adoption of regulations at least equal to federal regulations
2. Adoption and implementation of adequate enforcement procedures
3. Provision for emergency circumstances
4. Keeping adequate records and provide reports for the EPA

Appraisal. Next to oxygen, water is most indispensable for human existence. Yet, despite its importance, water can be a medium for the transmission of disease. It is commendable that lawmakers on the federal and state levels have provided the leadership in establishing safe drinking water programs. Human interrelations have been a key factor in the advancement in this program despite the fact that human relationships may well be man's greatest unsolved problem. The admonition of perpetual vigilance applies critically to community water safety.

QUESTIONS AND EXERCISES

1. To what extent is man creating a more hazardous environment at a more rapid rate than the development of his knowledge on how to control the environment?
2. If water is more important to man's health than any

drug, why should not water cost more than any drug?

3. What is meant by this statement: "Man must regenerate the environment"?

4. It is important to determine that a certain source of water is the vehicle for the transmission of typhoid fever, but why is it more important to determine who put the typhoid bacilli in the water?

5. Why do public health officials favor ground water as a community supply?

6. From your observations and other data who in the United States has the safest water supply, urban dwellers or rural people?

7. What is the source of your community's water supply and what are the merits and demerits of the water?

8. In one area ground water less than 30 feet below the surface is a safe water supply. In another area ground water more than 60 feet below the surface is an unsafe supply. Why the difference?

9. A student reported visiting a water plant that was in operation and finding no one there. How would you explain this paradox?

10. Locate some community where the fluoridation of the community water supply is a controversial issue and analyze the basic factors underlying the controversy.

11. Most community water supplies contain fluorides, in some cases up to 8 ppm. In the light of this, examine the contention that adding fluorides to water is medication.

12. Examine the contention that a community has the right to remove fluoride from water but no community has the right to add fluoride to water.

13. If the water in all the wells in a rural area is known to be contaminated, what is the responsibility of the county health department and the state health officials?

14. Appraise the potential value of the Safe Drinking Water Act of 1974.

15. How is it possible for water to be contaminated and still be safe?

16. Why is the bacteriological examination of water not directed at finding the typhoid bacillus?

17. Bacteriological examination indicated contamination of the ground water supply of a midwestern community. What are the possible sources of contamination?

18. Why should the state regulate community water supplies?

19. Why does not the community health department operate the community water system?

20. Propose a program of health education to interest people in the safety of their community water supply.

REFERENCES

Ackerman, B. A., and associates: The uncertain search for environmental quality, Riverside, N.J., 1974, The Free Press.

American Public Health Association: Standard methods for the examination of water and wastewater, ed. 13, New York, 1971, The Association.

Aylesworth, T. J.: This vital air; this vital water: man's environmental crisis, rev. ed., Chicago, 1974, Rand McNally & Co.

Berger, M.: The new water book, New York, 1973, Thomas Y. Crowell Co., Inc.

Bloome, E. P.: Water we drink, Garden City, N.Y., 1971, Doubleday & Co., Inc.

Cairns, J., Jr., and Dickson, K. L., editors: Biological methods for the assessment of water quality, Philadelphia, 1973, American Society for Testing Materials.

Ciaccio, L.: Water and water pollution handbook, vol. 3, New York, 1972, Marcel Dekker, Inc.

Cox, C.: Operation and control of water treatment processes, Irvington-on-Hudson, N.Y., 1964, WHO International Document Service, Columbia University Press.

Cross, F. L., Jr., editor: Water pollution monitoring, the Environmental Monograph, Westport, 1976, Technomic Publishing Co., Inc.

Culp, R. L., and Culp, G. L.: New concepts in water purification, New York, 1974, Van Nostrand Reinhold Co.

Dieterich, H. B., and Henderson, M. J.: Urban water supply conditions and needs in seventy-five developing countries, Public Health Papers No. 23, Geneva, Switzerland, Irvington-on-Hudson, 1963, WHO International Document Service, Columbia University Press.

Ehlers, V. M., and Steel, E. W.: Municipal and rural sanitation, ed. 6, New York, 1965, McGraw-Hill Book Co.

Elliot, S. M.: Our dirty water, New York, 1973, Julian Messner.

Flanagan, J. E.: Water supply and pollution control, Science **145:**840, 1964.

Fried, J. J.: Ground water pollution (developments in water science, vol. 4), New York, 1976, American Elsevier Publishing Co., Inc.

Gehm, H. W., and Bregman, J. I., editors: Handbook of water resources and pollution control, New York, 1976, Van Nostrand Reinhold Co.

Giefer, G. J., and Todd, D. K.: Water publications of state agencies, Port Washington, N.Y., 1972, Water Information Center, Inc.

Gloya, E. F., and Eckenfieldor, W. W., Jr., editors: Advances in water quality improvement, Austin, Texas, 1967, (Water resources symposium, no. 1), University of Texas Press.

Holden, W. S., editor: Water treatment and examination, ed. 8, Baltimore, 1970, The Williams & Wilkins Co.

Hopkins, E. S., and Bean, E. L.: Water purification control, ed. 4, Baltimore, 1975, The Williams & Wilkins Co.

Hopkins, E. S., Bingley, W. M., and Schucker, G. W.:

The practice of sanitation, ed. 4, Baltimore, 1970, The Williams & Wilkins Co.

Hynes, H. B.: Biology of polluted waters, Toronto, 1970, University of Toronto Press.

Johns Hopkins University, Department of International Health: The functional analysis of health needs and services, Baltimore, 1976, The John Hopkins University Press.

Kerns, F. R.: Simplicity of water purification, Ardmore, Penn., 1972, Dorrance and Co., Inc.

Maier, F. J.: Manual of water fluoridation practice, ed. 2, New York, 1972, McGraw-Hill Book Co.

McCaull, J., and Croseland, J.: Water pollution (Commoner, B., editor), New York, 1974, text ed., Harcourt Brace Jovanovich, Inc.

Overman, M.: Water: solutions to a problem of supply and demand, Garden City, N.Y., 1969, Doubleday & Co., Inc.

The struggle for clean water, Public Health Service Publication No. 958, United States Department of Health, Education and Welfare, 1962.

Van Dersal, W. R., and Graham, E. H.: Water for America: the story of water concentration, New York, 1956, Henry Z. Walck, Inc.

Velz, C. J.: Applied stream sanitation, New York, 1970, John Wiley & Sons, Inc.

Warner, D., and Dajani, J. S.: Water and sewer development in rural America, Lexington, Mo., 1975, Lexington Books.

World Health: European standards for drinking waters, ed. 2, Albany, N.Y., 1970, World Health Organization, Q Corporation.

Wrigley, D.: Water (Raintree editions), Milwaukee, Wis., 1976, Raintree Publishers, Ltd.

14 ▪ COMMUNITY WASTE DISPOSAL

*The soil is the great organ
in which toxic substances of all kinds
are neutralized or destroyed.*

Milton J. Rosenau

The task of community waste disposal has become increasingly more difficult with the rapid increase in population, the movement of people to the metropolitan areas, the mobility of modern life, the increase in outdoor recreation, and the expansion of industry.

COMMUNITY WASTES

Household wastes, commercial wastes, recreational wastes, and industrial wastes are the general sources of community wastes. These wastes are in the form of garbage, refuse, street cleanings, human discharges, kitchen wastes, scavenger wastes, commercial wastes, and wastes from manufacturing and processing plants. The sheer volume in a year would run into millions of tons and would make a mountainous stockpile. If each year's wastes accumulated, in a period of 20 years a community would be buried by its own waste products. Fortunately, the lowly bacteria are man's saviors. By decomposing animal proteins, bacteria not only reduce the great mass of wastes to a negligible volume but also make the invaluable nitrogen available for reuse. This process is customarily referred to as the nitrogen cycle as shown in Fig. 14-1.

Nitrogen cycle. Animal proteins begin decomposing by the action of bacteria that converts the proteins to amino acids. Another set of bacteria next converts the amino acids to ammonia. The ammonia combines with carbon dioxide to form ammonium carbonate, which in turn is converted to nitrites by a third type of bacteria. Nitrites combine with sodium and potassium, and the resulting nitrites are converted into nitrates by yet another group of organisms known as the *Nitrobacters*. Nitrates dissolved in soil water diffuse into the root hairs of plants, where they combine with carbon dioxide and water to form plant proteins. The plant proteins are consumed by animals and are converted into animal proteins, thus completing the nitrogen cycle.

Communities aid nature in this process of waste disposal by providing the beneficial bacteria with a favorable environment and by dilution, chemical treatment, and the burning of wastes. The task of disposing of wastes is a continual one that is both important and costly. Processes involved in getting rid of man's wastes are also processes for destroying or removing pathogens that can cause disease and death. In this category perhaps the most important of these processes is sewage disposal.

SEWAGE DISPOSAL

"Sewage" consists of the liquid wastes from household effluents, commercial effluents, and industrial liquid wastes. It is carried in a system of pipes and other means of conveyance called a "sewerage system." In some communities storm water is carried in the sewerage system, and in other communities a separate system of pipes carries off storm water.

Generally, community sewage will be about 99% water containing animal, plant, and mineral matter in solution and in suspension. Bacteria of many types, mostly nonpathogenic, are always present. Paper, sticks, grease, and other materials are in suspension.

199

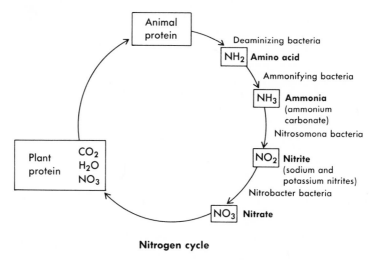

Nitrogen cycle

Fig. 14-1. Nitrogen cycle. The decomposition of organic material goes on continuously, thanks to bacteria that save communities from being buried by their own wastes.

The strength of sewage is measured by its biochemical oxygen demand (BOD), which is the quantity of oxygen required in a given time to satisfy the chemical and biological oxidation demands of the sewage. A high BOD means that an excessive quantity of oxygen is being used up by the biochemical action in the sewage, indicating a high sewage concentration.

While the primary purpose of sewage treatment is to prevent the spread of disease among human beings, for additional reasons the proper disposal of sewage is imperative in any nation, particularly one with a high population concentration. Sewage treatment protects water supplies, protects fish and other aquatic life, protects food by preventing soil pollution, protects livestock, and renders water fit for industrial use. Thus, in addition to the prevention of disease spread, sewage treatment returns water to such a condition that it can be reused with safety and with its general condition unimpaired.

SEWAGE TREATMENT

Treatment of community sewage is directed toward five factors: solids in suspension, organic matters in suspension, inorganic matters in suspension, organic matters in solution, and bacteria. A properly designed and efficiently operated sewage disposal plant will eliminate all five of these undesirable factors and leave an end product of clear, uncontaminated water that can be safely consumed.

A community sewage disposal plant that does the complete job of treatment involves the following five steps or processes.

1. Preliminary treatment to remove solids such as sand, sticks, paper, and other floating objects, and metal and plastic objects
2. Primary treatment to clarify the sewage by employing sedimentation to settle suspended particles and provide an environment devoid of free oxygen, so that anaerobic bacteria can digest the organic materials settling to the bottom of the clarifying tank
3. Secondary treatment to provide an environment in which the effluent comes in contact with air so that aerobic bacteria can oxidize putrescible material and thus reduce the oxygen demand of the sewage
4. Chlorination to decontaminate the effluent by destroying any bacteria that may remain

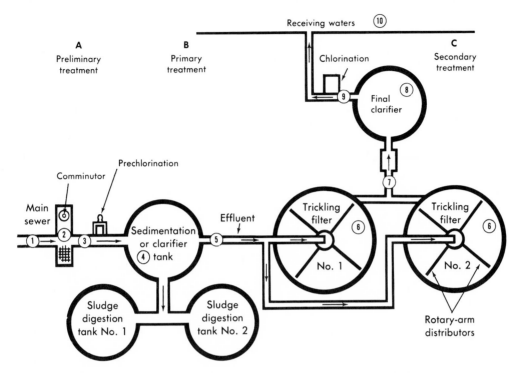

Fig. 14-2. Plan of a complete sewage treatment plant. After preliminary treatment, the sewage goes through primary (anaerobic) treatment, secondary (aerobic) treatment, and chlorination before being emptied into the receiving stream or lake.

5. Final disposal of the end product into a lake, river, canal, or other body of water

Sewage from about one-third of the population in this country is treated before final disposal, but only about 40% of this sewage is completely treated. Some communities have only preliminary and primary treatment, which could be acceptable. Other communities follow primary treatment with chlorination and, depending on conditions, the result may be acceptable to state sanitary authorities. Method of treatment depends on conditions. If the final effluent is to be discharged into a large body of water, less complete treatment may be necessary than if the discharge is into a small body of water. Complete treatment is the ideal, and more and more communities will be compelled to complete sewage treatment in order to protect human life and prevent stream pollution.

Preliminary treatment. Screens consisting of a series of parallel bars set at an angle of about 30 degrees from the horizontal permit sewage to flow through but intercept large suspended objects. Mechanically or manually operated rakes clean the debris and dump it into receptacles, where it is burned. This raking process may be continuous or intermittent. If fine screens are used, they must be continuously cleaned. Some plants use shredders or comminutors, which cut coarse material into fine enough particles to pass through with the effluent.

Grit chambers for preliminary treatment are tanks or basins in which sewage flow is reduced, causing gravel, sand, and other heavy materials to settle to the bottom. Two or more grit chambers are necessary so that one can be in operation while the other is being cleaned by manual labor or by mechanical means.

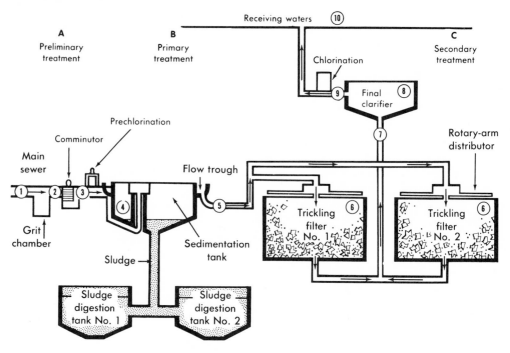

Fig. 14-3. Diagrammatic cross-section of a complete sewage treatment plant. Succession of numbers is used to show direction of flow. Tanks, pipes, and other segments are not necessarily in proper proportion as presented here.

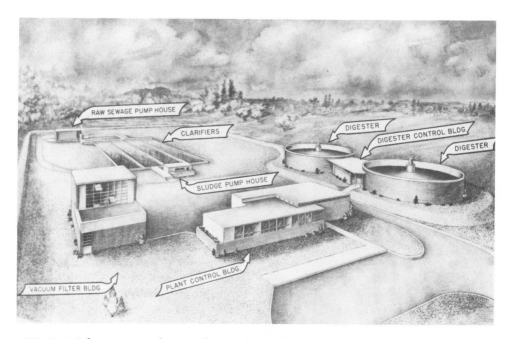

Fig. 14-4. Schematic reproduction of a complete preliminary, primary, and secondary sewage treatment plant. The plan here is similar to that shown in Figs. 14-2 and 14-3. (Courtesy CH₂M-Hill, Corvallis, Oregon)

Primary treatment. Sedimentation or clarifier tanks are either rectangular or circular and are about 10 feet deep. A concrete circular tank has many advantages and has become the prevailing choice. The effluent comes into the center of the circular tank through a pipe coming up from the bottom. This prevents agitation of the effluent in the tank and assures that the effluent is quiet, so that particles will settle to the bottom. To aid this sedimentation, chemicals are added to form a gelatinous floc that settles, carries suspended solids to the bottom, and forms sludge.

In some plants digestion of the sludge by anaerobic bacteria takes place in the sedimentation tank. This method has disadvantages because gas bubbles and other disturbances agitate the effluent and prevent settling. A better procedure is to pump the sludge from the bottom of the settling tank into concrete sludge tanks and permit the anaerobic bacteria to act there. Temperatures of about 85° to 95° will hasten digestion. Heat will result from the activities of the bacteria. In addition, the methane gas formed by the digestion process can be piped into water heaters and provide the sludge tanks with the necessary heat for the best sludge digestion. Not all sludge will be digested. Undigested sludge will be pumped out and hauled away to be used as fertilizer because it is high in nitrogen content. Sludge-drying beds will dehydrate the sludge. Fresh sludge is contaminated and is not safe for truck garden plots.

Because bacterial action is slow, scientists have been experimenting with chemicals as a replacement for bacteria. Their efforts have been fruitful and, while some expense is involved and the precipitate has to be disposed of, chemical digestion is fast-acting and will become the standard method of primary treatment.

Secondary treatment. In order to reduce the oxygen demand of the sewage, the secondary treatment requires aeration so that organisms can convert the organic matter in the effluent into stable nitrogenous products. Trickling filters serve admirably. Walls of the filters are constructed of concrete, brick, tile, or other building material. Underdrains of tile leading to central drainage channels are laid on the filter floor. Over this is laid a bed of gravel, crushed stone, or similar material, which provides good ventilation of the bed.

Effluent comes from the clarifier, or primary tanks, in pipes. Connected to these pipes is a series of equally spaced nozzles or spray heads, a foot or two above the surface of the stone bed. Automatic dosing devices permit one set of nozzles to spray effluent while the other is not operating. This method alternates spraying and being idle.

A gelatinous film that intercepts bacteria, algae, protozoa, worms, molds, and other forms of life forms on the stones as the effluent sprays over the stone bed. The organisms in this film convert dissolved, suspended, and colloidal materials into stable nitrogenous material. Excessive amounts of solids in the effluent coming from the primary treatment tank tend to clog the interstitial spaces.

Rotary distributors can be used instead of sprays. The liquid is layered over the surface of the stone bed as the rotary arm swings over the bed.

Intermittent sand filters are also used for secondary treatment. The underdrains are similar to those in the trickling filters. Surface distributing channels flood the effluent over the surface of the sand bed. Sand grains become coated with a gelatinous film, as do the stones in the trickling filters. In many respects, this is the slow sand filtration method used in water treatment; it is highly effective but rather slow-acting.

Sand filtration beds are alternated—one flooded, one idle. The surface of the sand bed must be cleaned and thus requires constant attention. The dry sludge is an effective fertilizer.

Tertiary treatment. Some community sewage treatment plants have used a third process to remove or reduce certain chemicals such as phosphates, nitrogen, and even carbon. Removal of these chemicals is desirable and even necessary because they can lead to eutrophication, a process that occurs in nature but normally requires thousands of years. However, the process is accelerated when excessive nutrients (such as nitrates and phosphates) stimulate marked growth of algae and other aquatic plants. The flourishing plants consume the oxygen essential to marine life and to the natural purification of wastes. This essentially has been the condition in Lake Erie.

Phosphorus compounds enter streams, lakes, and other bodies of water through synthetic detergents, domestic wastes, and precipitation from farm and other land runoff. Detergents are not the major source of phosphorus in the effluent of sewage treatment plants and this phosphorus is no more difficult to remove than that of other sources. In community sewage more than half of the total phosphorus comes from domestic wastes, detergents account for about 35% of phosphates, and the remainder comes from fertilizers used in farming and lawn care.

Removal of phosphorus is not too difficult. It can even be done as a phase of the usual primary treatment process. It involves the conversion of soluble phosphorus into insoluble forms and then precipitation of the insoluble forms, which is usually done by adding metal salts, for example, aluminum sulfate or ferrous chloride. Flocculants are then used to conglomerate solid particles, which fairly quickly sink to the bottom of the settling tank carrying the phosphorus compounds with them. When settled out, the phosphorus compounds are removed with the sludge, which is disposed of where it will not enter a body of water.

Nitrogen removal is not so simple. In the first place, the dose of metal salts used in phosphorus removal raises the effluent pH to about 11.5. This must be reduced to a pH of about 7.5, because with a high pH, ammonia is present as dissolved gas. Lowering the pH is accomplished by recarbonating the effluent through the addition of calcium carbonate.

One method for removing nitrogen utilizes a stripping tower from 25 to 50 feet high. The inside of the tower is laced with wooden slats about 2 inches apart. Effluent is pumped to the top of the tower and is distributed uniformly from a horizontal tray across the top of the latticework. As the falling water strikes a slat, droplets are formed. Droplet surface films are of minimum thinness, which favors the escape of ammonia gas from the droplet. Air in the tower enters through side louvers and, by completely surrounding the droplets, promotes a maximum transfer of ammonia from water to the air. The process of water falling and forming new droplets is repeated at least 200 times. Depending on the temperature of the air and the water, from 30% to 90% of the ammonia will be removed. This tertiary treatment vastly improves the efficiency of chlorination.

It becomes quite clear than tertiary treatment of most community sewage is imperative if America is to save its streams, lakes, and ponds. Ecology makes clear that all life on earth (man included) depends on good quality water. The cost of complete sewage treatment will be high, but compared with the alternative it will be essential.

Chlorination. Primary treatment of sewage may be all that is necessary when the effluent from community sewage is emptied into receiving waters that provide extreme dilution. In some instances, dilution is sufficiently great so that after secondary treatment it is safe to empty the effluent into the final disposal lake, river, or sea. However, when great population concentrations exist and available bodies of water are not great, a good safety measure is to chlorinate the effluent coming from the primary or secondary treatment unit. In some instances chlorination is necessary only during the summer months when available stream flow is low. Two-stage chlorination, in which chlorine is added to the grit chamber at the beginning of treatment and again to the final effluent, provides added safety.

Besides destroying organisms, chlorine reduces the BOD and odor of effluents. The chlorine injection mechanism is, similar to that used in water treatment plants.

Final disposal. The receiving waters into which the final effluent is emptied are usually public waters and, as such, are under the ju-

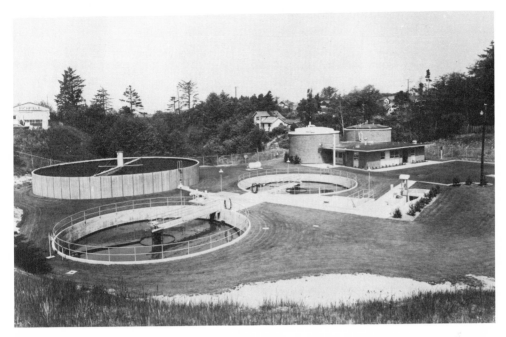

Fig. 14-5. A relatively complete sewage disposal plant. Controls are in the building near upper right of the picture, near the two sludge digestion tanks. The two tanks with catwalks are the sedimentation or clarifier tanks. A single trickling filter is identified by the rotary arms. (Courtesy CH_2M-Hill, Corvallis, Oregon)

risdiction and supervision of a state agency. Other communities and citizens have a claim to the use of the waters. The larger the body of receiving water the greater the safety factor. While the supervising state agency recognizes practical considerations, no community has the right to jeopardize the health of anyone. If a community is to be granted the privilege of disposing its wastes, it must take reasonable precautions to assure that its sewage effluent is not a threat to human life and welfare.

Lagoon treatment. Cost of a typical sewage treatment plant can be beyond the financial means of a small community. Raw sewage lagoons can provide economical and satisfactory treatment of community sewage. A lagoon is a shallow pond in which natural processes produce an acceptable purification.

A lagoon is usually located at least a quarter of a mile from residential areas, where seepage will not pollute groundwaters that may be used for domestic purposes. A lagoon is a rectangular excavation, at least half an acre in area and from 3 to 5 feet in depth. The soil at the bottom of the lagoon should be relatively impervious to prevent excess loss of effluent by seepage. Embankments prevent outside surface drainage from entering the lagoon. The inlet from the sewerage system should be near the center of the lagoon. Grinding objects in raw sewage will provide a desirable dispersal of the solids, prevent an accumulation of sludge deposits, assure better treatment, and help prevent odors.

Organic material that settles to the bottom of the lagoon is decomposed by bacteria and is converted into ammonia, carbon dioxide, and water. Algae feed on these soluble nutrients and, in the presence of sunlight, produce oxygen and thus maintain aerobic conditions and help prevent odor. If the lagoon freezes over, the ice shuts out sunlight and interferes with the treatment process. In addition, a low temperature slows down bacterial action.

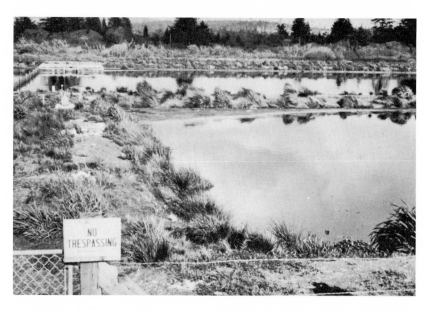

Fig. 14-6. Lagoon treatment of sewage. Raw sewage lagoons can provide economical and satisfactory treatment of community sewage. (Courtesy Lane County, Oregon, Department of Health and Sanitation)

Decontamination of sewage effluents may be necessary if they are being discharged into public waters, especially during the period between May and November. Raw sewage lagoon effluents are generally not discharged into public waters with less than 20 to 1 dilution.

Lagoon treatment may not be the equivalent of the standard methods of treatment, but it can be highly acceptable. It serves when the community concerned is not able to finance the more costly, more elaborate standard primary and secondary treatment plants.

Financing sewage treatment

Sewage treatment plants are costly but are a necessary community investment in protecting health, in maintaining an esthetic environment, and in disposing community wastes. No fully equitable method has been developed for paying the costs of treatment plant construction and maintenance. Virtually all payment methods are based on the volume of water citizens use from the community's water supply.

Most communities find it necessary to issue bonds for the construction of a treatment plant. The security for the bonds is the community's ability to collect fees and levy taxes to redeem the bonds when due. All establishments connected to the public sewerage system are charged a monthly sewer fee that is based on the amount of water the establishment used during the month. The practice is based on the assumption that the amount of water a household uses is a reasonable index of the extent to which the household uses the sewer service. During winter months the sewer fee is usually a higher percentage of water used than during summer, when the sewer rate is low to adjust to the fact that much of the water going through the meter is used for lawn sprinkling and does not go into the sewer lines.

What of the landlord whose property value is enhanced by having sewage treatment? He may pay nothing toward the construction and maintenance of a sewage treatment plant if his tenant pays all of the fee. This is an inequity that has been hard to correct. Some communities have a property tax to help defray the cost of the sewage treatment plant, and this equalizes the cost somewhat.

Regulation of sewage disposal

Construction and operation of sewage treatment facilities and disposal of the final effluent is the responsibility of the community, but the regulation of the community sewage treatment plants and disposal of final effluents is the province of the state. This authority may be vested in the sanitary engineering division of the state department of health or in a special state sanitary authority. There are advantages in having a special authority to regulate sewage disposal, largely because water pollution is increasing as a problem. In addition, a separate authority can deal with air pollution and other problems of the total environment.

The state can order a community to treat its sewage before emptying the final effluent into public waters. Courts have held this to be a proper function of the state and have ordered communities to raise the necessary funds to provide for proper sewage disposal. Plans for a community sewage disposal plant must be approved by state engineers, who also work with communities in an advisory role. Sewage disposal plant operators must pass state examinations to be certified operators. The operation of the sewage plant must meet state requirements and satisfy state sanitary authorities.

Septic tanks

A serious community health problem may exist when a residential area is not served by sewers. A septic tank for each domicile is the means used for sewage disposal in such areas. The fringes of a city or the outlying area just beyond the city limits are the usual sources of these problems.

A septic tank can be satisfactory for the disposal of household liquid wastes if the tank, drain tile, and seepage pit are properly constructed. When improperly installed, a septic tank can constitute a hazard to health and, esthetically, can be a severe nuisance. Sewage sporadically coming to the surface or,

during flooding, washing over a neighborhood can constitute a hazard to the well-being of everyone in the vicinity. There is a pattern that usually exists in such situations —first, a long-time toleration of the situation; then, protests to the health officials or others; then, perhaps, court action. The final solution is usually the installation of sewers as a part of the community sewerage system. When at all feasible, even at considerable cost, sewer lines rather than septic tanks should be the choice.

Cities without sewer systems

Many cities in the United States have inadequate sewerage systems, and the general public is concerned about the possible danger to health and life resulting from negligence. As a consequence pressures are exerted on officials and on voters to provide the necessary finances and plans for an adequate sewerage system for their community. Federal and state funding adds to the incentive to provide the community with an approved, safe means for the disposal of the community's wastes.

Americans generally have an appreciation of the importance of providing efficient, adequate sewerage systems almost without regard for what the cost may be. Yet throughout the world one can find cities of more than 1 million inhabitants without a sewer system. Tokyo, Japan, (with more than 10 million people) has the largest population of any city in the world. Yet Tokyo does not have a sewer system but depends on collection tanks and tanker trucks to collect and dispose of sewage.

Hiroshima was levelled by a nuclear bomb, which necessitated a complete rebuilding of the city. Environmentalists assumed that Hiroshima would begin by putting in a complete sewer system before erecting structures above the ground. The situation was ideal for this sequence. But no sewer system was built. The tank system apparently is the system of choice. This event could well cause Americans to ask themselves whether they have overemphasized

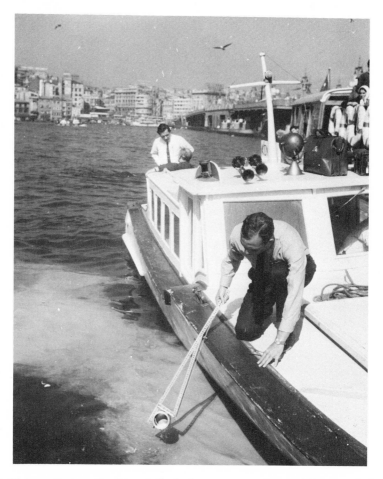

Fig. 14-7. Water pollution. Checking drift of submarine sewerage outfall in Istanbul. (Courtesy World Health Organization)

the necessity for all of the sewerage systems they have built. But America's experience wholly justifies its concern for the protection of the health and lives of its people. It is truly a concern for the common good.

STREAM POLLUTION

Stream pollution is the creation of objectionable conditions through the discharge of sewage or industrial wastes into natural waters. With the growth of cities and the expansion of industry, stream pollution has become a major concern in all states.

A single river may have many uses—navigation, power, swimming, boating, fishing, industrial waste disposal, domestic sewage disposal, industrial water supply, community water supply, and irrigation. Control of all conditions affecting a stream is as essential as it is demanding.

While stream pollution is generally thought of only in terms of a threat to human health, water pollution actually affects many factors of economic and other significance. It affects agriculture by altering the taste of milk from cows drinking polluted water. Polluted irrigation water represents possible dangers. Water fowl and other animals are exposed to botulism and cyanide poisoning. Turbidity of 6,000 ppm is lethal for fish. Thermal pollution can destroy marine life. Decomposition of nitrogen wastes forms nitrates and, because all of the oxygen is consumed, green plants die and anaerobic bacteria survive. Farther down the stream where little or no pollution exists, green plant life may be profuse and give off oxygen. Pollution may render water unsuitable for industrial use. Pollution with acids may cause dock deterioration. Pollution from such industries as mining and quarrying may interfere with navigation and thus require dredging of the stream.

It is apparent that stream pollution affects many factors, but its effect on use for domestic purposes is the most important. This holds priority over all other considerations. To reduce pollution to a point where streams are as clear as they were in their natural state would be an unrealistic ideal. If we can hold our own so that streams do not become more polluted, we will be doing very well.

Criteria of stream pollution

In the final analysis, the most reliable single index of stream pollution can be the biochemical oxygen demand (BOD), expressed as the quantity of oxygen required for oxidation or organic matter (expressed in pounds). The capacity of any body of water to oxidize wastes depends on the water's oxygen, oxygen resulting from photosynthesis in algae and other green plants, and the dissolved oxygen already in the water. If the oxygen utilization exceeds oxygen production, a negative oxygen balance occurs and an anaerobic condition results that provides for undesirable bacterial action. A stream need not be in a state of negative oxygen balance to be badly polluted. If the total oxygen demand exceeds the standard per capita demand from domestic sewage of 0.168 pounds of oxygen per day, the stream is likely loaded with excessive pollution.

Other criteria of pollution are also employed. Plankton are used as an index because pollution destroys the normal fauna and flora of a stream. By determining the populations of various species of plankton, it is possible to get an index of the degree of pollution. Other biological forms can also be used as indicators of pollution. A marked reduction in clean water species of life can be used as a criterion of severe pollution.

Classification of streams was established by the first state stream regulating agency, the Pennsylvania Sanitary Water Board, created in 1923. This board established standards for three classes of streams. Class A streams are those in their natural state, probably subject to chance contamination by human beings but unpolluted or uncontaminated from any artificial source. They are generally fit for domestic water supply after chlorination, will support fish life, and may be safely used for recreational purposes. Class B streams are those that are more or less polluted. The extent of regulation, control, or elimination of pollution from these streams will be determined by a consideration of (a) the present and probable future use and condition of the stream, (b) the practicability of remedial measures for abatement, and (c) the general interest of the public through the protection of the public health, the health of animals, fish, and aquatic life, and the use of the stream for recreational purposes. Class C streams are so polluted that they cannot be used as sources of public water supplies, will not support fish life, and are not used for recreational purposes. From the standpoint of the public interests and practicability, it is not necessary, economical, or advisable to attempt to restore them to a clean condition.

Other standards have been established by other stream pollution control boards. Some boards zone rivers. From the practical standpoint, perhaps, standards must be developed for each stream.

Control of stream pollution

The long-established principle of riparian rights holds that landowners have the right to have a stream come down to them with its quality unimpaired and its quantity undiminished. Most people agree that there should be an equitable distribution of water, particularly between states and between communities. Obtaining some degree of equitable distribution and protecting natural waters is a formidable assignment.

Control of pollution of interstate waters is a recognized function of the federal government, and Congress passed PL 845, the Federal Water Pollution Control Law, which went into effect in 1948. This act declared the pollution of interstate waters to be a public nuisance that must be abated. It protected the rights of the states in controlling water pollution. It also provided funds for surveys, investigations, and research. With the expiration of this law in 1956, the act was replaced by PL 660, which delegated to the United States Public Health Service responsibility for administration of the law.

The essence of the law is cooperation with all federal, state, and community agencies engaged in efforts to reduce or eliminate pollution of interstate waters and tributaries. As a supplement to the specifications of the law, provisions are made for personnel training programs, research, and grants to states and interstate agencies for administration purposes. Funds are made available for the construction of community sewage treatment facilities. PL 660 also provides for public hearings, conferences, and even abatement proceedings. This legal action may be taken on the request of any state affected by interstate pollution.

The 1965 Water Pollution Act passed by Congress provided that each state determine the uses of its lakes and rivers. This water-quality approach has much to recommend it but from the practical standpoint is difficult to administer. After 10 years, many states had not established water-quality standards, and other states were unable to reconcile the relationship between pollutants and water use.

In 1971 the Federal Water Pollution Control Act shifted from water-quality standards to direct effluent limits with the theoretical goal to be zero discharge. This act requires polluters to apply for a discharge permit from the Environmental Protection Agency. The first phase of this program ended in 1976, by which time all firms and agencies were obli-

gated to utilize the best available knowledge to control water pollution. The goal of the second phase, ending in 1981, is to achieve water clean enough for swimming and fish propagation. The goal for 1985 is the elimination of all effluents.

Both communities and industries find costs of effluent elimination to be the main hurdle. The National Council on Environmental Quality acknowledges that costs rise exponentially with the degree of cleanliness sought so that the last 1% of treatment could cost as much as the previous 99%. Because of prohibitive costs even with federal subsidies, zero discharge may be an unattainable goal. Perhaps zero discharge may not be necessary and something less can be satisfactory.

Some communities have developed land disposal systems in which wastes are routed through a simple treatment, then stored in lagoons, and finally sprayed over a wide acreage of land. Ecologists favor this approach because it returns invaluable nutrients to the soil. This type of simple approach may provide an acceptable, if not satisfactory, answer to the problem of effluent discharge.

Two or more states set up compacts when a stream is contiguous to more than one state. Some of these agreements are formal, others are informal. Usually, an interstate commission or water control council is created. Cooperation is the purpose for and the key to these programs for pollution control.

Within a state, pollution control may be vested in the state department of health; or some other agency will be responsible for general environmental health problems, including air pollution. The state agency may set up districts or drainage areas to provide control measures best suited to particular problems in specific sections of the state. The state sanitary authority may establish standards of pollution, conduct surveys, and take action to abate a pollution nuisance. However, cooperation is the reasonable approach, and only after all other measures have failed will the state agency resort to legal measures. There is a need for waste disposal and a need for water protection. To reconcile the two is the task that faces every community, every state, and the nation.

GARBAGE AND REFUSE

Community wastes consist of garbage, ashes, rubbish (boxes, papers, other scraps) street sweepings, trade wastes, and occasionally such things as dead animals. Leaves, grass, and shrub cuttings will often be considered wastes that must be disposed of. That communities vary in particular wastes is a common observation. Industrial wastes are normally not a community problem, because industries usually dispose of their own wastes.

Of the solid wastes of a community, garbage poses the most significant health menace because it provides feed for stray dogs, rats, and insects. In some sectors of the nation this may be a minor factor in health, but in some geographical areas dogs, rats, and mosquitoes are hosts of serious diseases and thus constitute a significant threat to health. Rubbish can also harbor rats and insects, but the removal of rubbish is more an esthetic

matter and one of convenience rather than health.

Collection. Both the collection and the disposal of garbage and refuse are accepted government functions. Some communities collect household and commercial garbage and rubbish without charge, the cost being met through general tax funds. Some have charges for garbage and rubbish collections. The responsibility for collection usually rests with the department of public works or some other comparable department, and responsibility for proper sanitation relating to garbage and rubbish usually rests with the health authorities of the community.

Some communities contract with private firms to collect garbage and rubbish. Specifications for collections are set up by the city council and bids are called for. The successful bidder is then granted a franchise for a period of about 5 years, when bids are again called for. The city council specifies what the charges will be and stipulates the frequency of collections. Each householder pays the disposal company for hauling garbage and

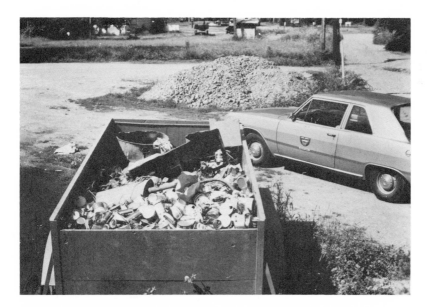

Fig. 14-8. An available container for disposal of household wastes is a first step, but a fly-tight covering is necessary to complete the operation. (Courtesy Environmental Health Division, Lane County, Oregon)

refuse. The garbage is usually collected at regular intervals, and the rubbish is hauled away only on the special request of the householder. Some cities have a can-exchange arrangement, in which the city provides a can, picks up the filled can, and leaves a clean, empty one at each collection. Garbage collections in residential areas vary from weekly to every other day. When ashes are kept separate, a weekly collection of ashes is frequently the pattern. Collections from commercial districts are made six times a week.

A 30-gallon container for garbage is usually adequate for a typical family. Community regulations specify that the containers must be of metal, be rubberized, or be of other special composition. The containers must be watertight, fly-tight, and easily cleaned. A tightly fitting lid is required. The householder is responsible for cleaning out the container and occasionally decontaminating it with some strong germicide such as Lysol. Some communities require that garbage and ashes be separated when incineration is the method of disposal. This may also be required when reduction or hog-feeding is the method of disposal.

Some communities require that garbage cans be lined with paper. Others require that garbage be wrapped either in ordinary paper or in wet-strength paper bags. Again, wrapped garbage is not desirable when hog-feeding or reduction is the method of disposal.

Enclosed trucks with hydraulic hoists for loading and unloading are both sanitary and economical. At least once a week the trucks are steamed and cleaned with detergents.

Disposal. Open dumps, sanitary land-fills, incineration, hog-feeding, reduction, and grinding are the recognized methods of garbage disposal. Most communities use dumps for the disposal of garbage and refuse. Burning at the dump creates a fire hazard and obnoxious smoke and odor. In addition, dumps are breeding grounds for rats and vermin. When the dump is in an isolated area and properly supervised, it could be an acceptable method of disposal.

Sanitary land-fills require a land depression or excavating a trench into which gar-

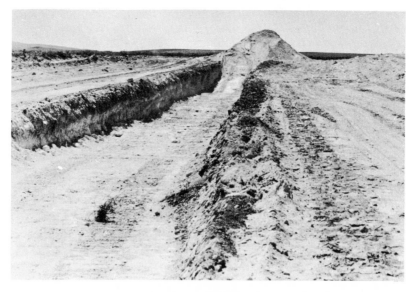

Fig. 14-9. Sanitary land-fill. Excavated trench 6 feet deep and 20 feet wide provides an approved method for disposing of solid wastes. When filled almost to the top, a covering of dirt is scraped over the fill. (Courtesy Idaho Department of Health)

bage is dumped and then covering the fill with dirt. This method serves to reclaim waste lands, does not require separation of ashes and garbage, can be virtually odorless, and can be free of rats and vermin. Availability of an acceptable area may be a problem.

Incineration is an expensive disposal method but is regarded as the most acceptable. Garbage and rubbish need not be separated. Ashes are excluded and, usually, magnetic separators remove cans and other metal objects. Incinerators are composed of a receiving bin, from which refuse is carried by conveyor to a hopper that feeds the refuse into a furnace. Oil, coal, or gas may be used as supplementary fuel for maximum combustion in the furnace. The final ash is removed from the bottom of the furnace and hauled to a dump or a land-fill.

Hog-feeding is an old method of garbage disposal still in use but not approved by health authorities. It requires both a separation of garbage from other wastes and a sorting of the garbage. An area of 2 acres and a ton of garbage per day for 100 hogs is the accepted standard. Even if the piggery is far removed from the community and even if it is well operated, feeding garbage to hogs is objectionable. Spreading garbage, raw and cooked, creates an environment where stench, flies, rats, and other objectionable factors exist. As a source of human trichinosis, garbage-fed hogs must always be regarded as a primary threat, even when an informed public cooks pork adequately before it is placed on the table.

Reduction consists in directly cooking garbage with steam or in steam-jacketed pressure kettles. Reduction plants are uneconomical, and the resulting odor can be highly objectionable. Grease, cattle feed, and other products can be salvaged, but their cash value would cover just a small portion of the cost of operating the reduction plant.

Grinding of garbage and disposal of it in the community sewage is both effective and practical. A large grinding plant receives garbage from the collection trucks and empties the ground garbage into the trunk sewer.

Experience indicates that ground garbage causes no serious interference with sewage treatment. Oxygen demand of the sewage is increased, but not to a degree that would have an adverse effect on the effluent of the treatment or on the terminal waters into which the sewage effluent is emptied.

Domestic garbage grinders attached to kitchen sinks are highly satisfactory although bones and other objects must be separated out. The individual householder can purchase his own grinder from a commercial firm, the city may install home grinder units on a citywide basis and resell to the householder on an installment plan, or the city may retain ownership and charge a monthly rental fee. The municipal sewage treatment plant can handle the ground garbage if the biochemical oxygen demand is in a controllable range. To take care of household garbage in this manner, the community rightfully makes a regular monthly charge.

Recycling certain combustible and noncombustible solid wastes is receiving increased attention by research agencies and community officials. Some states have passed legislation making mandatory a deposit on containers made of glass or metal. Whether this will reduce littering is still a matter of conjecture but certainly recycling merits further study and trial. Up to the present time recycling has not been financially self-sustaining, but the question remains whether recycling should not be continued even at some cost. In the meantime, further research may make recycling financially feasible and the chosen disposal method for certain solid wastes.

Reducing litter

However ugly litter may or may not be, it serves as a signal of a blight on the community that disregards the common good. It would indeed be difficult to establish a relationship between litter and physical health, but the effect of litter on mental health could be appraised although not in precise data.

A great deal is involved in litter reduction and any program to be effective must be based on organization of resources and professional leadership. On the national level the principal voluntary organization for the prevention of litter is *Keep America Beautiful, Inc.* (KAB). The program of this organization will be discussed in Chapter 17.

Oregon and Vermont have passed "bottle bill" legislation emphasizing the return of certain containers and responsibility for preventing and controlling litter. Total litter in Oregon has been reduced 10.6%. In Vermont total litter has been reduced by 14.6%. Both states report that though their programs are not perfect, results thus far have been highly satisfactory.

EVALUATION

Disposal of human wastes will become a spiraling problem demanding greater and greater investment in disposal plants and greater and greater expense in the process. It is a price that must be paid for progress. Man must conduct research to improve methods of waste disposal.

While the individual citizen has a personal responsibility in disposing of wastes, the very nature of waste disposal in a highly urbanized, highly populated nation makes it a community responsibility. It is through a cooperative community approach that this problem will be solved. Citizens must be willing to make the necessary investment for the protection of their health and for the creation and maintenance of an attractive, pleasant environment.

QUESTIONS AND EXERCISES

1. What problems of waste disposal have been created by the development of suburban areas?
2. Why is citizen resistance to change a barrier to community health agencies?
3. The Tokyo system for dealing with sewage appears to be effective. Why should not American cities adopt the Tokyo system?
4. What are the merits of having voluntary organizations initiate and support programs to keep communities clean and attractive?
5. Sewage from less than half the U.S. population is treated. What are the implications?
6. Under what circumstances would you agree that community sewage need not be treated?
7. Under what circumstances would you agree that community sewage should be treated but need not be chlorinated?
8. Appraise the so-called bottle bill as a measure for reducing litter.
9. A community of 10,000 people is considering a bond issue of $1,000,000 to construct a sewage disposal plant. What case would you present to justify the investment?
10. Why, under U.S. law, is a court justified in ordering a community to build and operate a community sewage disposal plant?
11. Locate a community that should construct a lagoon-type sewage disposal unit and explain the basis for your recommendation.
12. What is the most equitable method of charging for sewer service?
13. If communities are responsible for the erection and operation of their own sewage disposal plants, why should the state be the regulating agency?
14. We have had stream pollution with us for 50 years, so why all the concern now about it?
15. If you saw brown scum on a pond, what would you conclude?
16. It has been proposed that certain streams and lakes be abandoned for all purposes except as receiving waters for community sewage. What is your reaction?
17. What governmental agencies should contribute finances for the prevention and correction of stream pollution?
18. Why are garbage collection and disposal not regarded as functions of the health department?
19. Some communities permit householders to burn rubbish in metal incinerators in backyards. What are the pros and cons of such a practice, and what is your recommendation for the matter?
20. What type of garbage and refuse disposal do you recommend for your community, and what is your rationale?

REFERENCES

American Public Health Association: Standard methods for the examination of water and wastewater, ed. 13, New York, 1971, The Association.

American Public Works Association: Refuse collecting practice, ed. 3, Chicago, 1966, Public Administration Service.

Bartlett, R. E.: Surface water sewage, New York, 1976, Halsted Press.

Cargo, D. B.: Solid wastes: factors influencing generation rates (Research Papers Series No. 174), Chicago, 1977, University of Chicago Press.

Ciacco, L., editor: Water and water pollution handbook, vol. 1, New York, 1971, Marcel Dekker, Inc.

CSA Specialists meeting on water treatment, Pretoria, 1960 Proceedings, New York, 1961, International Publications Service.

Davies, J.: Politics of pollution, Indianapolis, 1970, Pegasus.

Ehlers, V. M., and Steel, E. W.: Municipal and rural sanitation, ed. 6, New York, 1965, McGraw-Hill Book Co.

Fair, G. M., and associates: Elements of water supply and waste-water disposal, ed. 2, New York, 1971, John Wiley & Sons, Inc.

Fried, J. J.: Groundwater pollution, New York, 1976, American Elsevier Publishing Co., Inc.

Hopkins, E. J., Bingley, W. M., and Schucker, G. W.: The practice of sanitation, ed. 4, Baltimore, 1970, The Williams & Wilkins Co.

Imhoff, K., and associates: Disposal of sewage and other waterborne wastes, rev. ed., Ann Arbor, Mich., 1971, Ann Arbor Science Publishers, Inc.

International Academy of Sciences: Disposal of low-level radioactive waste into Pacific coastal waters, Washington, D.C., 1962, National Academy of Sciences.

James, R. W.: Sewage sludge treatment, Park Ridge, N.J., 1972, Noyes Data Corporation.

Johns Hopkins University, Department of International Health: The functional analysis of health needs and services, Baltimore, 1976, The Johns Hopkins University Press.

Mara, D.: Sewage treatment in hot climates, vol. 2, New York, 1976, John Wiley & Sons, Inc.

Marx, W.: Man and his environment: waste, New York, 1971, Harper & Row, Publishers, Inc.

Mayall, K., editor: Advances in sewage treatment, Forest Grove, Oreg., 1974, International Scholarly Book Service, Inc.

National Academy of Sciences: Waste management and control, Washington, D.C., 1966, National Academy of Sciences.

Sinks, R. L., and Asano, T., editors: Land treatment and disposal of municipal and industrial wastewater, Ann Arbor, Mich., 1976, Ann Arbor Science Publishers, Inc.

Small, W. E.: Third pollution: the national problem of solid waste disposal, New York, 1971, Praeger Publishers, Inc.

Tchobanoglons, G., and associates, editors: Waste water management, a guide to information sources, vol. 2, Detroit, 1976, Gale Research Co.

Velz, C. J.: Applied stream sanitation, New York, 1970, John Wiley & Sons, Inc.

15 ▪ HOUSING

There is a growing recognition that in the modern complex social structure the public has a responsibility and must have an interest in providing, or making available by some means, acceptable housing for all citizens. This has cast a different light on the role of government in housing, yet it is a logical development, since government has always had an interest in the environment affecting its citizens.

Housing is a private concern, a public health responsibility, a matter of economics, and a measure of personal and family status. Housing is important in terms of physical, mental, and social health, but it also has implications for all phases of human existence.

RELATION OF HOUSING TO HEALTH

It is difficult to isolate the impact of housing on health, because many factors other than housing have a simultaneous effect on the people involved. Where there is top-level housing there is usually a top-level income, a high level of intelligence and education, availability of the best in medical care and hospital services, an excellent nutritional level, beneficial personal health practices, proper dental care, and a host of other factors related to health promotion and protection. Conversely, in poor housing, there tends to be other factors that threaten health and life. Yet it is valid to point out those factors in

housing that are directly and indirectly related to human health.

Physical health. Crowded living conditions increase the transmission of communicable diseases, as revealed by studies on the occurrence of infectious diseases in slum districts. The common communicable diseases occur earlier in slum childhood and the incidence is typically higher than is customary for the child in the general population. The incidence of tuberculosis rises with increased crowding. Communicable diseases may begin in a slum district but can spread to all strata of society.

Inadequate toilet facilities can be a constant threat to health. Lack of sunshine, inadequate artificial lighting, and deficient ventilation and heating can have an adverse effect on general physical well-being. Overcrowding in bedrooms can also affect well-being adversely.

Defective heating units produce hazards of carbon monoxide and fire. Defective floors, stairs, railings, and other structures account for a high accident rate.

Lead in paint has long been recognized as a danger to children, but this concern has increased in recent years as more children become seriously ill or die from eating or sucking on a chip of paint containing lead. Early symptoms and signs of paint poisoning are the skin appearing pasty, sallow, and pale, foul breath, anorexia, indigestion, abdominal pains, joint pains, malaise, fatigue, and weakness.

A program of prevention begins with the firms that produce paints. The industry has accepted its responsibility by producing lead-free paint, but paint 30 years old, which may contain lead, can be peeled off by youngsters and put into their mouths. Health education directed to parents must be a continual operation. Owners of rented property should be urged and even encouraged to scrape off or otherwise remove the paint containing lead and replace that paint with nonlead paint. Official inspections of rental property can be used as educational programs. Cooperation between tenants, landlords, and health officials is the formula for an effective program to protect children from the dangers of lead poisoning.

Mental health. Poor housing conditions promote a decline in pride and motivation, both of which are essential to optimum mental health. There frequently follows a carelessness in living practices, in personal grooming, and in self-growth. Social and esthetic decline results from the uncleanliness and disorder often associated with substandard housing. Confusion, noise, and a lack of privacy are not conducive to a feeling of self-esteem. Poor housing conditions can be depressing. A person living in substandard housing conditions very easily acquires a feeling of being a second-class citizen. From the standpoint of positive mental health, perhaps the lone contribution of poor housing is that it does challenge some individuals to rise above it.

CRITERIA OF SUBSTANDARD HOUSING

The Committee on the Hygiene of Housing of the American Public Health Association (1952) conducted an extensive study of the relationship of housing to health. Its findings and recommendations have been the standard for people in the health field. The Committee declared that if *any four* of the following criteria existed, the term "slum" applied:

1. Contaminated water
2. Water supply outside
3. Shared toilet or outside toilet
4. Shared bath or outside bath
5. More than 1.5 persons per room
6. Overcrowding of sleeping quarters
7. Less than 40 square feet of sleeping room per person
8. Lack of dual egress
9. Installed heating lacking in three-fourths of rooms
10. Lack of electricity
11. Lack of windows
12. Deterioration

Substandard housing is to be found particularly in the blighted areas of cities, that deteriorating section between the business center and the residential section of the community. This is the area on the fringes of the business section, where people live in retail store buildings that are no longer acceptable for commercial purposes. Owners put nothing back into the buildings in the way of maintenance. As a consequence, deterioration, rubbish, garbage, flies, vermin, rats, and fire hazards prevail.

BASIC PRINCIPLES OF HEALTHFUL HOUSING

The Committee on the Hygiene of Housing proposed minimum standards of housing based on fundamental human needs and necessary protection against hazards to health and life.

Fundamental physiological needs

Maintenance of a thermal environment that will avoid undue heat loss from the human body

Maintenance of a thermal environment that will permit adequate heat loss from the human body

Provision of an atmosphere of reasonable chemical purity

Provision of adequate daylight illumination and avoidance of undue daylight glare

Provision of admission of direct sunlight

Provision of adequate artificial illumination and avoidance of glare

Protection against excessive noise

Provision of adequate space for exercise and for the play of children

Fundamental psychological needs

Provision of adequate privacy for the individual

Provision of opportunities for normal family life

Provision of opportunities for normal community life

Provision of facilities that make possible the performance of the tasks of the household without undue physical and mental fatigue

Provision of facilities for maintenance of cleanliness of the dwelling and of the person

Provision of possibilities for esthetic satisfaction in the home and its surroundings

Concordance with prevailing social standards of the local community

Protection against communicable disease

Provision of a water supply of safe, sanitary quality, available to the dwelling

Protection of the water supply system against pollution within the dwelling

Provision of toilet facilities of such character as to minimize the danger of transmitting disease

Protection against sewage contamination of the interior surfaces of the dwelling

Avoidance of insanitary conditions in the vicinity of the dwelling

Exclusion from the dwelling of vermin, which may play a part in the transmission of disease

Provision of facilities for keeping milk and food from decomposing

Provision of sufficient space in sleeping rooms to minimize the danger of contact infection

Protection against accidents

Erection of the dwelling with such materials and methods of construction as to minimize danger of accidents due to collapse of any part of the structure

Control of conditions likely to cause fire or to promote their spread

Provision of adequate facilities for escape in case of fire

Protection against danger of electric shocks and burns

Protection against gas poisonings

Protection against falls and other mechanical injuries in the home

Protection of the neighborhood against the hazards of automobile traffic

These are the minimum basic requirements of good housing considered from the standpoint of health but also significant in economic, esthetic, and social terms. These basic housing needs may vary from one geographical location to another, from one community to another, and even from one section of a community to another. To provide good housing in Montana will be a different matter from providing good housing in Ala-

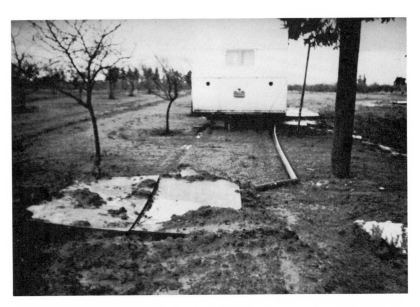

Fig. 15-1. New dangers from new modes of living. The recent trend toward mobile homes poses special health problems, particularly in sanitation. Sewage disposal of the type shown here is a community health hazard.

bama. Housing in the center of a metropolitan area may best be served by high-rise apartments, in the periphery by single unit dwellings. The criteria of housing requirements as set forth by the Committee on the Hygiene of Housing of the American Public Health Association (1952) can still serve as a guide wherever needed, regardless of the circumstances.

BUILDING REGULATIONS AND CODES

Regulations of the construction of housing has long been a recognized governmental function. In the community this authority is exercised through ordinances providing for building zones and for codes governing construction. Zoning is designed to control the type of building to be erected in a given section of a community. One zone may provide only for single-family structures. Another zone may provide for single- or two-family dwellings. Another zone may provide for single, double, or multiple dwelling structures. Another area may be zoned commercial and another one may be zoned industrial. Zoning protects the interests of those people having houses or other structures in an area against having their mode of life jeopardized and the value of their property reduced. Zoning provides a degree of uniformity in planning. In some communities a special planning commission considers matters of zoning and makes recommendations to the city council, which alone has the legal authority to enact local zoning ordinances.

Community building codes specify the type and quality of materials that may be used, standards of construction, quality and proper installation of plumbing fixtures, wiring specifications, and other provisions that will give the prospective dweller, the neighborhood, and the community assurance that the building will meet the needs of the inhabitants in terms of safe and secure living. Communities can enforce building codes by requiring a permit to build. The fee for the permit may be nominal, but in granting the permit the issuing community authority specifies that the permit is issued on the provisions of the building code. Plans for the building must meet zoning and code standards and must be followed in the construction.

The Committee on the Hygiene of Housing of the American Public Health Association has developed a model housing ordinance regulating supplied facilities, maintenance, and occupancy of dwellings and dwelling units. The International Conference of Building Officials has also developed a Uniform Housing Code. Both of these instruments can serve as excellent guides for health personnel and community authorities in developing ordinances or codes.

A building already erected before a building code was in effect will be bound by the requirements of the code if remodeling is to be done. Requiring a permit to remodel provides community officials with a means for requiring that the completed structure conform to code standards.

The housing problem of greatest general concern to the community and of particular concern to the health department is the house that was constructed years before a code existed but that now has deteriorated to a subminimal standard and will continue to decline. All of the objectionable aspects of deterioration will become progressively more apparent. It is doubtful that provisions of the building code can be enforced. Thus this avenue for relief may be closed. However, it is in this type of situation that health departments can play a vital role.

When, in the judgment of health officials, a particular dwelling is a threat to the health of the public, health officials can take necessary steps to abate the condition by negotiation and advisement with the owner or, as a last resort, court action to declare the condition a public nuisance. This approach is also extended to an area where inspections are made, hazards and other unsatisfactory conditions are reported, and a notice is issued to correct the unsatisfactory condition. Diplomacy and reasonable restraint are usually exercised by health officials. Legal measures

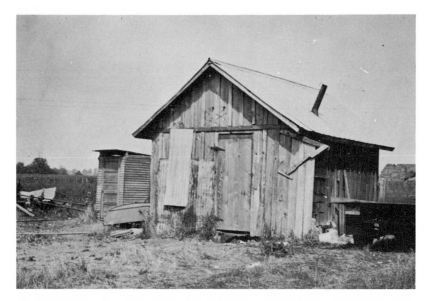

Fig. 15-2. Social engineering needed. Migrant workers living in substandard housing need more than better housing in order to attain an optimum level of health.

are taken only as a last resort. Public support, always essential to the health department, is not something that just happens. It is developed by a continuing program of public education, respect for the health staff earned by its exemplary professional conduct, and a high quality of service to the public.

COMMUNITY RESPONSIBILITY

People living in substandard housing sometimes become so discouraged that they do not recognize the deterioration going on about them. Tragically, children growing up under these circumstances can become so conditioned that they know nothing else, expect nothing else, and care for nothing else. Many people in substandard housing would like to get into something better, but their economic situation has them enslaved. A rising social consciousness has brought America to the realization that society has a responsibility to help these people to help themselves in obtaining acceptable housing. For decades housing was left to the individual or to private enterprise, but we have come to recognize that this was inadequate. A new partner has come into the picture—the governmen-

tal agencies. These are but a logical development if government exists to serve the public in fulfilling its needs. Certainly one of the primary human needs is that of adequate housing—adequate in terms of today's standards. Today we have individual initiative, business enterprise, and governmental agencies participating in the prodigious program of providing appropriate housing for all the American people.

FEDERAL GOVERNMENT HOUSING

In 1937 the federal government instituted a slum clearance and low-rent housing program by creating local housing authorities committed to slum clearance and to the construction of low-rent housing. Projects were initiated by community agencies, which also constructed and operated the housing. Federal funds made up 90% of the financing, with the remainder from municipal or private sources. Loans of federal funds at low interest rates were available. A community was obligated to eliminate a slum dwelling unit for each new low-cost dwelling unit.

The Housing Act of 1949 further extended

federal aid to housing by authorizing financial assistance to communities for the elimination of blighted areas and slums and for redevelopment sites. Federal financial assistance for housing was also given to private enterprise through local agencies. The Housing Act of 1949 also made provisions for area redevelopment. Funds were provided for clearing slums and blighted areas. The work was to be done by the community that possessed the right of eminent domain and could thus appropriate these properties at a fair price. Communities, in turn, could build on the sites or could interest private capital in purchasing the sites from the city and in building approved dwellings or other structures. Certain tax benefits have been granted to private purchasers and developers.

Urban renewal was established by the Housing Act of 1954 (Publication No. 560) as a combination of federal, community, and private resources to replace slum and blighted areas with adequate residential and business facilities. To qualify for federal aid, the community must agree to certain requisites, such as a comprehensive plan of development, and administrative organization, financial adequacy, citizen participation, and responsibility for adequately relocating persons displaced by urban renewal. Not all urban renewal leads to better housing, but the business and other structures that are erected are truly in harmony with the concept of urban renewal and contribute to the physical improvement of the community.

INSTITUTION LOW-COST HOUSING

Institutions with great financial reserves have moved into the housing field and have financed and established many housing developments. Insurance companies are classic examples of firms that have provided housing for low-income families. These have not been philanthropical enterprises but have been soundly financed and soundly operated business promotions. Low-cost apartment houses with low rental rates have been highly successful. Two-, three-, and even ten-story apartment houses have been constructed in

these programs and have given support to the contention that adequate low-cost housing is economically not only feasible, but profitable as well.

NEW APPROACH TO HOUSING AND HEALTH

In public health circles it has long been recognized that the existing static programs of housing and health must be replaced by a dynamic program that has a demonstrable effect on the dwellers, their health, and their mode of living. Elihu D. Richter and co-workers (1973) have come forward with a program modeled after the agricultural service approach. This certainly is one of the most forward-looking programs that has been developed in this area of human need.

Dr. Richter and colleagues point out that there has been a breakdown of the environment within the public domain. As a result of the breakdown, severe health and safety burdens are now imposed on people living in buildings that have every conceivable faulty condition. These authors define semi-public domain as the domain falling between the responsibility of the individual household family on one hand (for example, indoor cleanliness, safety, etc.) and municipal government on the other (public water supply, public sanitation, sewage disposal, etc.).

These investigators report that during the period of 1965-1968 in New York City owners abandoned 107,000 dwelling units housing 428,000 people. It was estimated that during the same period 10,115 low rent units housing 40,500 people were constructed. Dr. Richter and staff pointed out that poor maintenance was the primary problem and that buildings often are structurally sound but poorly maintained. If there is to be preventive maintenance, training of building superintendents is necessary. Building superintendents were poorly paid, with salaries ranging between $2,000 and $4,000 per year. This obviously was one factor in poor maintenance. An upgrading of the role of the tenement superintendent was in order. Dr. Richter points out that publicly subsidized tenement maintenance is a good health measure.

The East Harlem Environmental Extension Service, Inc. (a nonprofit corporation representing housing groups, owners, tenants, and job-training organizations working with the Department of Community Medicine of the Mount Sinai School of Medicine and New York City's Board of Education), is operating a training, stipend, and field service program for East Harlem residents. The Extension Service began its training programs in the winter of 1970. The program started three training cycles of fifteen men with ten more added. During training each participant received $80 per week, rising to $100. By the end of August, 1971, there were forty-one extension agents in the program, but lack of sufficient funding made it necessary to cut back the crew to twenty-five. Subjects taught were boiler maintenance, plastering, painting, electrical work, simple plumbing, carpentry, fire prevention, and rodent and pest control. Red Cross First Aid Training was a key part of the training. A field manual on health and safety was put to use. The program was linked with family health workers, public health workers, public health nurses, and community health guides.

A diversity of projects and proposed programs was introduced into the curriculum. For example, consideration was given to the community provision of steam heat, which would assure residents of home heating without air pollution. What the program did for the trainees was to give them assurance that they now had a vocational skill and service that gave them a place in the employment field.

Perhaps not all communities could operate a program such as that in New York City, but this pioneering project shows the way and encourages other communities to take a look at their situation and to develop a program that will provide improved housing for its citizens. Community leadership is offered an opportunity to initiate and develop housing betterment. A similar concept with inner-city youth was demonstrated in Baltimore by

Virginia Wang and associates (1975), activating the youth enrolled in a community pediatric center to repair broken windows in their neighborhoods.

QUESTIONS AND EXERCISES

1. What is the probability of reaching the goal of adequate housing for all citizens of this nation?
2. Explain this statement: "The effects of substandard housing on health are subtle effects."
3. Explain how the health conditions in the slum can affect the health of all strata in the community.
4. What can be the layperson's contribution to the improvement of housing in a community?
5. Some outstanding men and women have come out of slum areas. What is the explanation and why do not all people in the slums rise above their circumstances?
6. What single deficiency in housing would you regard as the greatest threat to health and why?
7. What causes a "blighted" area to develop?
8. What factors in substandard housing have an adverse effect on mental health?
9. In a substandard house, who in the family is likely to be most affected—the parents, teenagers, or young children?
10. Why would housing tend to be of low quality where tenants move frequently?
11. Poor maintenance is more than poor business, but what other effects does poor maintenance cause?
12. Objections are made to the government providing housing for private citizens, the contention being that this is socialism. What is your reaction?
13. People moving from the center of big cities to the suburbs in many instances create housing problems in the big city. What is the nature of the problem that is created?
14. Explain this statement: "It is not possible to draw up a universally applicable housing code."
15. If an inhabited house in a well-kept neighborhood becomes dilapidated and an eyesore, what factors and interests must be considered in solving the problems involved?
16. To what extent should governmental agencies become involved in housing problems?
17. If an uninhabited house in a well-kept neighborhood becomes dilapidated and a community liability, what steps should be followed to deal with the problem?
18. Various community organizations sponsor home clean-up and paint-up campaigns. What community health implications are involved and what should be the role of health people in such campaigns?
19. In a community controversy involving zoning, what should be the role and position of the official health agency of the community?
20. Analyze your home community in terms of factors

that will affect future housing conditions, and indicate the community health implications.

REFERENCES

American Public Health Association: Basic principles of healthful housing, ed. 2, Washington, D.C., 1950, The Association.

American Public Health Association: Appraisal method for measuring the quality of housing; 1, Nature and uses of the method; 2, Dwelling conditions; 3, Appraisal of neighborhood environment, Washington, D.C., 1952, The Association.

American Public Health Association: Proposed housing ordinance, Washington, D.C., 1952, The Association.

American Public Health Association: Committee on the hygiene of housing: planning the neighborhood, rev. ed., Washington, D.C., 1960, The Association.

American Public Health Association: Guide for health administrators in housing hygiene, Washington, D.C., 1967, The Association.

Beyer, G. H.: Housing and society, New York, 1965, The Macmillan Co.

Clinard, M. B.: Slums and community development, New York, 1966, The Macmillan Co.

Curran, W. J.: Recent Supreme Court decisions on health and housing inspections, American Journal of Public Health **57:**1714, 1967.

DeLeeuw, F.: The distribution of housing services, Washington, D.C., 1972, Urban Institute.

Grier, E., and Grier, G.: Privately developed interracial housing, Berkeley, 1960, University of California Press.

Guomo, M.: The crisis of low-income housing, New York, 1974, Random House, Inc.

Halperin, L.: Cities, New York, 1967, Reinhold Publishing Corp.

Hartman, C.: Housing and social policy, Englewood Cliffs, N.J., 1975, Prentice-Hall, Inc.

Helper, R.: Residential segregation and the real estate broker: ideology and action, Minneapolis, 1968, University of Minnesota Press.

Hepler, D. E., and Wallach, P. I.: Housing today, New York, 1965, McGraw-Hill Book Co.

Kaufman, M.: Housing of the working classes and of the poor, Totowa, N.J., 1975, Rowman & Littlefield.

Kleevans, J. W.: Housing and health in a tropical city, Detroit, 1972, International Book Center.

Lansing, J.B.: New homes and poor people, Ann Arbor, 1969, University of Michigan Press.

Lansing, J. B., and associates: Planned residential environments, Ann Arbor, 1970, University of Michigan Press.

Mandelker, D. R.: Managing our urban development, Indianapolis, 1971, The Bobbs-Merrill Co., Inc.

Mandelker, D. R.: Housing subsidies in the United States and England, Indianapolis, 1973, The Bobbs-Merrill Co., Inc.

Mandelker, D. R., and Montgomery, R.: Housing in America: problems and perspectives, Indianapolis, 1973, The Bobbs-Merrill Co., Inc.

Mascai, J., and associates: Housing, New York, 1976, John Wiley & Sons, Inc.

Meehan, E. J.: Public housing policy: convention versus reality, Edison, N.J., 1975, Transaction Books.

Musson, N., and Heusinkveld, H.: Buildings for the elderly, New York, 1963, Reinhold Publishing Corp.

Paulus, V.: Housing: a bibliography, New Brunswick, N.J., 1975, Center for Urban Policy Research.

Phillips, B. G.: Building law illustrated: a guide to practice, ed. 4, New York, 1967, Barnes & Noble, Inc.

Richards, B.: New movement in cities, New York, 1966, Reinhold Publishing Corp.

Richter, E. D., and associates: Housing and health—a new approach, American Journal of Public Health **63:** (10):878-883, October, 1973.

Senn, C., and associates: Housing—basic health principles and recommended ordinances, Washington, D.C., 1970, American Public Health Association.

Smith, W. F.: Housing, the social and economic elements, Berkeley, 1970, University of California Press.

Starr, R.: Housing and the money market, New York, 1975, Basic Books, Inc., Publishers.

Thomson, B., and Coplan, N.: Architectural and engineering law, ed. 2, New York, 1967, Reinhold Publishing Corp.

Wilner, D. M., and associates: Housing environment and family life, Baltimore, 1962, The Johns Hopkins University Press.

Wolman, H. L.: Housing and housing policy in the United States and the United Kingdom, Lexington, Mass., 1975, Lexington Books.

Wood, E. E.: Slums and blighted areas in the United States, College Park, Md., 1970, McGrath Publishing Co.

16 ■ COMMUNITY FOOD PROTECTION

I aimed for the public's heart and hit it in the stomach.

Upton Sinclair

Dr. Harvey W. Wiley, leader in pure food and drug legislation in America, carried on a long battle to have the first Pure Food and Drug Act passed by Congress in 1906. The Act was directed primarily at food adulteration and was supplemented by the Copeland-Tugwell Act of 1938, which aimed at proper sanitation in processing and handling of foods. The final Act was considerably watered down from the original proposal as the result of lobbying by manufacturers with vested interests. Yet the Food and Drug Administration has ample authority to protect the interests of the public. In addition, other agencies and persons have responsibility for the sanitation and safety of foods.

Legally, the producer, processor, or manufacturer of foods is responsible for sanitary and safe food, which means food that is clean and safe for human consumption. This has long been referred to in common law as the implied warranty or guarantee that the product is safe. Ignorance of the fact that food is contaminated or otherwise objectionable is not a valid defense. Regulatory control of foods sold to the public is still necessary, and the closer this control is to the consumer the more effective the control. On the state level, the department of agriculture as well as the department of health has responsibility in controlling foods. On the community level, the county or city health department has this responsibility.

DISEASE TRANSMISSION BY FOODS

No normal person wants to consume dirty or decomposed food, even though there may be no threat to health. Food must be sanitary and safe in that it is not a vehicle for the transmission of disease. Food can be a source of disease by four different means —inherently harmful characteristics, ptomaine poisoning, toxin transfer, and infection transfer.

Inherently harmful foods. "Food poisoning" is a term so generally used that it encompasses a spectrum of digestive disorders, but distinction should be made between a food that is itself poisonous and a food that merely serves as a vehicle for the transmission of pathogens to man. Certain types of mushrooms are inherently poisonous to all people. Yet these poisonous plants are not a serious community health problem because the general public is quite well informed in this regard. Commercial producers of such foods as mushrooms have both the knowledge and the legal responsibility for providing the market with safe foods.

A food may also be classed as poisonous for a person who is allergic to it. By "allergy" is meant a condition of altered tissue reaction, in which reexposure to a substance produces disturbing effects. About 30% of Americans exhibit food allergies. Rarely does a person have an allergy to a single food. From the community health standpoint, it is important that, through public health education, the public know that food allergy may cause rhinitis, asthma, gastrointestinal disturbances, cardiovascular disturbances, and various skin disorders. The logical corollary is for the informed citizen to seek medical services to determine whether allergies exist.

Ptomaine poisoning. A ptomaine is a toxin formed in the decomposition of protein through bacterial action. Meat that is sufficiently decomposed to possess ptomaines would be totally unpalatable to the human. Even though the meat were this badly decomposed, if it were well cooked before being eaten there would be no harmful results because the heat would break up the protein chains that compose the ptomaines. It is doubtful that anyone in America dies of ptomaine poisoning. The public needs education regarding the question of ptomaine.

Toxin transfer by food. Food occasionally serves as the vehicle for transferring toxins to the digestive system of man. Normal cooking processes usually disintegrate toxins but, because of a lack of understanding, people fail to take precautions necessary to protect themselves against poisoning by toxins carried on food.

Botulism is caused by a toxin produced by the spore-forming organism *Clostridium botulinum,* which is found in alkaline and neutral soils throughout the United States. Raw vegetables have vast numbers of the organism on them but are harmless because the organism is an anaerobe and does not produce toxin in free air. A human being eating raw beans, peas, beets, or other vegetables would not be affected. However, if these vegetables in canning are subjected to an ordinary boiling temperature of 212° F (100° C), the spores withstand that temperature and the organism survives. Placed in the anaerobic conditions of a can or jar, the organism produces toxin. If the vegetables are cooked before they are eaten, the toxin is destroyed. If the vegetables are eaten without being brought to a boil, the toxin can be fatal as it is one of the most potent of known poisons. About 24 hours after the toxin has been ingested, gastrointestinal symptoms may appear. This being a neurotoxin, an acute poisoning of the nervous system becomes apparent and paralysis of the respiratory system occurs or the muscles of swallowing are affected.

Polyvalent antitoxin is given intravenously. Antitoxins are available for two more known types. The important thing is that the antitoxin should be administered as soon as possible to be effective.

Commercial canners using pressure cooking at 248° F (120° C) have the problem solved. The community health problem is that of educating the public of the need to use pressure cookers for canning or to use tyndallization. That means bringing the kettle to a boil (212° F) on 3 consecutive days before canning. The public should know that, regardless of the method of home canning, the best security measure is to bring the vegetables or meat to a boiling temperature before they are eaten.

Infection transfer by food. A food cannot transfer pathogens unless the following favorable conditions exist:

1. The organism must be virile and exist in large numbers.
2. The time interval from reservoir to a new host must be short.
3. The temperature must be favorable (in the neighborhood of 100° F, which is optimum for pathogens of man).
4. Moisture must be available.
5. Very little light can be present.

Many pathogens of man are not transferred by food. Except for a few respiratory diseases transferred via milk, virtually all infectious diseases of man transferred by food are those of the digestive system—amebic dysentery, salmonellosis, tapeworm, trichinosis, typhoid fever, and viral hepatitis. Because cow's milk can be an excellent medium for pathogens affecting the respiratory and other systems of man, a few other diseases also transferred by milk must be mentioned —bovine tuberculosis, brucellosis, diphtheria, human tuberculosis, Q fever, and streptococcal infections. Protection of food is primarily directed toward the prevention of food becoming a vehicle of pathogen transmission, a task that can be accomplished by preventing pathogens from reaching food and by destroying the organisms that have reached food.

CONTROL OF MILK AND MILK PRODUCTS

Pathogens can enter milk from many sources, but there will likely be only two reservoirs—the cow, and human beings who handle the milk. Accordingly, all cows should be tested for tuberculosis, brucellosis, and mastitis, and all reactors should be culled out. Even though pasteurization would destroy the organisms causing these diseases, it would be foolhardy not to use the added safety of preventing pathogens from entering the milk to be consumed by human beings.

Clinical examination of dairy personnel is of questionable value. A history of tuberculosis or typhoid fever would be a significant factor. Most important are knowledgeable personnel who know how disease may be transmitted by milk and who remain off the job during an illness and until a physician has declared the illness to be no longer communicable.

Milk processing. With the use of modern equipment, milk can go from the cow's udder to the bottle without ever being exposed to light. Yet even with the finest equipment, the key factor in milk processing is the quality of the operating personnel. Crews on the farm and in the milk plant who have both know-how and pride are the important link in providing the public with sanitary and safe milk.

Well-constructed stables with cement gutters and outfloors, ample light, and well-maintained ventilation are essential. Fly control should be effective. A separate milking room has merit from the standpoint of sanitation. Whether hand milking or machine milking is used, there should be decontamination of all objects that might conceivably contaminate the milk.

The milk house should preferably be at least 50 feet away from the stable. This applies whether it is merely a producing farm or one that bottles its milk for retail sale. The milk house should be ample in size and should have a cement floor and excellent drainage. Ample ventilation, light, and screening should be provided. An adequate supply of potable water is required, and facilities for providing hot water are necessary for sanitizing all equipment and utensils. All equipment must be noncorrodible and in good condition. Producing farms should filter, or strain, all milk and cool it to 50° F immediately after milking.

Pasteurization is the best available safeguard against transmission of disease via milk. Pasteurization consists in heating a medium to a certain temperature over a period of time, which will destroy pathogens of man but will not appreciably affect the quality of the medium. In the "holding" method of pasteurization, the milk is heated to 143° F and is held at this level for 30 minutes. This method destroys pathogens but does not affect taste, proteins, fats, sugars, or salts. Vitamin C is reduced, but milk is not relied on as a source because the vitamin C content of milk is normally low. The "flash" method of pasteurization does the same job by heating the milk to 161° F for 15 seconds. Modern pasteurizers with extremely sensitive thermostats hold the temperature stable and thus assure dependable pasteurization.

Underpasteurization can be detected easily, because 96% of the milk enzyme monophosphoesterase is destroyed in pasteurization and the ability of the enzyme to liberate phenol is reduced by that amount.

Cooling and bottling should be done immediately after the pasteurizing. A temperature of 50° F should be maintained. Paper containers have advantages and are in wide use.

Regulation of milk supplies. In some states the regulation of milk supplies is a function of the state agricultural department. In other states the agricultural department regulates economic factors and the health department regulates sanitation of milk supplies. Some states have a milk control board. State regulations are essential, but it is on the local level that the most effective control can exist. Accordingly, on the recommendation of the city health department, cities pass milk ordinances regulating the sale of milk in the community. A county, through its health department, can pass and regulate the sale of milk within its jurisdiction. These regulations can exceed state standards but cannot be lower than state standards.

The United States Public Health Service has developed a model ordinance governing the marketing of milk. Communities adopt ordinances that are modifications of the model but that retain the essentials of the model.

Health authorities favor the pasteurization of all milk sold to the public, but in a small village where a milkman may be selling only 20 or 25 quarts a day, the price of a pasteurizer would be prohibitive. However, a milk-borne epidemic of typhoid or dysentery would be far more costly.

The model ordinance recognizes two grades of milk to be sold to the public. In addition to specifications dealing with farm facilities, processing methods, and other essentials, the ordinance sets up laboratory examination criteria of grades of milk. (See chart below.)

Obviously, pasteurized milk with a bacteria count of 50,000 would be much safer for human consumption than raw milk with the same count. These bacteria are harmless to man but they are in index of the sanitary handling of milk. The ordinance also recognizes grade C milk for manufacturing purposes only.

Enforcement of regulations is effected through the issuance of a permit to sell milk following approval of the farm, the processing facilities, and other factors. Inspections by sanitarians from time to time will apprise the dairyman of the sanitary quality of his operations. A health department, after reasonable warnings, may order a dairyman to discontinue the sale of milk. He has the right to appeal to the governing health board or to the courts, or the department may refuse to renew the permit when it expires.

The competitive economic system does much to give Americans high-quality milk products. The dairyman who cannot meet the quality standards of competitors soon falls by the wayside.

Milk-borne epidemics are relatively rare in America, but they can happen. Knowledge and vigilance will continue to protect the community.

Milk products. Manufacture of milk products has become big business, with processes controlled to a degree where the public is well protected. State regulation is supplemented by local supervision. Epidemics or endemics originating with milk products are rare but are always a possibility.

Ice cream mixes are pasteurized. Freezing is usually with chilled brine, and storage is at 10° F. Contamination would come from containers, dippers, and dispensers.

Butter requires pasteurization at higher levels than market milk. Temperatures between 155° and 160° F for 30 minutes are used. The fat is promptly cooled and then held in vats for churning.

Cottage cheese should always be pasteurized and stored at 40° F; otherwise, this medium could easily transmit pathogens of man. Most producers of cottage cheese pasteurize their product.

Cheese, because its curing process kills most pathogens, is relatively safe. "Green" cheese (not time-cured) can transmit pathogens such as typhoid bacillus. Some cheese

| | Sold as raw milk | Sold as pasteurized milk | |
		Raw milk	Pasteurized milk
Grade A			
Maximum bacteria count	50,000 per ml	200,000 per ml	30,000 per ml
Grade B			
Maximum bacteria count	200,000 per ml	1,000,000 per ml	50,000 per ml

manufacturers take the precaution of pasteurizing the milk they use, but most cheese makers do not deem this necessary.

Frozen desserts processing comes under the same official scrutiny as dairy products, generally. Constant supervision is necessary, although the management of most processing plants take pride in their business and can be relied on to produce a safe product. The relationships between processors and inspectors is usually harmonious. Inspectors serve in an advisory capacity on sanitation as well as in a regulating role. Legal measures to control dairy product sanitary standards are usually employed only after all other means have been exhausted.

MEAT PRODUCTS

Meat products are cured or cooked before being consumed. As both processes destroy the pathogens of man, it is natural to ask why there should be a need for governmental regulation of meat production. The answer is that the public rebels against eating the meat from diseased animals. Even though cooking may kill pathogens of man, there is always the possibility that biochemical changes in the animal can give the meat a foul taste and even produce illness in man. In addition, how meat is processed after slaughter affects its palatable and nutritional qualities. Improper canning can also be a danger to man in that pathogens conveyed to the meat can survive and harm man. In addition the public should be protected against the adding of corn meal or other grains to ground meat or other meat products.

Training of personnel, health education, demonstrations, and conferences have been more effective in proper meat processing than has been the use of legal authority. There remains a need for governmental inspection of meat on the federal, state, and local levels, nevertheless.

The Meat Inspection Service of the United States Department of Agriculture was inaugurated by the Meat Inspection Act of 1906. The agency responsible for the administration of the law is the Meat Inspection Division of the Department of Agriculture. The purpose of the Act was to safeguard the public by eliminating diseased or other bad meat from distribution, to supervise the sanitary preparation of meat and meat products, and to prevent the use of false or misleading names or statements on labels. Technically, the authority of the federal agency extends over meats and meat products shipped in interstate or international commerce. In recent years, however, courts have interpreted "interstate" so broadly that virtually all transported meat is being classed as "interstate." This has caused some conflict between federal and state inspection, particularly in those states with decidedly inadequate meat inspection programs. In general, the large meat plants have been under federal regulation and the local plants have been under state or community regulation.

In 1967 Congress passed the first substantive legislation on meat inspection since the original Act of 1906. The new Act provides that, within 2 or 3 years, the states must have "at least equal" requirements or the United States Secretary of Agriculture is authorized to take over interstate meat inspection in states falling below the federal standards. Title I of the Act greatly broadens the scope of the inspection, so that more than 500 additional plants come under federal inspection.

Fresh meats. Some slaughterhouses limit their activities to slaughtering and the necessary cold storage, but many meat packing plants combine slaughtering, cold storage, freezing, smoking, and pickling. Most states supplement the federal meat inspection program by having their own inspection services for those slaughterhouses and packing plants not under federal inspection. However, in many instances the small slaughterhouses are not checked by any agency.

Antemortem inspection of animals before slaughter serves to detect any disease or other adverse conditions. Killing, bleeding, and the care of the hides, organs, and carcasses are observed. Postmortem inspections of the carcasses and organs will detect gross pathology. Tissue examination will further detect disease conditions. Questionable carcasses are condemned, although the meat may be used for some purposes. A "grade" stamp on meat designates the grade quality of the meat, while the "inspection" stamp indicates that the meat has been passed as being safe.

Immediately after slaughter, beef is placed in a cooler at 34° F, where it will be stored from 4 to 6 weeks. This storage improves flavor and texture because of the autolysis that occurs. Beef frozen at −15° F can be stored for more than a year. Pork, veal, and mutton are usually held for 3 days before being cut. Deep freezing and storing at −15° F will keep these meats for long periods.

Curing of such products as bacon, ham, and frankfurters calls for chilled meat that is moderately moist, pickle and brine, and a covered vat to prevent any possible contamination. Cured meats are not necessarily completely protected against spoilage or deterioration. Proper storage is always necessary.

In today's market, luncheon meats pose the greatest danger of all meats and meat products. The usual processing of luncheon meats does not assure the destruction of all pathogens. Packaging and storage under inadequate refrigeration can provide a medium in which pathogens of man can readily multiply; once the package is opened, after handling, the remaining meat may be left at room temperature for some time, and then, in many instances, placed in refrigerators with temperatures considerably above 50° F.

Canned meats. Canned meats are first cooked. High temperatures and pressures are used without seriously affecting the quality of the product. Bacterial contamination can occur, the *Clostridium botulinum* being one of the pathogens that might survive. However, the likelihood is slight with modern methods of meat canning.

Fish is processed much like beef products. Fish can be held at a temperature of 40° F

for 2 weeks and be in excellent condition. Quick freezing of fish, followed by a dip into clean water, produces an airtight coat of ice around each fish. All equipment used in processing fish should be decontaminated daily.

Poultry should be observed for a few days before killing. Poultry is quick frozen at −30° F and stored at −10° F. Canned poultry is processed under steam pressure of about 15 pounds per square inch, which should kill the *Salmonella* organism that fowl may harbor. If cold turkey or chicken is eaten without having been refrigerated since being served hot, salmonellosis transmission might occur.

Because of modern refrigeration and cooking facilities, there is no excuse to transmit disease via meat. Cold meats handled by a person who is an active case or carrier of one of the food-borne diseases is a likely mode of disease transmission via meat. People who know how to prevent the spread of disease via meat can feel secure in their knowledge. The need is public health education to make consumers knowledgeable in disease prevention.

EATING ESTABLISHMENT REGULATIONS

Perhaps no valid proof exists that if dust or other dirt gets on food, persons who eat the food will have their health impaired. Likewise there may be no overwhelming evidence that a person coughing on food will produce illness in a person who eats the food. Yet the public is entitled to sanitary and safe food when it eats in a public eating establishment. *Salmonella* infection and viral hepatitis acquired in public eating places is more common than is generally realized. Amebic dysentery and typhoid fever can also result from eating in restaurants.

A citizen walking into a public eating establishment may be neither qualified nor in a position to judge the sanitation of the place. He has to depend on the expertise and vigilance of the community health staff. Yet, a better informed public could be a positive aid to the health staff by looking for restaurant ratings and by insisting that all public places practice sanitation standards set forth by the health department.

Control measures

Licensing of public eating places is the instrument of control. In order to qualify for a license, the establishment must satisfy the equipment and operating requirements of the health department. Once the license has been issued, health department sanitarians make periodic inspections. Frequency and timing of inspections will depend on the known conditions of the restaurant and the available sanitarians.

Rating of restaurants is usually made following the first inspection. Numerical scores are used for ratings, but sanitarians find such precise rating to be difficult. Some health departments give grades A, B, or C ratings. Other departments give a rating of "approved." A restaurant that is not approved following an inspection will be given a probationary period in which to correct the deficiencies shown on the inspection form. Renewal of the operating permit will be denied if the establishment has failed to correct its faults. The owner may appeal to the community board of health and, in the event of an adverse decision, may appeal to the courts.

Inspections

Many of the factors covered in the inspection of eating establishments are inferentially related to health. For example, it would be difficult to show that a restaurant floor had to be constructed of smooth and nonabsorbent material in order to protect patrons. Yet each item checked in an inspection contributes to the overall image of good construction, good maintenance, and good operating practices.

Clinical examinations of new employees, even accompanied by laboratory tests, are of limited value as a means for preventing spread of disease via the restaurant. A more effective measure is to have employees well informed on the nature of disease spread. They should not come to work when they may have a communicable disease. Workshops for food handlers are held periodically by health departments. This is one of the key factors in protecting the patrons against infectious disease.

A second key factor in the protection of the public is a safe water supply. A third factor is proper toilet and lavatory facilities, with approved methods of waste disposal. Proper refrigeration and storage of food are highly important. Corrosion-proof utensils and equipment should be properly sanitized with detergents, decontaminants, and hot rinse water. All other factors are significant but perhaps not as vital as those enumerated. Many sanitarians contend that rodent control is important.

A meaningful overview of a full inspection can be garnered from the items of inspection of eating and drinking establishments required for its sanitarians by the Oregon State Board of Health. These items are not intended to be listed in the order of importance, but for inspection convenience.

1. Floors
   ( ) Cleanable, good repair
   ( ) Smooth, nonabsorbent
   ( ) Cleaned properly
2. Walls and ceilings
   ( ) Clean, good repair
   ( ) Finished, light color
   ( ) Washable to level of splash
3. Lighting
   ( ) Adequate light: working surfaces, storage rooms, preparation areas
   ( ) Fixtures clean
4. Ventilation
   ( ) Adequate ventilation
   ( ) Free from odors, condensate
   ( ) Stove-hoods and ventilators, adequate design
5. Toilet facilities
   ( ) Clean, ventilated
   ( ) Convenient, ample number
   ( ) Proper construction, good repair
6. Water supply
   ( ) Adequate supply and pressure
   ( ) Approved construction

( ) Safe, complies with state standards

7. Lavatory facilities
   ( ) Adequate, convenient to kitchen
   ( ) Hot and cold water
   ( ) Soap, sanitary towels
   ( ) Clean
   ( ) Good repair

8. Construction—utensils, equipment
   ( ) Cleanable construction
   ( ) Self-draining, no corrosion
   ( ) Free from cracks, chips
   ( ) No open seams
   ( ) No toxic utensils

9a. Cleaning of equipment
   ( ) Clean cases, counters, shelves, tables, meat blocks, refrigerators, stoves, hoods, can openers, freezers, and so on
   ( ) Clean cloths used

9b. Cleaning of utensils
   ( ) Single service used only once
   ( ) Dishwasher, sinks, drainboards, approved and maintained
   ( ) Kitchenware, tableware clean
   ( ) Dishwashing procedures approved

9c. Bacterial treatment—utensils
   ( ) Approved sanitization, time, temperature, chemical concentration
   ( ) Machine properly operated
   ( ) Kitchenware adequately treated
   ( ) Dishtowels not being used

10. Storage—handling of utensils
   ( ) Protected from contamination
   ( ) No handling of contact surfaces
   ( ) Single serviceware properly handled
   ( ) Dippers kept in running water

11. Disposal of wastes
   ( ) Approved liquid waste disposal
   ( ) Plumbing complies with state code
   ( ) Approved garbage cans
   ( ) Covered pending removal
   ( ) Clean and in good repair
   ( ) Garbage storage and removal approved

12. Food temperatures
   ( ) Cold perishable food below 45° F
   ( ) Hot perishable food above 140° F
   ( ) Ice storing, handling approved
   ( ) Thermometer in each refrigerator
   ( ) Refrigerators maintained

13a. Wholesomeness of food
   ( ) Clean, no spoilage, safe
   ( ) Approved sources

13b. Wholesome milk products
   ( ) Milk, milk products approved
   ( ) Milk dispensed properly

13c. Wholesomeness of shellfish
   ( ) Approved sources
   ( ) Stored in original containers

14a. Preparation and storage of food
   ( ) No contamination by immersion, leaking, or condensation
   ( ) Neat storage, off floor

14b. Display—serving food, drink
   ( ) Minimum manual contact
   ( ) Food wrapped or covered
   ( ) Cafeteria front protected

14c. Vector control
   ( ) Fly control approved
   ( ) Roaches, insects controlled
   ( ) Rodents under control
   ( ) Structure rat-proof
   ( ) No animals or fowls
   ( ) All poisonous compounds stored away from food, proper use

15. Cleanliness of employees
   ( ) Clean outer garments
   ( ) Clean hands and nails
   ( ) No spitting, no tobacco used in rooms where food prepared

16. Housekeeping
   ( ) Site, premises neat and clean
   ( ) No operations in private quarters
   ( ) Adequate clothing lockers and dressing rooms kept clean
   ( ) Storage of soiled clothing, linens, mops, and so on

17. Control
   ( ) No person at work with any communicable disease, sores, or infected wounds
   ( ) ORS 624.080 and washing sign posted in all toilets

In the final analysis the integrity of the management and the quality of the employees are the true keys to sanitary and safe food in eating establishments. Restaurant personnel who are aware of their responsibility to the public and who know how to prepare and serve food properly represent the best safeguard the public has when it dines out.

Bakeries and confectioneries. Safeguards in producing bakery and confectionary products are similar to those essential to restaurant operations but somewhat less demanding. Employee exclusion as a communicable disease control measure, safe water supply, proper waste disposal, protection against rodents and insects, refrigeration, and utensil sanitizing are all important. The use of sanitary ingredients and the exercise of sanitary precautions during manufacture are also significant. The use of wrapping and other sanitary provisions are essential in handling and storing the finished product. Cleanliness is the very nature of the bakery and the confectionery and, while sanitary inspections should be made at intervals, these establishments are rarely a source of problems for the sanitarian and even less rarely a vehicle of disease spread.

Retail food stores. Safety of food is a first consideration in protecting the public. Refrigeration and storage are of first importance. Elimination of all spoiled foods should be prompt and complete. Employees who are convalescing from an infection of the digestive tract should not handle uncovered foods, even though it would be difficult for organisms they may put on lettuce or tomatoes to survive the customer's journey home and infect a family member who later eats the vegetable. The risk, though slight, should not be ignored. Safe water should be used for all store purposes.

Cleanliness is a second consideration. Because of modern packaging, the customer is usually assured of clean food, especially because self-service methods give customers an opportunity to do some inspecting themselves. Yet the cleanliness of the whole store is desirable, and store managers know they will not be in business long if their store is not clean.

Community health departments do not find retail food stores a great problem. Occasionally the health department will have complaints against a market. Failure to dispose of discarded produce does pose a problem when employees are lax. A written warning by the health department sanitarian usually produces the necessary results.

APPRAISAL OF FOOD CONTROL MEASURES

Constant vigilance by health officials is essential to protect the public against foodborne diseases. The busy citizen cannot make an inspection of restaurants, dairies, slaughterhouses, or canneries. He must depend on the technical expertise of officials paid from taxes. Yet citizens can aid their own cause by being knowledgeable and by cooperating with public officials who are protecting the public.

From many technical fields mankind has been the recipient of methods and procedures for protection against the transmission of disease and poisons. Freezing as an alternative to canning is both convenient and safe. Chemical additives have been a protection as well as a danger. Legislation has protected consumers against the indiscriminate use of ingredients such as soybeans in hamburgers. Legislation protects the public by requiring sanitation and proper food handling in the retailing business. This has become increasingly important with the growth of food chains and franchise marketing. The "natural food" fads have required some degree of official supervision largely in the area of fair trade rather than as vehicles of disease spread.

Despite all the technical advances in safeguarding the food the public eats, there is always present the need for individual citizens to contribute to their own protection. Such self-supervision requires public health education to be fully effective. Constant, well-formulated health education will be valuable to all health programs.

QUESTIONS AND EXERCISES

1. Why do manufacturers lobby against proposed legislation that is designed in the public interest?
2. In terms of health protection, what is the value of home freezers?
3. Why are most cases of food-borne infections to be found in the lowest economic, social, and educational groups in the nation?
4. Why should or should not food allergy be regarded as a community health problem?
5. To what extent is the prevention of food-borne disease a matter of community health education?

6. Botulism occurred from eating lake fish produced by a commercial cannery. What is your explanation of how this happened?

7. Why are respiratory diseases not transmitted via solid foods such as vegetables, fruits, and baked goods?

8. If pathogens are destroyed by pasteurization, why are cows with brucellosis, tuberculosis, or mastitis culled out as producers?

9. A dairy inspector once remarked that a certain dairyman could not produce satisfactory milk if he had the best equipment in the world. What was meant and what is the significance?

10. If the bacteria count of milk is not of pathogens, what is the significance of the bacteria count?

11. Why is more attention given to underpasteurization than overpasteurization of milk?

12. When some cases of disease, such as typhoid, are traced to pasteurized milk, what are some possible breakdowns in the milk processing that account for the disease transmission?

13. Why are knowledgeable dairymen so eager to do everything possible to prevent the spread of disease via the milk they sell?

14. Why is prepackaged meat displayed in open cases an important factor in the sanitary handling of meat?

15. Should governmental officials prohibit adding ingredients to meats or permit adding ingredients under governmental inspection and control?

16. In a certain junior high school, thirty-one cases of viral hepatitis occurred. Propose a hypothesis on the source and transmission of the disease.

17. Which is more important in restaurant sanitation —what is done in the dining area or what is done in the food preparation area, and why?

18. In restaurant rating, which do you prefer—an A, B, or C rating or an "approved" or "not approved" rating, and why?

19. In a certain bakery, one of the bakers was under treatment for syphilis. Appraise the situation and indicate what the community health department should and should not do.

20. If a community health department has a shortage of sanitarians, where should inspection be concentrated or emphasized by the available sanitarians?

REFERENCES

Bigwood, E. I., and associates, editors: Food additives tables, New York, 1976, Elsevier Scientific Publishing Co.

Brisco, A.: Your guide to home storage, Bountiful, Utah, 1974, Horizon Publishers.

FAO-WHO Expert Committee on Food Additives, Geneva, 1975, World Health Organization.

FAO-WHO Exports on Pesticide Residues, Rome, 1975, Pesticide residues in food, Report, Geneva, World Health Organization.

Food Protection Committee of the Food Nutrition Board: Evaluating the safety of food chemicals, Washington, D.C., 1976, National Academy of Sciences.

Inglett, G. E., editor: Symposium: sweetness: proceedings, Westport, Conn., 1974, Avi Publishing Co.

Jernigen, A., editor: Iowa State Department of Health, Food sanitation study course, Ames, Iowa, 1971, Iowa State University Press.

Leitch, J. M., editor: Food science and technology in five volumes, New York, 1966, Science Press, Inc.

Longree, K.: Quantity food sanitation, New York, 1967, John Wiley & Sons, Inc.

Marr, J. S.: The food you eat, New York, 1973, M. Evans & Co., Inc.

Roth, J.: Complete book of canning and freezing, New York, 1976, David McKay Co., Inc.

Sullivan, G.: Additives in your food, New York, 1976, Cornerstone Library, Inc.

U.S. Public Health Service: Food service sanitation manual, including a model food service sanitation ordinance and code, Public Health Service Publication No. 934, 1963.

Verrett, J. and Carper, J.: Eating may be hazardous to your health, Garden City, N.Y., 1975, Anchor Press, Doubleday and Co., Inc.

Whelan, E. and Stare, F. J.: Panic in the pantry, Boro of Totowa, New York, 1975, Atheneum Publishers.

17 ■ OTHER ENVIRONMENTAL AND OCCUPATIONAL HEALTH PROBLEMS

Away, then, with crowded cities, the 30 feet lots and alleys, the artificial reservoirs of filth, the hotbeds of atmospheric poison. Such are our cities. They are great prisons built with immense labor to breed infection and hurry men prematurely to the grave.

Noah Webster, 1799

Ecology and "general environment" are convenient descriptive terms in daily communication but of only theoretical value to the health scientist. Effective community health practice dictates that efforts and actions be directed to specific things in the environment. Health personnel deal with specific conditions in the environment and, while it is practical to speak of air pollution, noise, insect control, and rodent control, specific problems exist within each of these categories. Factors in the environment affecting health, welfare, and life itself must be dealt with as specific entities.

Air pollution, noise, and other aspects of environmental health are not new. These are conditions that have been with man through the centuries. It is a matter of degree and public redefinitions of acceptable conditions that is the concern in dealing with these factors in environmental health.

OCCUPATIONAL HEALTH

The objective of occupational health is the personal health of the worker and, logically, also involves environmental health. Modern occupational health promotion has been extended to include nonoccupational as well as occupational factors that affect the health of workers.

Management usually has a legal responsibility for factors affecting the health of workers, but in many instances management goes beyond legal requirements. Indeed, frequently management concerns itself not only with the well-being of workers but with the welfare of their families as well. This policy may be regarded as benevolence by some people and is criticized as paternalism by others. Yet, at times, it is necessary to extend the health program beyond the plant to the home. A classic example is the migratory worker whose home conditions may be a far greater menace to health than is the occupation.

Because many workers are overlooked in the promotion of industrial health, the community must be concerned. This concern extends itself beyond mere legal requirements to the sphere of whatever measures are essential for the protection and promotion of the health of every worker.

An occupational health program properly goes beyond the prevention of hazards to physical and mental health and extends into the positive promotion of the health of workers. Health education, rest, recreation, treatment of sudden illness, optical services, and even diagnosis of ailments are aspects of modern occupational health promotion. A competent, trained worker is a valuable asset in industry. The same worker possessing a high level of health is an even more valuable asset. Management is interested in the quality of health possessed by its employees for economic reasons, which include concerns with absenteeism, productivity, and satisfaction with working conditions.

Attempts to promote the health of workers should be encouraged, not as a legal requirement, but as a product of collective bargaining if not as the self-initiating action of management. The protection of workers by preventing hazards of occupations however, is of such public concern that it must be translated into legal codes recognizing minimum responsibility for reducing hazards in occupations. Most managements accept this responsibility willingly and go beyond legal stipulations, but some are governed entirely by the requirements of the law in dealing with occupational health and safety.

Hazards of occupations

Some hazards to health are always present in any occupation, operation, plant, or industry. It is a matter of degree with which we deal. Some hazards are so extreme that they must be eliminated or markedly reduced, while others are somewhat innocuous and are of minor concern.

Accidents. Injuries are an immediate concern in virtually all occupations. Industries alert to their responsibilities in injury control, particularly in those hazardous conditions peculiar to their particular industry, and are concerned almost entirely with the safety of their own employees. However, in some industries, such as transportation, the problem is extended to possible injuries to others as well as employees.

Prevention of injuries is an employee, as well as an employer, responsibility. Safe workers carry a certain degree of responsibility for other workers, but such responsibility cannot logically be far-reaching. Because unsafe practices loom so important in occupational accidents, identifiable accident-prone workers must be shifted to jobs that they are qualified to do safely.

Systematic plant inspections are conducted for the detection of hazards that can

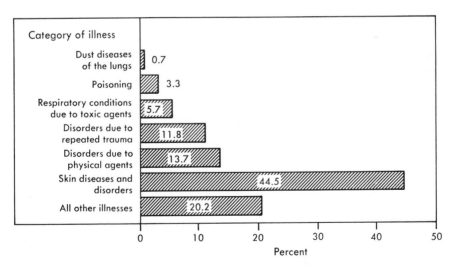

Fig. 17-1. Percent distribution of illness by category of illness, 1973. More than 200,000 occupational illnesses in the United States were reported in 1973. The largest number of reported illnesses was occupational skin diseases. (From Bureau of Labor Statistics, U.S. Department of Labor, unpublished data, 1973; and American Public Health Association, Washington, D.C., 1975)

cause either disease or injury. Safety engineers or other experts carry out these inspections. Rules are formulated to safeguard all employees as well as to promote maximum production. Through their safety committees, workers can participate in the establishment of rules of safety and thus are more responsive to compliance with regulations.

Practices of the workers are most important in industrial safety, but management can supplement their efforts by providing conditions and devices that will afford protection. Guards, goggles, helmets, and other protective clothing may appear to be of little significance but at a particular moment may be the difference between sight and blindness or even between life and death.

First-aid instruction for key employees is a recognized arm of an industrial safety program. On-the-job training in first aid is an investment in the prevention of further harm or even death. The psychological benefits of the first-aid training program can be considerable.

Dusts, gases, and fumes. Dusts, gases, and fumes can be a hazard to the general public as well as to employees. Fortunately, means are available to reduce these hazards to tolerable levels. At conferences of Government Industrial Hygienists, maximum allowable concentration values for various industrial poisons have been adopted. These standards refer to average concentrations that can be tolerated 8 hours per day continuously without impairment to health immediately or in the future.

Dusts are generally classed as inert, irritating, and toxic. Inert vegetable and animal dusts are present in paper making, weaving, spinning, and other manufacturing processes using wool and similar raw materials, but the dangers are not great. Mineral and metallic dusts are more dangerous. Stonecutters, drillers, miners, grinders, and polishers encounter respiratory damage resulting from inert dusts. Granite and quartz dust cause damage to the lungs resulting in a condition termed *silicosis*, which is fatal unless the con-

dition is recognized early and exposure to dust is prevented.

Dusts pose two problems: The first is that of concentration, which can be measured by devices such as the Greenburn-Smith impinger. The second is the important matter of particle size, which can be measured by photographic techniques, microprojectors, filar micrometers, and other devices.

Inert and irritating dusts usually can be reduced and removed. Wet processing reduces the production of dust. Enclosing work that creates dusts, combined with the use of exhaust systems, can reduce dust to a level below the danger point.

Toxic dusts, gases, and fumes such as arsenic, mercury, lead, iron oxide, sulphuric acid, carbon monoxide, and manganese pose specific problems of control. Management is usually alert to hazards of this type and is constantly devising procedures to reduce and eliminate these dangers. Research, often with an assist from governmental agencies, is developing measures for the prevention of these industrial hazards. While the immediate concern is for the worker within the plant, management also has a concern for possible effects on the general public. It is generally conceded that no industrial process hazardous to human health is so indispensable to the economy that it could not be eliminated if it cannot be altered sufficiently to protect the health of workers.

Excessive temperature or humidity. Blast furnaces, smelters, kilns, tanneries, textile mills, laundries, and breweries are examples where the industrial process itself makes atmospheric control difficult. Dermatitis, gastrointestinal disturbances, eye inflammations, and even exhaustion result from atmosphere extremes. Air conditioning can bring atmospheric conditions to tolerable levels. Some workers are physiologically not equipped to tolerate even moderate atmospheric change.

Excessive noise. Industry recognizes that noise is more than a health hazard, as it affects production. Noise is measured in decibels. The lowest sound the human ear can detect is one decibel (db). Loudness is expressed as multiples on a logarithmic scale of the smallest distinguishable sound. Thus, a sound of 10 decibels is ten times louder that 1 decibel. A sound of 20 decibels is 100 times louder than the lowest sound. This logarithmic expression is used as a convenience in avoiding the use of numbers in four or more figures. Long doses of 90 decibels can cause hearing loss. Higher levels can be injurious to hearing, and lesser levels can be disturbing. Annoyance threshold for intermittent sounds is 50 to 90 db, discomfort is at 110 db, and pain threshold is in the vicinity of 120 db. A short exposure to a noise of 150 db can cause permanent hearing loss.

Decibel levels obviously vary: whisper, 10 db; quiet street, 50 db; normal conversation, 50 to 60 db; truck, sports car, 90 db; pneumatic jackhammer, 95 db; loud outdoor motor, 100 db; loud power mower, 105 db; siren, 125 db; riveting, 130 db; jet takeoff, 150 db. Rock music bands have adversely affected the hearing of its members, indicating a hazard of that occupation.

Infections. Infections are a latent hazard in all occupations and are a particularly serious hazard in some industries. Slaughterhouse employees, dairymen, and others who handle livestock or hides are exposed to such diseases as brucellosis and anthrax. Other workers handle substances that serve as media for pathogens of man. The use of disinfectants and sterilizing methods should prevent most infections in these categories. Medical attention to all suspected infection is necessary in industry as well as elsewhere.

Poisons. Harmful substances other than gases and fumes can be present in industry. Chemicals used in plant operations can cause harm to the skin. Chronic poisoning can occur in workers improperly handling materials in routine operations. Knowledge of the presence of these hazards and proper regulations governing their handling reduces or virtually eliminates the danger. Legal regulations and management alertness combine

to make poisoning rather rare in modern industry.

Radiation. Health hazards of radiation are not a new concern. Luminous paints containing radioactive compounds were recognized as a hazard more than 50 years ago.

Today, the use of radioactive products commands special precautions of shielding and the use of personal safety measures such as protective clothing. A necessary safeguard is the use of meters for recording the amount of exposure to radiation. Standards for maximum permissible concentration (MPC) of radiation have been established.

Monitoring, shielding, and other safeguards are practiced constantly. Disposal of radioactive wastes is in conformity with standards set by the U.S. Atomic Energy Commission. Sufficient knowledge on radiation hazards is now available, and industry is applying this knowledge to prevent any radiation danger to employees or to the general public.

The current opposition to reactors is partially the usual clamor when new developments are introduced, according to those who work with radioactive materials. But the concerns are related to environmental effects as much as to health effects.

Sanitation. Proper sanitation measures have long been a concern and accepted responsibility of industry. Industrial sanitation programs are designed to provide conditions that will safeguard the health of employees as well as provide for maximum production.

A safe and adequate water supply is a first requisite. Industries usually obtain their water from an approved municipal supply. If a private source is used, it should be free from turbidity and contamination and should be tested regularly. A daily test would be called for when a threat of contamination is present. Once a week can be ample at other times. About 20 gallons per worker per day is necessary for all purposes, although the amount varies with the kind of industry involved. Approved-type drinking fountains are placed in convenient locations, the number depending on the number of workers and the nature of their work.

When an auxiliary water supply is used for fire protection, flushing, and other such purposes, this second supply should be safe for human consumption or so controlled that there will be no possibility that workers will use the unsafe water for drinking or handwashing purposes. Using red or other color on faucets or fixtures is a common safeguard.

An approved type of sewerage system for liquid wastes is an indispensable sanitation need. If the plant sewerage system cannot be connected to a community system, then provisions must be made for plant sewage disposal.

Toilets and washrooms must be of good construction with adequate toilets and washbasins. The number of toilet units varies from one per ten workers to one for thirty workers. When urinals are installed, only two-thirds as many units are needed.

Washing faucets may be preferred over washbasins because they are less likely to be a means of infection spread. Automatic control of temperatures at 125° F is possible with the mixtures of hot and cold water running from the same faucet. Liquid soap is preferred merely because bar soap too easily finds its way to the floor. Shower-bath heads are attached to the wall usually just below average worker chin level.

Illumination. Lighting meeting recom-

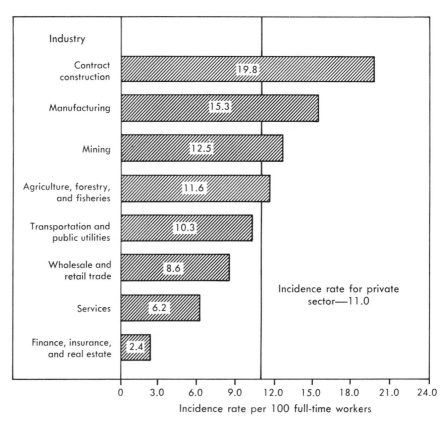

Fig. 17-2. Injury and illness incidence rates, by industry division, United States, 1973. The incidence rates for occupational injuries and illnesses per 100 full-time workers were highest in the contract construction industry. (From Bureau of Labor Statistics, U.S. Department of Labor, unpublished data, 1973; and American Public Health Association, Washington, D.C., 1975)

mended standards reduces accidents and eyestrain and improves efficiency and productive output. Where high detail and speed of vision is required, as much as 100 footcandles are recommended. Illumination of 50 footcandles is required. Along hallways, or where no great visual discrimination is called for, from 10 to 20 footcandles can be adequate. It is always important to avoid great contrasts in degree of illumination. A ratio of 5 to 1 is preferred with 10 to 1 the outside limit.

Ventilation. Properly, ventilation of industrial plants is designed to provide physical comfort by controlling the temperature, humidity, and movement of air. Either natural or artificial means are employed. Removing body heat and moisture in the summer and providing circulation and moderate temperature in the winter are the customary goals. Temperature between 66° and 72° F with a relative humidity of 50, combined with movement of air, provides for physical comfort.

Some industries have the problem of removing dusts, gases, vapors, and fumes, for which exhaust systems are employed. If air is recirculated, the ventilation system must be operating efficiently at all times. This requires competent maintenance.

Responsibility for occupational health. Management, workers, unions, local government, state government, and the federal government all have responsibilities in occupational health. Local health departments are rarely equipped to provide the highly technical professional services that occupational health problems command. Whether the local health department can provide extensive or decidedly limited service, the whole approach must be that of cooperation between all persons concerned with a particular occupational health situation. Health departments do not enter these situations as policemen but as public servants ready to assist with health problems that exist. Only when industrial management fails to live up to established and accepted standards will the force of legal authority be exercised.

A state occupational health division may be in the state department of health or the state department of labor. In either arrangement, the purpose of the occupational health staff is to assist all industry with health problems unique to the industry, to conduct surveys, and to enforce regulations relating to occupational health. Teamwork between industry, workers, and official occupational health personnel is the key to effective programs for the promotion of ˙occupational health.

On the federal level the National Institute for Occupational Safety and Health was created by the Occupational Safety and Health Act of 1970 (PL 91-596). Congress declared as its purpose and policy in this Act "to assure so far as possible every working man and woman in the Nation safe and healthful working conditions and to preserve our human resources"

1. By encouraging employers and employees in their efforts to reduce the number of occupational safety and health hazards at their places of employment, and to stimulate employers and employees to institute new and to perfect existing programs for providing safe and healthful working conditions
2. By providing that employers and employees have separate but dependent responsibilities and rights with respect to achieving safe and healthful working conditions
3. By authorizing the Secretary of Labor to set mandatory occupational safety and health standards applicable to business affecting interstate commerce and by creating an Occupational Safety and Health Review Commission for carrying out adjudicatory functions under the Act
4. By building upon advances already made through employer and employee initiative for providing safe and healthful working conditions
5. By providing for research in the field of occupational safety and health, including the psychological factors involved, and by developing innovative methods, techniques, and approaches for dealing with occupational safety and health problems
6. By exploring ways to discover latent dis-

eases, establishing causal connections between diseases and work in environmental conditions, and conducting other research relating to health problems, in recognition of the fact that occupational health standards present problems often different from those involved in occupational safety

7. By providing medical criteria which will assure insofar as practicable that no employee will suffer diminished health, functional capacity, or life expectancy as a result of his work experience

8. By providing for training programs to increase the number and competence of personnel engaged in the field of occupational safety and health

9. By providing for the development and promulgation of occupational safety and health standards

10. By providing an effective enforcement program which shall include a prohibition against giving advance notice of any inspection and sanctions for any individual violating this prohibition

11. By encouraging the States to assume the fullest responsibility for the administration and enforcement of their occupational safety and health laws by providing grants to the States to assist in identifying their needs and responsibilities in the area of occupational safety and health, to develop plans in accordance with the provisions of this Act, to improve the administration and enforcement of State occupational safety and health laws, and to conduct experimental and demonstration projects

12. By providing for appropriate reporting procedures to help achieve the objectives of this Act and accurately describe the nature of the occupational safety and health problem

13. By encouraging joint labor-management efforts to reduce injuries and disease arising out of employment

AIR POLLUTION

Community air pollution is generally regarded as the presence in the ambient (surrounding) atmosphere of substances put there by the activities of man in concentrations sufficient to interfere directly or indirectly with one's comfort, safety, or health, or with the full use of one's property. In general it does not refer to the atmospheric pollution incident to employment in areas where workers are employed, nor is it concerned with air-borne agents of communicable disease, nor with overt or covert acts or war. It does not deal with natural air pollution such as dust from deserts or barren areas, gases from volcanoes or geysers, sea spray, or pollution from other sources to which man has been exposed. From the earliest of times man-made pollution has been the concern and the problem.

Man-made pollution comes from industrial exhausts, home heating, incineration, open fires, open dumps, dust from roads such as blacktop roads, engine exhaust, crop spraying, construction debris, and other sources. Pollutants may be in the form of solids, liquids (vapors), and gases. Perhaps there is no such thing as a typical area, but the atmosphere of a representative industrial area will have about 22% of its pollutants from industrial sources, about 10% from commercial sources, and the remaining 68% from public sources. It must be pointed out that pollution is not a problem unless there is a receptor—essentially, human beings adversely affected by the pollution.

Smog is the result of the photochemical reaction of hydrocarbons and sulfur oxides produced by sunlight. Nitrogen dioxide acts as a photoreceptor and is decomposed to nitrogen oxide and atomic oxygen. This reactive form of oxygen attacks hydrocarbons, and a further chain of reactions results in a complex mixture of toxic substances. Smog thus tends to have both an irritating and a direct toxic effect on human beings.

As a threat to human well-being, the most devastating effect of air pollution results when a temperature inversion occurs. The Los Angeles area is particularly plagued by this problem. Warm air normally rises, but a layer of warm air resting on top of relatively cool air pins the cool air down much like a lid on a kettle. The topography formed by the mountains to the east prevents winds

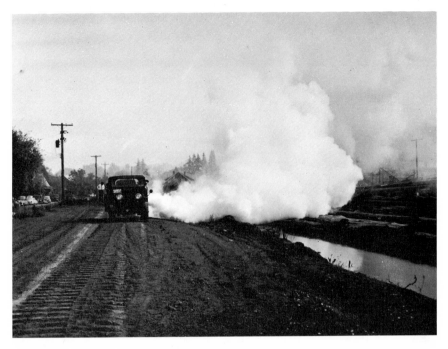

Fig. 17-3. Insect eradication. Solving one problem can create another problem. Eliminating mosquitoes by spraying can create air pollution. Solving the energy crisis may create additional pollution. (Courtesy Lane County, Oregon, Department of Health and Sanitation)

from driving off the immense amounts of smoke, fumes, and other pollution.

Health aspects. More research is necessary before precise statements can be made on the specific effects of pollution on human health. Sufficient empirical evidence does exist to alert communities to the possible dangers of air pollution. Some effects are acute and can be fatal, while some effects are delayed and may be apparent only after years of exposure.

Three cities have experienced air pollution disasters. In the Meuse Valley, Belgium, in 1930, sixty people died as the result of heavy air pollution. In Donora, Pennsylvania, in 1940, a reported twenty people died from pollution. In London in 1952, during a 2-week period of air pollution, about 4,000 more people died than normally. In all of these cities a heavy fog settled over the area and did not lift, but retained the air pollutants. In all three cities most of those patients who died had had chronic respiratory or circulatory diseases. A large portion were the elderly.

People with asthma and other respiratory diseases have their condition aggravated by air pollutants. Eye, nose, and throat irritation may be mild, moderate, or severe, depending on sensitivity and specific air pollutants. Irritation of the lungs may make individuals more susceptible to lung infections. Carbon monoxide poisoning may affect heart action adversely and have delayed adverse effects on a person. Gastrointestinal disturbances, especially in children, appear to be more prevalent during periods of heavy air pollution.

Economic and esthetic aspects. Air pollution can damage trees, shrubs, and flowers and ruin crops. Cattle become ill from air pollutants. Air pollution causes damage to residences and other structures. It can soil and damage clothing. It can interfere with the enjoyment of an otherwise attractive environment. Air pollution properly can be declared a nuisance on esthetic as well as health grounds. Economic damage has been adjudicated on a monetary basis. Persons who believe that they have been harmed or inconvenienced or have suffered monetary loss can obtain redress in court. A suit for damages against the firm or persons creating the objectionable air pollution can result in a judgment of monetary compensation for the damage to the plaintiff's person or property. Courts have awarded compensation for harm to cattle resulting from air pollution caused by industrial plants producing aluminum products.

Pollution control

In the absence of precise air quality criteria, the *usual* approach has been to control the *sources* of pollution even though such control measures must rely on empirical methods. To control and regulate air pollution by solid particles is not difficult. Various smoke-inspection devices are available for measuring the density of smoke and other particles in the air.

With established means for measuring smoke pollution, cities have passed ordinances limiting the emission of smoke to periods of 6 minutes in 1 hour for industrial plants. Proper firing and design of coal furnaces eliminates 90% of smoke from industrial plants.

Control of pollution by smoke is relatively easy. Unfortunately most serious air pollutants are sulfur oxide, nitrogen oxide, and motor vehicle pollution, and these are more difficult to measure.

Sulfur oxide pollution arises principally from the combustion of sulfur-containing coal and fuel oil and is highly injurious to human health, to property, and to vegetation. The increased use of sulfur-containing fuels threatens a fourfold increase in sulfur oxide pollution by the end of this century. Use of low-sulfur fuels or removing sulfur from fuels before they are burned will reduce pollution. Natural gas is somewhat free of sulfur and is preferable to other fuels in terms of reduction of air pollution. Coal is still the nemesis, because only a fraction of its sulfur content can be removed before burning. Efforts are now directed toward removing the sulfur oxides from the combustion gases before they escape into the air.

Nitrogen oxides are a by-product of all combustion processes, including those from automobiles. At present, nitrogen oxide pollution is not as serious a problem as sulfur oxide pollution; but, as fuel combustion increases, the nitrogen oxide pollution problem will increase proportionately unless control methods are discovered.

Motor vehicle air pollution is more extensive than sulfur oxide and nitrogen oxide pollution, but motor vehicle air pollution is yielding to newly developed control techniques. Among the methods effective in reducing tailpipe emissions are the modification of motors to achieve more complete combustion, the injection of air into the exhaust system to oxidize the gases before they reach the tailpipe, and the passage of exhaust gases through afterburners before they are released into the air. Some of these methods were applied by American automobile manufacturers in the form of catalytic converters and exhaust gas recirculation to comply with the standards established by the Secretary of Health, Education and Welfare, as authorized by the Clean Air Act adopted in 1965. The Secretary has authorization to revise standards in accordance with the increase in knowledge of the nature, effects, and control of motor vehicle air pollution. With 110 million motor vehicles on the highways, just keeping up with the air pollution problem will require extensive research and drastic control measures, but the energy crisis is now making it difficult to adhere to some of them.

Legislation. Back in the era when air pollution meant smoke pollution, community ordinances could be enacted to control the problem because the smoke constituted an obvious nuisance. In addition the degree of smoke pollution could be measured with some precision. Today, air pollution is more subtle and can no longer be regarded as a localized, strictly community concern. Air pollution is a national problem that recognizes no geographical or political boundaries. Pollution originating in one state can affect people in an adjoining state. It thus becomes evident that air pollution must be regarded as a national problem dealt with on a national scale in which cooperation and mutual assistance rather than coercion is the approach. Regional and local planning are essential, but such planning must be coordinated with all related programs.

The first identifiable federal air pollution control program was established in 1955 as a consequence of the action of Congress, which passed PL 84-159 in order "to provide research and technical assistance relating to air pollution control." The act directed the Secretary of Health, Education and Welfare to prepare research programs on pollution control, encourage cooperative state and local activities, collect and disseminate information, conduct research and surveys, and make grants for training, research, and demonstration projects.

With the adoption of the Clean Air Act in 1963, Congress acknowledged that federal financial assistance is essential for the development of programs to control air pollution. Matching funds encouraged state and local governments to initiate air pollution control programs. The Act encouraged area-wide interjurisdictional control of air pollution on a regional basis. The Act included legal regulatory authority on the federal level for the abatement of specific pollution problems with respect to the following two types of situations:

1. When pollution originating in one state affects persons in another state, the Secretary of Health, Education and Welfare may initiate formal abatement proceedings.
2. When pollution of an interstate nature occurs such that air pollution affects persons, the Secretary may invoke formal abatement proceedings only on request from designated officials in the state involved.

In 1967 Congress passed and the President signed the Air Quality Act, authorizing $428.3 million for federal air pollution control efforts in fiscal years 1968, 1969, and 1970. Of the total authorization, $125 million was earmarked for research. The Act provides that the federal government can step in to control air pollution when the state fails to act. No national emission standards for specific pollutants were set up, but provisions were made to study the problem of standards. The Secretary of Health, Education and Welfare was authorized to designate air quality control regions throughout the nation, and the Act provided funds for regional control commissions. All of these Acts have had further amendments and will continue to be amended as knowledge and conditions change.

State programs. While states were slow to initiate pollution control programs, the stimulation of federal legislation and funding had changed this picture so that by 1965, forty states had pollution program budgets of $5,000 or more. The recognized minimum per capita expenditure for an adequate state program is set at $0.25, and few states have reached this level, indicating that most state programs are not yet in that stage where effective control measures can be taken.

An effective state air pollution control program requires the following basic factors:

1. A sanitary authority with status, funds, and research including field studies
2. Regional approach to air pollution control
3. Calculated program to reduce pollution each year
4. Licensing of new industries and new operations based on realistic appraisal of all factors involved
5. Industrial zoning based on an intensive study of all factors involved, including the economic benefits to be gained for each proposed industrial installation
6. Impartial application of regulations, but with a policy permitting changes in regulations, as dictated by experience

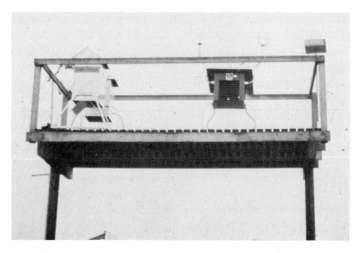

Fig. 17-4. Air pollution recording devices. Working automatically these instruments provide a 24-hour record of air conditions. (Courtesy Lane County, Oregon, Health Department)

Community programs. Local and regional air pollution control programs in few cities or counties are spending the recognized standard of $0.40 per capita on air pollution control.

On all levels—federal, state, and local—programs are being developed, but many communities have a more serious pollution problem today than they had 5 or 10 years ago. It must be conceded that not until reliable and valid standards of pollution are established can there be fully realistic enforcement of pollution control. To wait for such measures would be foolhardy. Even though present empirical source emission standards for pollution control are not totally adequate, they do have merit and should be applied until new and more precise standards are developed.

Leaders in industry and business are becoming more responsive to the need for air pollution control, yet there are still countless sources of air pollution that could be controlled with existing technology. There are other problems of control for which technological know-how is not available. Improvement of control technology is the responsibility of both government and industry. Control will require continuing research, education, cooperation, legislation, and enforcement.

The United States will be forced to make some difficult choices between energy needs and environmental pollution.

Radioactive pollution

Man has always been exposed to natural sources of chemical activity and cosmic radiation. This is referred to as background radiation. All people are exposed to a harmless amount of about 0.1 R (roentgens) per year. Not until man split the atom did radioactive atmospheric pollution become a problem.

The use of radioactive materials for treatment, research, and other purposes must always be regarded as a potential hazard, but these possible sources of radioactivity are usually well controlled and are not a danger to the general public. The immediate danger is to those people working with radioactive materials, and they have the necessary knowledge to take proper shielding and other precautions to protect themselves.

When nuclear weapons are tested, explosions spray the atmosphere with radioactive particles. These particles, such as strontium^{90} and cesium^{137} with half-lives of 28 years, settle to the earth. This represents a threat to human life, because penetration of body cells by radioactive particles causes ionization of the atoms of cells, particularly cells undergoing division. The extent of damage depends on the dose received and whether the dose is received externally or internally. For doses received or applied externally, the unit of radiation is known as a roentgen, which means radiation that causes two ionizations per cubic micron. An adult exposed to 1 R would receive about 10^{17} ionizations over the whole body. A dose of less than 100 R produces no symptoms or signs in a person, but 500 R in one dose will be fatal. The Atomic Energy Commission reports that the average external dose from fallout is from 0.001 to 0.005 R per year, less than 5% of the background radiation. Internal dosage is expressed by the Sunshine Unit (SU), which is equivalent to 0.003 R per year to bone tissue. Internal doses result from ingesting radioactive water, milk, and other foods. Internal effect of radioactivity is a greater health concern than is external exposure. Strontium^{90} is chemically similar to calcium and thus is deposited in bone. In young children, strontium^{90} is distributed throughout the bones. Localized high doses may cause malignancies. In adults the cancellous bone is usually affected causing acute poisoning.

Maximum permissible concentration (MPC) has not been established to the satisfaction of scientists in the field of radiation. The National Academy of Sciences has proposed 50 SU as the MPC, but the National Committee on Radiation sets the standard 25% higher.

Fallout is greater in the United States than anywhere else, yet the United States Public Health Service, with monitoring stations distributed throughout the nation, keeps a close surveillance of atmospheric radiation and takes all possible action to control sources of radiation. On the state and community level, detection and correction of radiation "leaks" in x-ray machines, fluoroscopic equipment, and other sources of radiation is a continuous effort by health officials and special agencies set up to safeguard the public. At present, the general public is relatively safe from radiation hazards, but constant vigilance is imperative.

Energy needs of the nation are increasing at a rate faster than the rate of population growth, and it is apparent that fossil sources are inadequate to meet rising energy needs. The next available source is nuclear energy, which can be converted to electrical energy. To obtain this additional electrical power the federal government and public utility companies have developed plans for nuclear reactors. Protesters have raised objections to the proposed plant sites and even to the construction of such plants. The objections are that there may be constant emissions from the reactors, thermopollution from heated water emptied into streams, unsafe disposal of radioactive wastes and, foremost of all, accidents that would saturate the atmosphere with lethal radioactive ions.

Emissions are controlled by shielding and the use of other proved controls. Water is cooled before being discharged into streams, and wastes are buried, disposed of in the ocean, or otherwise rendered harmless to human beings. Accidents are virtually on the order of zero. Those who work at these nuclear plants are the most exposed to any possible danger and the most knowledgeable. These experts who understand the situation see little reason for fear. When solar energy is tapped the need for nuclear reactors and fear of some of the public will be reduced.

Aerosol spray

For some time health scientists have recognized that fluorocarbon propellants can produce atmospheric effects harmful to human health. Some American investigators have done research in this field, but Russian and German scientists have been doing a major share of the on-going research.

Fluorocarbon propellants from spray containers do not decompose chemically in the lower atmosphere because they do not react with any other gases. Rainwater does not remove these propellants from the air. Fluorocarbons drift slowly into the upper regions of the stratosphere and release chlorine after being subjected to ultraviolet rays. Released chlorine atoms react with ozone molecules to

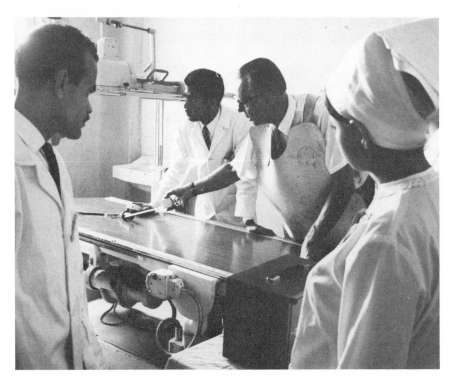

Fig. 17-5. Radiation protection demonstration. Special methods have been developed to assure radiation safety of patients and medical and auxiliary personnel exposed to ionizing radiation in the course of diagnosis and therapeutic procedures. (Courtesy World Health Organization)

produce chlorine oxide and oxygen. This in turn reduces the amount of ozone, eventually reducing the ozone equilibrium concentration by as much as 4%. Recovery to normal levels of ozone may take more than 100 years even if the fluorocarbon release were stopped this year.

When the ozone level is lowered, more ultraviolet rays reach the earth, which could result in such effects as cancer, particularly of the skin. In addition it must be recognized that the human respiratory tract can be directly affected by fluorocarbons. In the nonciliated part of the nasal junction fluorocarbon particles move slowly. Particles deposited in the ciliated tissue move more rapidly. Thus there can be an immediate threat to the health of exposed citizens as well as possible long-term effects from atmospheric changes created by fluorocarbons.

Fortunately, from the public health standpoint, the elimination of this hazard in the environment is relatively easy. At least forty-four products on the market in the United States use fluorocarbon-driven propellants in spray cans. These propellants can be replaced by different types of spray cans such as pump or water-driven sprays. The federal government could require that industry either label containers as being dangerous to human health or completely ban these propellants.

Some states have taken action through legislation that bans the sale of containers using fluorocarbon propellants. The State of Oregon law provides that violation of the propellants ban is a class "A" misdemeanor, a criminal violation punishable by fines up to $1,000 and 1 year in prison.

However, members of the public health

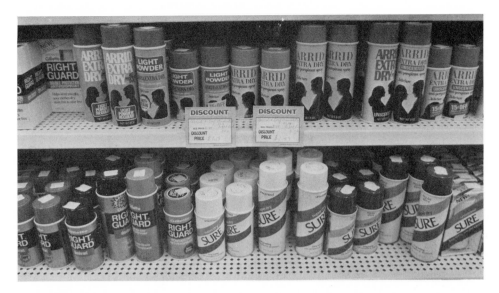

Fig. 17-6. Types of containers using fluorocarbon-driven propellants. Retailers are phasing out existing stocks on their own initiative, and producers are converting to safe containers. Here is an excellent example of solving a health problem without resorting to legal means. (Photograph by Paul Colvin)

profession readily see that this problem is primarily a matter of health education, rather than legal measures. When people understand the problem they will take the steps necessary to ban the use of fluorocarbon. Manufacturers will use other sprays, retailers will refuse to sell products using fluorocarbons, and consumers will refuse to purchase spray cans containing the objectionable propellants. Health educators have an opportunity to serve the public through an education program if it is designed and implemented immediately. Within a relatively short time this hazard to health can be eliminated.

NOISE

Noise is increasing in significance as a public concern. The increasing magnitude and complexity of society has brought with it increases in noises to a degree that calls for programs to relieve people of distress. Not all sound is objectionable, nor is all sound classed as noise. Technically, noise is any disturbing sound that interferes with work, comfort, or rest. It is doubtful that death has ever been caused by noise, yet noise can have an adverse effect on health, particularly mental health. Objectionable noise is not protested on health grounds, but because the noise disrupts and interferes with the normal enjoyment of tranquility.

The urgency of the problem created by noise depends on the frequency of the occurrence, the absolute as well as the relative loudness, and whether the noise is necessary or unnecessary. The honking of an automobile horn may be objectionable, but the siren of a fire truck may not be. A sound may be objectionable but nevertheless must be accepted. As much as the public objects to the boom when jet planes break the sound barrier, citizens in certain locations have had to learn to live with this noise.

Industry noise control. In many industries noise represents a problem of some significance. Exposure to high noise levels can cause deafness. Noises of lower levels can affect workers' efficiency and be otherwise objectionable. Industry usually makes surveys of noise intensities and takes necessary corrective measures. Segregation of noisy operations, insulating for sound, redesigning machinery, and changing operations are among corrective measures. Where noise intensity cannot be avoided, providing workers with ear protectors will safeguard their hearing.

Community noise control. Certain noises in the modern community such as the noise of traffic, street work, construction work, locomotives, and certain industries may be ever-present. The public generally accepts a certain noise intensity from these sources, but, when these sources rise above a certain level of intensity, complaints will be lodged.

City planning, including restricting industrial or commercial operations to particular zones, is a first measure. Cooperation resulting from communication between all parties concerned is the key to dealing with noise problems that arise and that are not covered by existing ordinances. Community organization efforts should precede court action, but if all other efforts fail, court action resulting in an injunction will prohibit the offender from continuing the noise nuisance or will command the offender to reduce the noise to a defined, tolerable level.

SWIMMING FACILITIES

Recent developments in swimming pool construction and natural bathing areas have caused health officials to extend their programs for regulating public swimming facilities. This regulatory function of state and community health departments is directed to those facilities that serve the public. This authority extends to pools and natural bathing areas of motels, hotels, resorts, parks, and other enterprises serving the public.

Health aspects of swimming facilities. On the positive side, swimming can promote both physical and mental well-being. On the negative side, accidents represent the greatest threat to health and life. In recent years, unsupervised motel pools have taken a frightful toll of lives by drowning. Slipping on slick walkways and in shower and locker rooms has been a source of serious injuries. Accidents related to diving have also taken lives and have been a source of injuries.

Disease spread via swimming facilities is always a possibility, but the general public harbors many misconceptions about the role of swimming facilities in disease spread. It is extremely doubtful that respiratory diseases are ever spread by water in a pool or other swimming facility. No tangible evidence exists that such diseases as the common cold, influenza, tuberculosis, or poliomyelitis are spread via pool water. The close social contact of swimmers themselves may be a factor in the spread of respiratory diseases, but the pool itself is not a vehicle of spread. Pink eye is not spread by pool water, but swimmers using the same towel or other article may thus communicate conjunctivitis.

Diseases of the intestinal tract are most likely to be transmitted via water in swimming facilities. Typhoid fever and bacillary dysentery may be conveyed by water, but it is doubtful that salmonellosis is thus ever transmitted to an individual. However, if water in a swimming pool is chlorinated properly, the danger of typhoid fever and dysentery spread is zero.

Certain skin infections are transmitted from swimmer to swimmer by physical contact associated with activities at the pool, the locker room, or the shower room, or by handling common objects. Athlete's foot (tinea pedis), boils (furunculosis), and impetigo contagiosa can be transmitted through contacts associated with swimming activities. Swimmer's itch (schistosomiasis) can be a threat in natural swimming waters harboring schistosomes. However, dragging a bag of copper sulfate around a lake behind a boat will rid the waters of schistosomes.

Swimming pools. The presence of competitive pools, diving tanks, instructional pools, recreational pools, and pools for other purposes indicates that many types of pools are being built. Yet, as specified by the American Public Health Association (1970), there are certain common construction needs—materials impervious and permanent for walls, bottom, vertical ends and sides, inlets submerged in a safe place, outlets synchronized with inlets, overflow gutters all around to allow slight overflow, and nonslip walkways at least 5 feet wide all around the pool. Showers and locker rooms should be well lighted, well ventilated, and clean.

Artificial pools are classified on a basis of quality control.

1. Fill-draw means the pool is filled and emptied at regular intervals. Timing is determined by the physical appearance of the water and the bathing load. This type of pool can be acceptable when properly operated. However, whether this type is used depends on the cost of water and the nature of pool use. Fill-draw pools are acceptable where limited bathing use occurs but are used very little today.

2. Flow-through means there is a continuous passage of water in and out of the pool and the chlorine content is controlled. This type of pool is highly acceptable, but the cost of water makes this class of pool highly uneconomical.

3. Recirculating means that pumps remove the water from one part of the pool; after being filtered and decontaminated by chlorination, the water is returned to the pool. Using the water over and over again is economical. In addition, the water quality is excellent. For these two reasons, this type of pool is most frequently constructed.

Decontamination of water in swimming pools is usually attained by chlorination, although bromine and ozone are also used. Bromine is more stable and tenacious than chlorine, but bromine fumes are highly irritating to the eyes and respiratory tract. Ozone is extremely expensive and little used, except for pools on ships, on estates, or at clubs.

When chlorine is used, a chlorine residual from 0.4 to 0.6 ppm should be maintained. This chlorine level may be irritating to the eyes of some swimmers. An alkalinity of the water should be maintained at a pH between 7.2 and 8.2. Not more than 15% of water

samples should contain more than 200 bacteria per milliliter, as determined by the standard agar plate count, or show more than 1.0 coliform organism per 50 ml of sample.

Wading pools. Much less sanitary than swimming pools, wading pools are frequently little more than cesspools. The usual practice is to add water constantly, using a standard of 0.5 ppm chlorine residual for decontamination purposes. Under moderate or heavy use, a wading pool should be drained and refilled at least twice a day.

Natural bathing areas. Lakes, rivers, and ponds used for swimming purposes are frequently dangerously polluted. Sewage, cesspool drainage, and other effluents pollute and contaminate the lake or river water. Many public swimming areas are unsupervised, but even those that are supervised are not always safe.

Supervision of natural bathing areas consists of identifying and preventing all possible sources of pollution and then keeping a close check on the degree of contamination. A permissible maximum coliform count of 1,000 per 100 ml is standard. Areas are also classified by the following average coliform index:

Class	Coliforms per 100 ml
A	0-50
B	50-500
C	500-1000
D	Over 1000 (unacceptable)

Because of the danger of typhoid, dysentery, and staphylococcus infections, even a relatively low coliform index does not make the swimming area safe. For this reason, health officials, using other data, close down swimming areas that may have been used for many years without any apparent mishaps.

Regulations. All public swimming pools are subject to official regulation. A pool is classed as a public pool if it is used by others than the owners or their families. Whether a charge is made for the use of the pool is not a consideration in classifying a pool as public. Authority to regulate public swimming facilities rests with the state. However, if the state

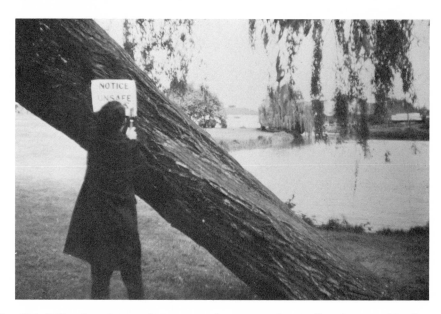

Fig. 17-7. Polluted pools in parks. Even in the apparently unpolluted water of family picnic grounds, contamination is possible. (Courtesy Environmental Health Division, Lane County, Oregon)

legislature has granted home rule to a county or city, the county or city thus has authority to regulate public swimming pools within its territorial jurisdiction.

State regulation of public swimming facilities is usually vested in the state department of health. Permits to operate a public swimming facility are issued annually to those individuals or organizations having pools that meet all state specifications relating to construction and maintenance. A nominal fee is charged for the permit. Annual renewal is contingent on the operation and the maintenance of conditions acceptable to the state inspectors, who make periodic inspections.

Community regulation of public swimming pools is based on an ordinance and related regulations. Many communities use as a guide the *Suggested ordinance and regulations covering public swimming pools*, a model developed by the Joint Committee on Swimming Pools of the American Public Health Association in cooperation with the United States Public Health Service. This model ordinance is a guide to be used in the design, construction, operation, and mainte-

nance of public swimming pools. Provisions are reasonable and are not restrictive or punitive. The ordinance begins by requiring submission of plans and specifications and specifies acceptable materials and construction. This includes specifications for dressing rooms, showers, and toilet facilities. Suggestions for supervision of bathers and pools, including safety requirements and lifesaving equipment, are included. In all respects, this proposed ordinance is a model that can be adapted to all situations and can serve admirably for communities accepting their responsibilities in regulating public swimming pools.

The community health department is customarily charged with responsibility for enforcement of the swimming pool ordinance. This would mean either the county or city health department. Health department sanitarians include this function in their regular responsibilities. In addition, sanitarians provide a consulting service for citizens requesting information or advice relating to private residential pools. Sanitarians also make regular inspections of conditions involving natural bathing areas and take such action as is necessary to protect the public against hazards. Much of the work in swimming facilities regulation goes unnoticed, yet is becoming a progressively more significant public health function as the population and its recreational activities expand.

VECTOR CONTROL

In community health practice the term vector is not limited strictly to forms of the class Insecta but includes allied arthropods such as ticks and mites. The health interest in these forms is in their role as vectors of organisms pathogenic to man. Virtually all of these are biological vectors in that the pathogen passes through part of its life cycle in the intermediate invertebrate host. The common housefly is strictly a mechanical vector. Some biological vectors, under certain circumstances, can be mechanical vectors and transfer pathogens on their wings, feet, or body.

In some geographical areas vectors are not a great community health concern. This is particularly true in some of the northern states in America. Yet the tick and the common housefly may transfer pathogens of man even in the northern climes. Man everywhere does have to contend with the annoyance of mosquitoes, flies, lice, and other arthropods, but the significant health problem is in their role as vectors of disease.

Transmission of disease by vectors can be visualized in these patterns:

Man—vector—man
Man—vector—lower vertebrate—vector—
man
Lower vertebrate—vector—man

In epidemiology all three of these patterns must be considered as possible routes over which the disease is transmitted.

Vector-disease relationships. Known vector-disease relationships indicate that a specific pathogen is transmitted via a specific vector. To say that the mosquito transmits yellow fever is not a complete statement. Only the specific *Aedes aegypti* mosquito serves as the intermediate host for the pathogen causing yellow fever. For present purposes, however, a list will serve that identifies the type of vector with the disease or diseases it transmits to man.

> Mosquitoes—yellow fever, malaria, encephalitis, filariasis
> Fleas—bubonic plague, murine typhus
> Ticks and mites—Rocky Mountain spotted fever, tularemia
> Biting flies—tularemia
> Lice—epidemic typhus, relapsing fever
> House flies—salmonellosis

Roaches have been suspected of transmitting enteric diseases, and bedbugs have been suspected of conveying relapsing fever.

Control measures. The first principle of vector control is to identify the specific vector and plan control measures accordingly. When the tick is the known vector, control measures will differ from measures taken when a mosquito is the intermediate host. Yet, three factors must always be considered —elimination of breeding places, destruction of the insect or its larva, and protection of possible human hosts by preventing the vector from reaching human beings.

Mosquito control presents the classic example of insect control, whether the particular species is a vector or simply represents a general annoyance. In either event three factors must be considered:

1. Elimination of breeding places
   a. Destroying and emptying containers holding water
   b. Filling water holes
   c. Draining ponds, marshes, and swamps
   d. Rendering bodies of water unsuitable for breeding by use of larvicides, releasing water at high velocities, and fluctuating the water level
   e. Diverting stream flow
   f. Trimming the banks of ponds, lakes, and streams to prevent swamps
   g. Introducing natural antagonists of mosquito larvae, such as fish (*Gambusia*)
2. Destroying adult insects
   a. Insecticide sprays in areas inhabited by mosquitoes

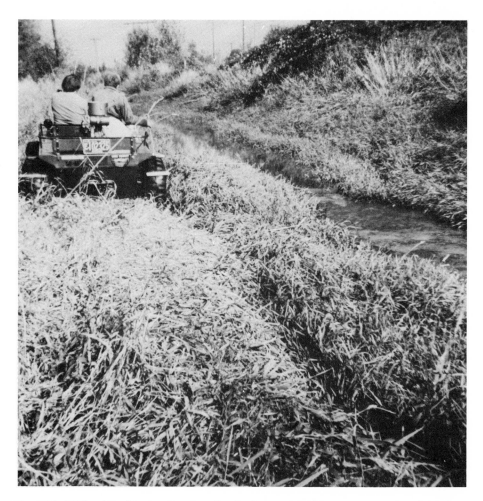

Fig. 17-8. With a bit of ingenuity virtually all places concealing vectors can be cleaned out. (Courtesy Environmental Health Division, Lane County, Oregon)

　　b. Insecticide-impregnated sawdust spread on surface of flowing streams
　　c. Oil solution insecticide over rain barrels and other water containers
3. Protecting human beings against contact by mosquito
　　a. Screening
　　b. Clothing
　　c. Nets
　　d. Repellents

It must be recognized that insecticides can have harmful as well as beneficial effects. Man himself, lower vertebrates (wildlife especially), and vegetation (food) can be harmed if the insecticide solution is too highly concentrated. The controlled use of insecticides is imperative. While *Silent Spring*, by Rachel Carson, overstated the case, there is considerable support for the theme the book presented—overuse of insecticides is destroying wildlife. Because insecticide effects at best are temporary, it is necessary to spray or otherwise apply the insecticide about once a week. A certain degree of air pollution can be created by insecticides.

The community has a responsibility to reduce vector populations in its area. This is usually a function of the community health department and is carried out in cooperation with state agencies. Community authorities also have a responsibility in regulating the use of insecticides by private citizens. This is primarily a problem of public education directed to specific groups or individuals. Research on insecticides is being carried on by federal agencies and by scientists in universities and colleges throughout the nation. Permissible concentration of insecticides is the immediate problem, but the long-range objective is that of developing insecticides that destroy insect life but are harmless to man, other animals, and vegetation.

RODENT CONTROL

Strictly speaking, the term "rodents" encompasses all animals belonging to the order Rodentia and includes squirrels and other forms as well as rats and mice. The ground squirrel can harbor the pathogens that cause Rocky Mountain spotted fever and tularemia in man and can transmit rabies directly. A vector must transmit most pathogens from the rodent to man—the tick for Rocky Mountain spotted fever and the horsefly for tularemia. Control of squirrels is essentially a state and federal problem, and both the federal and state governments have extensive programs to eliminate ground squirrels. Field teams using guns, traps, and poisons carry on a constant campaign to eliminate ground squirrels in regions with endemic Rocky Mountain spotted fever and tularemia.

In communities the rodent problem is essentially confined to rats and mice. These rodents are responsible for economic loss, create esthetic problems, and transmit disease. Rats and mice destroy and eat poultry and eggs, grains and sprouts, and corn. They also destroy merchandise. Despite the enormity of this economic loss, it is as a carrier of disease that the rodent poses the greatest threat to man.

Rat-borne diseases. Rodents harbor several pathogens of man. In many instances the rat dies of the disease. In other instances the rat remains a carrier of the disease over a considerable period of time. Although many misconceptions exist regarding the relationship of rats to human disease, at least six diseases of man are definitely known in which the rat serves as a reservoir of infection.

Murine typhus: rat—rat fleas—man
Bubonic plague: rat—rat fleas—man
Weil's disease (infectious jaundice): urine of rat
Salmonellosis: feces of rat and house mouse
Rat-bite fever: bacteria via bite
Rickettsial pox: house mouse—mite—man

Obviously, not all rats harbor pathogens of man, but the greater the rat population the greater the potential reservoir.

Varieties of rats in America. Three types of rats and the house mouse are of health concern in the United States. The black rat lives in walls and between floors. It has a pointed muzzle, slender body, long tail, and a sooty color. The roof rat is more brown but otherwise resembles the black rat and usually lives off the ground. The brown rat is also called the sewer rat, wharf rat, and Norway rat. It is a large rodent with a blunt head, short ears, and short tail. It burrows and nests in the ground. The house mouse lives in walls, furniture, and other protective places.

Control measures. A community rodent control program must begin with a well thought out plan based on surveys and participation by residents. Education of the public is essential to the success of the control program, because an informed public can provide the type of cooperation on which a successful program must be based. When all residents make their premises rat-free, the task of community officials is not a difficult one.

A community program has five aspects: surveys, elimination of food sources, elimination of nesting and breeding places, rat-proofing, and killing of rats. Each aspect involves certain measures.

1. Surveys
   Poor sanitation areas
   Slums
   Tenements
   Railroad areas
   Areas near dumps
2. Elimination of food sources

Placing all food in rat-proof containers

Covering garbage cans

Prohibiting dumping food wastes in open areas

3. Elimination of nesting and breeding places

Disposing of debris

Burning trash and rubbish

Prohibiting piles of building materials

4. Rat-proofing

Closing external openings

Placing screens and metal over cracks and openings

Eliminating all possible passages

5. Killing of rats

Trapping

Use of approved rodenticides with all possible safeguards

Fumigation with warning signs and other safeguards

Droppings of infected rats and mice on food consumed by man transmit disease. Keeping all food where rats and mice cannot reach it is of primary importance. Of secondary importance is the practice of all possible safety measures when using rodenticides and fumigation to kill rats. Eliminating mice by trapping is relatively simple.

SANITATION SURVEY

A systematic inventory of environmental conditions in a community can serve to tabulate adequate conditions as well as hazards. It can point up strengths in community health and can place a finger on those conditions that need attention. Such a survey should preferably be conducted by some qualified person not a resident of the community. A qualified citizen of the community can conduct an objective sanitary survey directed toward specific environmental factors such as water supply, sewage disposal, refuse disposal, milk supply, restaurants and food establishment, public buildings, housing, swimming pools, insect and rodent control, air pollution, health department, and government.

APPRAISAL OF GENERAL SANITATION

As society becomes increasingly complex, the need to control adverse environmental factors becomes more urgent. No one has the right to jeopardize the welfare of one's neighbor by making the environment annoying and even threatening to health. The community must impose requirements on each of us for the best interest of all. Besides the authority of the community represented in legislative requirements, community officials must provide services that will assist citizens in maintaining the best possible environment from the standpoint of health. Equally important, each citizen should understand the responsibility for a healthful environment and be motivated to assume responsibility for the quality of the environment the community has. A "blitz" program or clean-up campaign may be justified on occasions but should not be the regular mode of community effort. Constant efforts in promoting environmental health is the effective prescription.

ENVIRONMENTAL PROTECTION AGENCIES

With the growing concern about environmental health problems it was logical that special agencies should be created and serve as the responsible agency to safeguard the interests of the general public in the protection and promotion of environmental quality. These agencies are found at all levels of government and basically are regulating agencies. At the federal level is the Environmental Protection Agency. State agencies are variously named, but a common designation is Department of Environmental Quality. Some metropolitan areas have environmental control departments, but the nature of environmental quality, being geographically broad rather than localized, dictates that the state agency serve all state needs in matters of environmental control. (See Chapter 21).

A state department of environmental quality is usually governed by an unpaid lay commission appointed by the governor. The Commission appoints a full-time professional director who appoints the professional staff subject to approval by the commission. Usually the state is divided into districts, and members of the professional staff are assigned to the different districts. Responsibilities of the staff in each district usually are as follows:

1. Air quality: investigation of complaints of air pollution and obtain necessary corrections; surveillance of air quality problems in the district; conducting surveys and collecting samples of air; reviewing and preparing permits for air quality emissions.

2. Water quality: investigation of complaints of water pollution and develop necessary controls and enforcement to protect the state's water standards; investigate and review proposed waste treatment plant locations and prepare waste discharge permits for plants; surveillance of existing sewage treatment plants and sewage collections systems and preparation of waste discharge permits for plants; conducting inspections and surveillance of existing industrial treatment facilities and waste discharges with preparation of permits; conducting water quality basin surveys.

3. Solid wastes: investigation of solid waste disposal sites, evaluation of proposed sites, and preparation of solid waste disposal facility permits.

4. Community and interagency responsibilities: provision of technical assistance and advice to local health departments and officials on such matters as sewage disposal, solid waste disposal, industrial waste disposal, water quality surveys; consulting with the public, industry representatives, city, county, state and federal officials, engineers, and others regarding plans and programs related to waste discharge permits, the design, construction and operation of sewage treatment facilities, industrial waste treatment facilities, air treatment systems, and solid waste disposal systems; providing public information to local groups on all aspects of environment quality.

While these state environmental quality agencies are separate from the state health departments, cooperation and a close relationship exists. The magnitude of environmental health problems in modern society makes imperative the creation of a self-contained agency to be responsible for environmental quality. Health departments still carry on their traditional functions, perhaps more effectively after being relieved of the many tasks inherent in environmental health programs.

Congress has passed a solid waste management bill that creates broad new programs to deal with the growing solid waste management problem facing our cities and states. The Resource Conservation and Recovery Act calls for the establishment of comprehensive hazardous waste regulations, incentives for better state and regional solid waste planning, acceleration of solid waste research and development, and a greater emphasis on materials conservation and resource recovery. Specific provisions include:

1. Grants totaling $70 million in fiscal year 1978-1979 for states initiating solid waste management plans in compliance with the guidelines of the Environmental Protection Agency (EPA). The EPA is also required to furnish technical assistance when necessary.

2. The authorization of $50 million in fiscal year 1978-1979 for hazardous waste control grants at the state level. The Act requires the EPA to establish mandatory federal standards for regulating the generation, transportation, storage, and disposal of hazardous wastes.

3. In fiscal year 1978 $30 million is authorized for grants to states, cities, or regional agencies for research, development, and demonstration programs designed to improve methods of extracting reusable materials and energy from waste. The EPA will conduct research in specific areas such as small-scale re-

source recovery systems for smaller cities.

4. Grants amounting to $30 million in fiscal year 1979 to assist in the planning of solid waste facilities.

5. Over the next 2 years $50 million is authorized in grant assistance to rural communities for solid waste management. Open dumping is banned, with the states administering a 5-year phaseout of this disposal process.

6. The EPA is also required to conduct special studies of solid waste problems including resource conservation, glass and plastic recovery, the composition of the solid waste stream, and the handling of sludge and mineral wastes.

Another important environmental measure was the Toxic Substances Control Act. The purpose of this Act is to permit the EPA to test and screen chemicals considered potentially hazardous to public health or to the environment prior to commercial production and distribution. Ninety days before marketing a new chemical or using an old chemical for a significant new use, the manufacturer will be required to supply the EPA with enough information on the substance to allow the EPA to evaluate its safety.

Pesticides represent a special category of toxic substances. Congress has extended the Federal Insecticide, Fungicide and Rodenticide Act (FIFRA), thereby continuing authorizations for the EPA's pesticide programs.

A clean environment cannot be measured only in economic terms or as a function of expended energy resources. Legislation dealing with the environment must weigh the effect of solutions to all problems in the environment.

Voluntary organizations interested in ecology and related health problems have added impetus to the development of official environmental health programs. Voluntary organizations can supplement and complement the work of the official agencies and thus contribute tangibly to the preservation and promotion of environmental quality.

KEEP AMERICA BEAUTIFUL, INC. (KAB)

A unique and effective voluntary organization for improving the environment, Keep America Beautiful, Inc., was founded in 1953 with headquarters in New York City* and a National Field Office in Grand Prairie, Texas.† The organization is primarily a consulting and educating medium that seeks to encourage communities to initiate their own programs of environmental improvement. KAB is available for guidance and other services. Keep America Beautiful, Inc. (KAB) is

1. A national, nonprofit, nonpartisan, public service organization

2. A staff of communications, field service, and program development experts encouraging and guiding individuals from citizen groups, government, and industry in controlling littering as a first step toward overall environmental improvement

Founded in 1953, KAB

1. Is supported by individual citizens and more than 100 companies, trade associations, and labor unions representing a cross section of industry in the United States

2. Receives information and guidance from a National Advisory Council composed of 100 service, youth, conservation, and professional groups and federal agencies

3. Works through thirty-five state affiliates, some 7,000 local groups, KAB's members and contributors, National Advisory Council members, and their chapters

4. Cooperates with organizations and agencies in thirty-seven countries through Clean World International, established in 1974

KAB's clean community system

1. Is the first local-level program to reduce littering through application of behavioral science concepts

---

*99 Park Avenue, New York, New York 10016.
†PO Box 1476, Grand Prairie, Texas 75050.

2. Adapts the normative systems change process to improve individual waste control attitudes and handling practices in participating communities
3. Is based on action research and field tests in three cities where a sustained litter reduction of up to 65% was achieved at sample measurement sites

Other major KAB programs include

1. Consulting services: KAB provides advice and counsel for business firms, trade associations, government agencies, and civic organizations that want to develop their own environmental improvement programs
2. Events: regional, annual, and national meetings, open to the general public; Keep America Beautiful Day, held annually in late April
3. Information: how-to guides for community organizations, informational periodicals, educational publications, guides for youth leaders, and a slide presentation are among the materials available from KAB headquarters
4. National awards program: KAB has sixteen award categories for state, county, and community programs. Included in KAB's recognition for outstanding achievement in environmental improvement are: a KAB Federal Highway Administration award to state highway departments; the Mrs. LBJ Award, for outstanding women volunteers in the area of community improvement
5. Public service advertising: through The Advertising Council, Inc., KAB sponsors a national series, featuring Iron Eyes Cody, the famous "crying Indian," which has reached millions of people. The ads run on television and radio and in newspapers and magazines. The theme, "People Start Pollution. People Can Stop It," is carried by the various media, totaling 1.4 billion network television impressions in addition to local television spots, radio play, and donated space in newspapers, magazines, and mass transit stations and vehicles

KAB promotes ideas and programs. An example is the list of suggested ideas associated with the promotion of a "Day" Program. The list is impressive.

"Idea inventory" for KAB day

Improve and beautify *airports*—terminals, access roads, parking lots, etc. Establish frequent policing of *beaches* to eliminate litter and unsupervised pets. Construct *birdhouses* and place them in public parks and near reservoirs. Create and maintain *bird sanctuaries*, with assistance from public agencies. Beautify *downtown areas* and place litter cans on sidewalks at frequent intervals; establish a public information center. Aid the *elderly* in yard cleanups and house painting. Improve and landscape the *entrances* and *exits* to your town; place signs at them, listing local antipollution ordinances and sites of interest. Help stop *erosion* by planting shrubs, vines, and grasses in eroded areas. Plant vegetable and flower *gardens* and maintain them. Remove *graffiti* from walls, mass transportation vehicles, sidewalks, and elsewhere. Create *herb gardens* at historic sites and other locations. Beautify municipal *hospitals* and landscape grounds. Distribute *litterbags*.

Where are the volunteers?

A KAB Day project will increase in effectiveness if it is a joint project between two or more organizations—government departments, businesses, civic groups, and schools. Sources of volunteers vary from community to community, but these and other civic groups are likely to offer their assistance to the KAB Day undertaking:

Boy Scouts	Military installations
Girl Scouts	Chambers of Commerce
Garden clubs	Veterans organizations
Jaycees	and their auxiliaries
Colleges	Volunteer fire and
Fraternal societies	ambulance corps
Church groups	High school ecology
Women's clubs	clubs

Citizens who want an improved community would do well to contact KAB. The necessary information and motivation that KAB can provide often makes the difference between action and inaction. The same applies to county and state action programs.

QUESTIONS AND EXERCISES

1. Why has there been an increased interest in environmental health despite the great advances in the understanding and control of environmental health conditions?
2. Explain this statement: "Occupational health programs are concerned with more than occupational diseases."
3. Why should not employers alone be responsible for all occupational health promotion?
4. Explain this statement: "Air pollution is increasing at a faster rate than man's understanding of the nature, prevention, and control of air pollution."
5. Which is the greater threat to human welfare, stream pollution or air pollution?
6. When farmers burn their fields in the fall in order to destroy parasites, should this be regarded as objectionable air pollution? How can it be controlled?
7. Why must air pollution be regarded as a regional problem?
8. If an industrial firm that will employ 1,000 people wishes to set up in your community a plant that will cause a great deal of air pollution, what would be your reply and what would be the rationale of your stand?
9. In the past year, to what radiation dangers have you been exposed?
10. Explain this statement: "What is music to one person may be noise to another person."
11. What requirements would you make of motel and hotel swimming pools in order to safeguard guests and others?
12. What measures can be taken around a swimming pool to prevent the spread of skin diseases such as "athlete's foot"?
13. What are the responsibilities of home owners who permit neighborhood families to use their residential pool?
14. How can the common housefly be a vehicle for the transmission of salmonellosis?
15. How is it possible for an insect to be both a biological vector and a mechanical vector?
16. To what vector-borne disease is your community exposed?
17. Under what circumstances should a person be immunized against vector-borne diseases when such immunization is available?
18. What can be the value of the Federal Environmental Protection Agency to your state?
19. How can the voluntary organization Keep America Beautiful, Inc. (KAB) be of service to your community?
20. Will the environment in the future be more hazardous to human welfare than the environment of today?

REFERENCES

American Association for the Advancement of Science: Global effects of environmental pollution, a symposium, Amelia, Ohio, 1968, D. Reidel Publishing Co., Inc.

American Public Health Association: Suggested ordinances and regulations covering public swimming pools, New York, 1964, The Association.

American Public Health Association: Swimming pools and other bathing places: recommended practices for design, equipment and operation, ed. 10, Washington, D.C., 1970, The Association.

Andrews, W.: Guide to the study of environmental pollution, Englewood Cliffs, N.J., 1973, Prentice-Hall, Inc.

Anerbach, I. L.: The importance of public education in air pollution control, Journal of Air Pollution Control Association 17:102, 1967.

Ashford, N. A.: A crisis in the workplace: occupational disease and injury in a report to the Ford Foundation, Cambridge, Mass., 1976, M.I.T. Press.

Berthouex, P. M., and Rudd, D. F.: Strategy of pollution control, New York, 1977, John Wiley & Sons, Inc.

Bragdon, C. R., editor: Noise pollution, a guide to information sources, Detroit, 1976, Gale Research Co.

Burns, W.: Noise and man, Philadelphia, 1973, J. B. Lippincott Co.

Bush, V. G.: Safety in the construction industry, Englewood Cliffs, N.J., 1975, Prentice-Hall, Inc.

Clayton, K. M., editor: Pollution abatement, Pomfret, Vt., 1974, David & Charles, Inc.

Committee on Medical and Biological Effects of Environmental Pollution, Division of Medical Science, National Research Council: Medical and biologic effects of environmental pollution series, Washington, D.C., 1976, National Academy of Science.

Cross, F. L., Jr.: Handbook of swimming pool construction, maintenance and sanitation, Wesport, Conn., 1974, Technomic Publishing Co., Inc.

Davies, C. N., editor: Aerosol science, New York, 1968, Academic Press, Inc.

Davies, C. N., and associates: Effects of abnormal physical conditions at work, Baltimore, 1967, The Williams & Wilkins Co.

Grey, J.: Noise, noise, noise (Franklin Institute Book), Philadelphia, 1976, The Westminster Press.

Gunningham, N.: Pollution, social interest and the law, South Hackensack, N.J., 1974, Fred B. Rothman & Co.

Hirschborn, H.: All about rats, Neptune, N.J., 1974, T.F.H. Publications.

Hopkins, E. J., Bingley, W. M., and Schucker, G. W.: The practice of sanitation, Baltimore, 1970, The Williams & Wilkins Co.

Hutchins, B. L., and Harrison, A.: History of factory legislation, Fairfield, N.J., 1968, Augustus M. Kelley, Publishers.

Jaffee, L. S.: The biological effects of photochemical air pollution on man and animals, American Journal of Public Health 57:1269, 1967.

Kavaler, L.: Noise, the new menace, New York, 1975, John Day Co., Inc.

Klainer, A. S., and Geis, I.: Agents of bacterial disease, New York, 1973, Harper & Row, Publishers, Inc.

Kroeber, F. V: Public swimming pools: a manual of operation, Cranbury, N.J., 1976, A. S. Barnes & Co., Inc.

Leh, F. K., and Lak, R. K.: Environment and pollutions: sources, health effects, monitoring and control, Springfield, Ill., 1974, Charles C Thomas, Publisher.

Lipscomb, D. M.: Noise: the unwanted sounds, Chicago, 1974, Nelson-Hall Publishers.

Magrab, E. M.: Environmental noise control, New York, 1975, John Wiley & Sons, Inc.

Malsky, S. J.: A two year radiological institute: five year summary and future trends, American Journal of Public Health 60:2102, 1970.

Miller, R. K.: Handbook of industrial noise management, Atlanta, Ga., 1976, Fairmont Press.

National Agency for International Publications: Basic safety standards for radiation protection, New York, 1967, The Agency.

National Safety Council Staff: Accident prevention manual for industrial operations, ed. 7, Chicago, 1974, National Safety Council.

National Safety Council Staff, McElroy, F. E., editor: Handbook of occupational safety and health series, Chicago, 1975, National Safety Council.

Navarra, J. G.: Our noisy world: the problem of noise pollution, Garden City, N.Y., 1969, Doubleday & Co., Inc.

Olishifski, J. B., and McElroy, F. E., editors: Fundamentals of industrial hygiene, Chicago, 1971, National Safety Council.

Prohansky, H.: Environmental psychology: man and his physical setting, New York, 1970, Holt, Rinehart & Winston, Inc.

Shimkins, D. B.: Man, ecology and health, Archives of Environmental Health 20:111, 1970.

Smith, R. S.: The occupational safety and health act: its goal and its achievements, Washington, D.C., 1976, American Enterprise Institute for Public Policy Research.

Still, H.: In quest of quiet, Harrisburg, Pa., 1970, Stackpole Books.

Stilley, F.: One hundred thousand dollar rate and other animal heroes for human health, New York, 1975, G. P. Putnam's Sons.

Strobb, M. A., editor: Understanding environmental pollution, St. Louis, 1971, The C. V. Mosby Co.

Symes, C. B., and associates: Insect control in public health, New York, 1962, American Elsevier Publishing Co., Inc.

Taylor, R.: Noise, ed. 2, New York, 1975, Penguin Books.

Thuman, A., and Miller, R. K.: Secrets of noise control, ed. 2, Atlanta, Ga., 1976, Fairmont Press.

Waldbott, G. L.: Health effects of environmental pollutants, St. Louis, 1973, The C. V. Mosby Co.

Woolsey, T. D.: The health of the American worker, Journal of Occupational Medicine 9:456, 1967.

PART V

Health services

18 ▪ PERSONAL HEALTH SERVICES

One of the first duties of the physician is to educate the masses not to take medicine.

Sir William Osler, M.D.

Despite the quality of training for physicians, dentists, nurses, pharmacists, medical technologists, and other health personnel in America, and despite our investment in clinics, hospitals, and other health facilities, America does not have the greatest life expectancy or the highest level of health. This paradox is largely attributed to two factors. The first is the tendency of Americans to expose themselves to unnecessary risks. The second has been the difficulty in bringing together the citizen who needs medical, dental, and other health service and the professions that provide the necessary service. The people who need help the most are not getting it (Roemer, 1976; Weaver, 1976).

EDUCATION OF THE PUBLIC

Knowledge of when and how to use medical, dental, and other services is invaluable to human well-being, but millions of Americans are victims of ignorance in matters relating to self-care and the use of medical services. Health superstitions, fads, hopelessness, recklessness, and folklore must be replaced by knowledge and responsibility. The gullibility of the public, as represented in the acceptance of drug advertising, extravagant claims, and outright quackery, must be replaced by confidence in scientific fact and personal responsibility. A primary requirement is a recognition that health does not come in a package or in a clinic. It comes with a style of life (Fuchs, 1974).

Danger of quackery. Defrauding and robbing the healthy as well as the sick, quackery is a parasite of the nation. Quackery can be defined as a false medical claim, fraudulently used to prey on the public by professing to cure disease by useless, ineffective procedures, remedies, nostrums, and diagnostic and therapeutic devices. A nostrum is a secret or patented device for which false therapeutic claims are made. Some "patent medicines" or "proprietary drugs," as contrasted with ethical drugs, are examples (Editors of Consumer Reports, 1974).

Where a certain segment of the population is inadequately educated in matters of health protection, quacks are able to operate because many people have emotional needs not adequately met by physicians and clinics.

Classifications of quackery are drug and cosmetic, food and nutrition, and electrical and mechanical. Some quacks use all three, but others operate only one form of quackery so long as it is profitable.

Drug and cosmetic quackery is perhaps the most widely practiced. In the United States more than a billion dollars a year is spent on patent medicines, many of which are worthless and some of which are actually harmful. Many of these proprietary drugs mask pain and distress and thus delay the time in which the person goes to a physician. This delay can be critical. Drug quackery exists in many forms—rejuvenation nostrums, blood purifiers, cancer cures, hay fever remedies, cold cures, breast developers, sex vitalizers, nerve tonics, kidney cures, liver cures, and concoctions that "cure" the whole spectrum of ailments. Cosmetic quackery appears as skin "foods," hormone creams, skin restorers, geriatric cosmetics, salves, tablets, and every conceivable potion. These nostrums usually do nothing. They could do harm.

Nutrition quackery yields over half a billion dollars a year in sales in the United States. For more than half a century in the United States, "health foods" have been sold in the form of natural foods, organic foods, exotic foods, miracle foods, bee products, and other dietary cure-alls. "Nutrition experts" and "health lecturers" write books on food fads that find ready sales. Somewhere schools have failed in nutrition education when food and nutrition quackery find a clientele ever eager to pay exorbitant prices for foods that can be purchased at regular food markets at one-fourth the cost.

Electrical and mechanical nostrums are frequently only leased rather than sold. This can be a clever bit of strategy from the legal standpoint as well as from the sales angle. Charms, "galvanic" belts, amulets, "radionized" water, radioactive ore, electron o-ray, deploray, and other devices with equally mysterious designations are offered to the public and readily purchased or rented by desperate patients and hypochondriacs. It is tragic but true that the more emphasis on the term "electronic" the more acceptable the device is to the public.

Most quacks use advertising and testimonials, but not in reputable scientific journals. The basis of most quack treatment is "secret," the name of a high-sounding foundation is used, and supporters may be actors, writers, and politicians. Quacks generally refuse inspection, contend that "the medical trust" is persecuting them, and, when challenged, promise to make their methods or drugs available to health authorities—but they seldom follow through on such a promise. Cultists, hypnotists, arthritis specialists, and purveyors of devices use "health lectures," "clinics," and demonstrations that can be highly dramatic. Communication media permit the advertising of products without sufficient regard for consumer interests.

Protection of consumers. An informed and alert public is the best protection against fraud and quackery. The low-income groups in particular need health education. The informed citizen will not be a prey of quacks. Yet all citizens are entitled to protection from their governmental agencies so that they are not victims of the fraudulent claims of health charlatans. This protection is afforded by legal agencies and by professional organizations that help set standards and offer mechanisms of "quality control."

In 1906 Congress passed the Pure Food and Drugs Act, regulating the interstate exchange of drugs and adulterated food. Additional provisions were enacted in subsequent years, and in 1931 the enforcement agency was given its present name of Food and Drug Administration (FDA). In 1938 the Food, Drug, and Cosmetic Act was passed to further protect the public against hazardous, worthless, and mislabeled drugs and cosmetics and adulterated, misbranded foods.

Nutritional labeling of food. Consumer protection laws have seen good times in Congress in recent years, but one law that may have particularly important long-range implications for community health is the landmark FDA legislation on nutritional labeling, which was an outgrowth of the White House Conference on Nutrition in 1969. Even if the food companies comply fully with this law, however, labeling does not stand alone in its current Latin and numerical form. Apart from understanding the language in its present form, there remains the problem of motivation. A survey in 1973 revealed that 80% of shoppers were aware and said they were familiar with product labeling information, but only 37% said they use nutritional labeling, open dating, or unit pricing in their purchasing decisions. Consumer educational programs are needed, especially among diabetic persons and homemakers.

Nonprescription drugs. The pharmaceutical industry obtains over $4 billion each year from over-the-counter sales of medications that have been determined by the

FDA to be largely ineffective. Vitamin pills, mineral supplements, laxatives, sleeping pills, and analgesics (painkillers) are massively promoted in advertising campaigns sponsored by the pharmaceutical industry but ultimately financed by the public that purchases the products. Three-fourths of the American public, according to a recent FDA survey, believe that extra vitamins provide more pep and energy. One-fifth of the public is convinced that cancer, arthritis, and other such diseases are caused, at least in part, by vitamin and mineral deficiencies. Over 37% of Americans accept the validity of advertisements for health products on the belief that they must be factually correct or such agencies as the FDA and FTC would not permit them to appear.

The Food and Drug Administration. The FDA conducts over 50,000 inspections and about 1,500 court actions per year in connection with seizure of harmful products and requests for injunctions restraining persons from continuing a product or practice hazardous to public health. This agency also tests products, sets standards, passes on claims, investigates imports, and cooperates with state and local officials in matters of food and drug production, marketing, adulteration, and contamination.

The Federal Trade Commission (FTC). The FTC has authority over false advertising and deceptive practices. Following complaints, the Commission investigates and may issue orders to the offending person or firm to cease and desist from continuing the practice.

Post Office officials prevent the use of the mail service in promoting the shipment and sale of deceptive, adulterated, contaminated, or fraudulent foods, drugs, cosmetics, or devices. A citizen complaint is sufficient to initiate an investigation, followed by legal action when warranted.

Other professional and voluntary agencies. The American Medical Association has a Bureau of Investigation, a Council on Foods and Nutrition, and a Committee on Cosmetics. These agencies work through state medical associations and together carry out the following measures in the public interest:

1. Determination of the nature of treatment
2. Interviewing of participants and reviewing their backgrounds
3. Examination of clinical evidence
4. Examination of experimental evidence
5. Examination of biopsy or autopsy data
6. Securing of some of the drug for analysis
7. Consultation with other investigators
8. Summarizing and reviewing findings

The American Public Health Association, the American Cancer Society, Inc., and the Arthritis Foundation are other agencies that alert the public to fraudulent health claims. Patients with cancer or arthritis are prime targets of quacks, and special vigilance is essential in order to protect these patients from the ruthless frauds who prey on them. The National (and local) Better Business Bureau also is alert to health frauds and provides protection to the public.

All of these official and voluntary agencies are valuable in protection against quackery, but it is the individual citizen who can do most to put quackery out of business. Education concerning recognition of symptoms and self-medication is the first measure. The second need is to select and to use wisely the available medical, dental, and hospital services when necessary, and safe forms of self-care at other times (Levin, 1976).

MEDICAL, DENTAL, AND HOSPITAL NEEDS

No one should be denied the medical, dental, hospital, and other health services he or she needs, but making these services available is a most formidable problem. People vary in their knowledge of how to use medical services, in their economic ability to obtain medical service, and in the quality and quantity of medical and hospital services available to them. To bring together people and the medical services they need is the task of society, health pro-

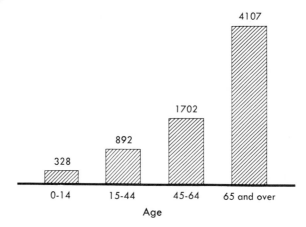

Fig. 18-1. Number of short-stay hospital days per 1,000 population, by age, 1974. (From National Center for Health Statistics, Hospital Discharge Survey)

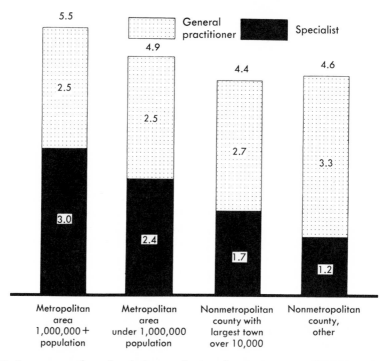

Fig. 18-2. Average number of ambulatory physician's visits per person per year by type of physician and place of residence, 1973. (From National Center for Health Statistics, Health Interview Survey)

fessions, local communities, and individuals (Kennedy, 1972).

The medical needs of people and their ability to pay for medical services are determined largely by their age, income, and the location of their community. In any year 20% of the population will bear 60% of all medical and hospital costs. Although averages serve as a guide, the most meaningful data are frequently in comparisons, as shown in Figs. 18-1 and 18-2.

Families in the lower income brackets gen-

Table 18-1 ■ Number of physician's visits per person per year and percent of the population with no physician's visits in the past 2 years by poor and not poor status and by color for all ages: United States, 1964 (before Medicaid and Medicare) and 1973 (after Medicaid and Medicare)

	Total		White		All other	
	Poor*	Not poor	Poor*	Not poor	Poor*	Not poor
	Number of physician visits per person per year					
1964	4.3	4.6	4.7	4.7	3.1	3.6
1973	5.6	4.9	5.7	5.0	5.0	4.3
	Percent with no physician visits in past 2 years					
1964	27.7	17.7	25.7	17.1	33.2	24.7
1973	17.2	13.4	16.8	13.2	18.5	15.3

From National Center for Health Statistics: Data from the Health Interview Survey, summarized in Health, United States, 1975, Rockville, Md., DHEW Publication No. (HRA) 76-1232, 1976.
*Definition of poor is based on family income—under $3,000 in 1964; under $6,000 in 1973.

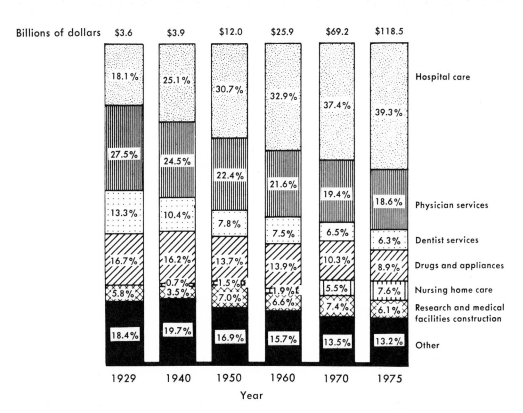

Fig. 18-3. Percent distribution of aggregate national health expenditures by type of expenditure, selected fiscal years, 1929 to 1975. (From Social Security Administration, Office of Research and Statistics)

erally have a poorer level of health and a greater need of medical services than do families in the upper income groups. Yet before Medicaid and Medicare, people in the higher income brackets used most medical services to a greater extent than did people in lower income groups. Data from the National Health Survey show that the utilization differences have been offset by these federal programs (Table 18-1), but the differences in health remain.

The lesson learned from this experience, as in Canada where the installation of a universal health care system also equalized access to medical care without substantially improving health (Lalonde, 1974), has been to recognize the importance of life-style, behavior, and environment. These factors have emerged throughout the preceding chapters as the most effective points of intervention to improve community health. This bears particular emphasis here because the provision of personal health services in the form of medical care alone is an extremely expensive and not very productive way of improving community health. The alternatives of health education, preventive medical services, and environmental health programs have not had proportional investments, as can be seen by the shrinking percentage of "other" expenditures in Fig. 18-3.

PROFESSIONAL PERSONNEL

The United States has more than 4.4 million employed people in some phase of health work. This includes some 3 million professional and technical workers. Reports from the Public Health Service show that in the United States in 1973 there were 333,300 medical physicians. In the same year there were 12,000 with the degree of Doctor of Osteopathy (Health Resources Statistics, 1974). The American Medical Association (1974) estimates one physician for every 562 people. Certainly this would be an adequate number of physicians were it not for two factors. The first is the uneven distribution of physicians. A tendency of physicians to

congregate in the metropolitan areas is a problem not unique to America, because other nations have the same experience. A second factor lies in the inclination of most physicians to become specialists. In this respect, the trend from 1950 to 1973 is of interest (Cambridge Research Institute, 1976).

With only 30% of physicians in general practice the result is that primary medical services are not available for many citizens. It must be pointed out that in the category of medical specialists, many are internists who, in practice, are available for primary care service. Having 70% of practitioners in the specialties also creates financial problems. If, in a particular specialization, there are twice as many physicians as necessary in a location, fees likely will be adjusted upward to guarantee specialists an income commensurate with what they think they should have. A new specialty of general practitioners, which is called family practice, is developing in response to these needs.

In the academic year 1976-1977 total enrollment of the 116 accredited medical schools was 57,236, and 11,613 seniors were graduated (Crowley, 1975). Again, if less than 30% of these graduates go into general practice, the general public will be no better off in terms of physician services than they have been. How to make general practice attractive is the problem that must be resolved or the cry will continue that there is a physician shortage when, in fact, it is merely a shortage of general practitioners. The new programs in family practice have attracted some students, and the number of family practice residency programs in hospitals has increased from sixty-two in 1970 to 219 in 1974 (Stimmel, 1975).

Some communities have been able to attract a physician by building a small but adequate hospital, providing office facilities, and guaranteeing a minimum salary. A second problem is the inefficient use of physician services. Too many physicians are taking too much valuable time doing tasks that

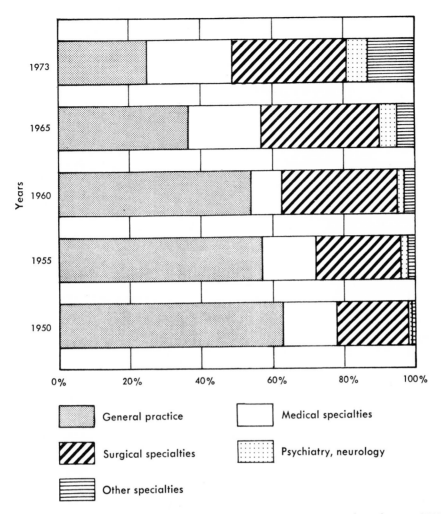

Fig. 18-4. Specialization of nonfederal physicians in private practice, selected years 1950 to 1973. (From Dickerson, O.D.: Health insurance, Homewood, Ill., 1968, Richard D. Irwin, Inc., p. 77; U.S. Department of Health, Education and Welfare, Office of the Assistant Secretary for Planning and Evaluation: Health, education and welfare trends, 1966-1967 edition, Washington, D.C., 1968, U.S. Government Printing Office, pp. 5-48; American Medical Association, Center for Health Services Research and Development: Distribution of physicians in the United States, 1973, Chicago, 1974, The Association, p. 76; and Cambridge Research Institute, 1976)

others could do or should be trained to do. Others can be trained to take family and personal histories. Nurse practitioners can be trained for further duties. In addition others can relieve the physician of certain time-consuming tasks. Examples are physicians' assistants, accredited record technicians, medical secretaries, medical transcriptionists, physical therapy aides, inhalation therapists, surgical technicians, and darkroom technicians. Training of paramedical personnel is gradually taking hold (Otten, 1974).

In 1973 the United States had 105,400 active dentists. While 11,142 dentists were specialists, all of these directly served the public as the following specialist titles indicate:

Specialties	Number in specialty
Endodontists	585
Oral pathologists	120
Oral surgeons	2,714
Orthodontists	4,566
Pedodontists	1,225
Periodontists	1,114
Prosthodontists	702
Public health dentists	116

Assuming that the 97,970 civilian dentists provide direct service to a civilian population of 207,313,000, we arrive at a figure of one dentist for every 2,120 people. Authorities in the field maintain that the optimum ratio should be one dentist for every 1500 people. Using this standard as a base, the United States has a shortage of 40,000 practicing dentists (Health Resources Statistics, 1974).

In the academic year 1972-1973, the fifty-six dental schools in the United States had an enrollment of 18,376. One of these schools is in Puerto Rico. Dentistry attracts fewer students than does medicine, partially because the cost of an education in dentistry is almost as high as that in medicine. To supplement the supply of dentists coming from America's schools of dentistry, between 200 and 300 qualified dentists immigrate to the United States each year.

The federal government is attempting to offset the shortage of dentists by encouraging the use of dental hygienists, dental assistants, and dental laboratory technicians. In 1972 some 21,000 dental hygienists were in practice. Dental hygienists receive at least 2 years of education at the college level and usually are admitted to the program following high school graduation. In 1972 thirty-four of the 148 schools offering dental hygiene programs required some college preparation. In 1972-1973 these 148 schools had 9,193 students and graduated 3,410. A bachelor's degree was offered by forty schools and the remaining 108 schools offered only the as-

sociate degree or certificate in dental hygiene (Health Resources Statistics, 1974).

Nurses are assuming expanded roles in personal health services. Their numbers increased faster than the increase in physicians or in population, more than doubling between 1950 and 1973. Registered nurses (RNs), as shown in Fig. 18-5, numbered 815,000 in 1973. An additional 459,000 practical nurses and 910 nursing aides, orderlies, and attendants have relieved RNs of many direct patient care functions, leaving them more time for supervision, administration, and patient education. The ratio of one nurse for every 256 people in the average community allows nurses greater time than physicians have with patients. They have used this time increasingly to help patients cope with emotional and learning aspects of self-care and rehabilitation. The potential for nurses to bring a humanizing and preventive orientation back into our highly technological health care system gives them a most promising and central role in the future of community health.

The Health Professions Educational Assistance Act of 1976. This law (PL 94-484) extends health manpower training authorities through 1980 with significant changes to meet national needs. The law, which amends Title VII of the Public Health Service Act, is designed primarily to produce more primary care practitioners and improve health services in manpower shortage areas. It provides support for the training of health professions including medicine, osteopathy, dentistry, veterinary medicine, optometry, pharmacy, podiatry, public health, and allied health manpower.

New student assistance programs of insured loans to health professions students, scholarships for first-year health professions students of exceptional need, and Lister Hill Scholarships for medical students are established. Authorizations are greatly increased for National Health Service Corps Scholarships. Health professions student loan and loan repayment programs are continued on a more restrictive basis. Unconditional Health

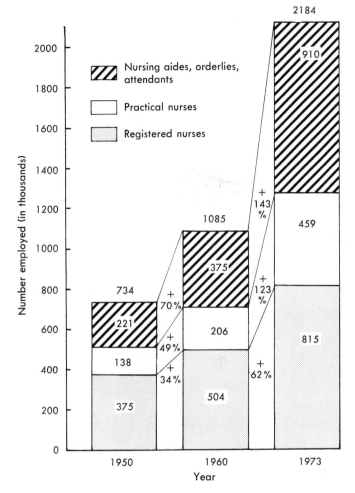

Fig. 18-5. Number of persons employed in nursing and related services, by type of personnel, 1950, 1960, and 1973. (From U.S. Department of Health, Education and Welfare, National Center for Health Statistics: Health resources statistics, 1974, Rockville, Md., 1974, pp. 197, 201, and 209. Also 1970 edition, p. 149, and 1969 edition, pp. 11, 145, 146, and 152)

Professions Scholarships and Physician Shortage Area Scholarships are being phased out.

Institutional grant support is broadened to include public health schools, and the conditions of participation are changed. Medical schools are required to train specified percentages of residents in primary care. The construction grant program is amended to provide authority for construction of ambulatory primary care teaching facilities.

Special projects grants provided in eight categorical areas reveal federal priorities. Categorical programs include new authorities for Area Health Education Centers; family medicine departments; family medicine and general dentistry training; general pediatrics training; assistance to disadvantaged; physician assistant; expanded function dental auxiliary and dental auxiliary and dental team practice support; and occupational health training centers. Start-up, financial distress and interdisciplinary training programs also are authorized.

Restrictions are tightened on the entry of foreign medical graduates. Special project authority is provided for medical and osteopathic schools to assist in the transfer of United States students from foreign medical schools.

Support is continued for allied health, public health, and health administration programs with purposes more specifically targeted on training in biostatistics, epidemiology, health administration, health planning, health policy analysis, environmental health, occupational health, and dietetics or nutrition. For further information students may write to The Office of Communications, Bureau of Health Manpower, 9000 Rockville Pike, Bethesda, Maryland 20014.

Other health professions provide personal health services. Not all such occupations will be listed, but categories from the report for 1974 include:

Dietitians and nutritionists	45,000
Health educators	2,500
Hospital administrators	17,000
Opticians	11,000
Optometrists	18,400
Pharmacists	132,900
Podiatrists	7,100
Psychologists, clinical and other health	27,000
Therapists, occupational	7,700
Therapists, physical	16,500
Therapists, speech and hearing	26,500

The distribution of minorities and women among the health professions is an indication of the problems of access. For example, less than 3% of physicians and dentists but over 20% of dietitians and practical nurses and

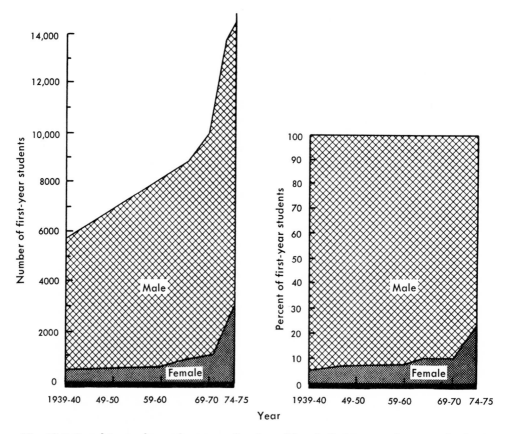

Fig. 18-6. Trend in number and percent of male and female first-year students in schools of medicine in the United States, selected academic years 1939-1940 through 1974-1975. (From Forward plan for health FY 1978-82, DHEW Publication No. [OS]76-50046, p. 24)

40% of lay midwives are black. Nurses, mostly women, are unevenly distributed around the country; in the south central states there is one nurse for every 400 to 500 people, whereas the New England states have one nurse for every 150 to 210 people (Health, United States, 1975). There has been a recent increase in the number and percentage of minority and female admissions to medical schools (see Fig. 18-6).

HOSPITAL FACILITIES

Consideration of community hospital facilities must be centered on short-term general and special hospitals and their bed capacity. It is the bed capacity that is the key factor. Actually, the number of short-term general and special hospitals in the United States was greater 50 years ago than it is today. Half a century ago, because of limited transportation, almost every little hamlet in the nation had its fifteen- or twenty-bed hospital, poorly equipped, poorly serviced, and poorly administered, but accessible. With modern transportation it is altogether logical to have fewer hospitals and maintain only those hospitals with a large enough bed capacity to warrant extensive equipment and well-trained personnel. There is no longer a need for every town to have a hospital. As a result large, well-equipped, well-staffed, and well-administered hospitals are erected in the large centers of population. These large hospitals serve communities for regions as defined and planned by Health Systems Agencies.

The standard of four and one-half general hospital beds for every 1,000 inhabitants is attained in many metropolitan areas, but there are many communities that have but half this number. The uneven distribution of hospital beds was partially corrected by the federal Hill-Burton program, which made more than $4.1 billion in grants to hospitals in all of the states during the 29 years of its existence and added 496,000 beds to the nation's hospital system. These grants were made to local government hospitals, church hospitals, and nonprofit hospitals. Nearly 4,000 communities were aided in the construction of 6,549 public and nonprofit medical facilities.

A short-term general hospital is one in which the average patient stay is 30 days or less. Of these hospitals, about 5% are federal hospitals, 27% are local government hospitals, 14% are church hospitals, 40% are nonprofit hospitals, and 14% are proprietary hospitals. Average occupancy of short-term general and special hospitals is about 80%. In the winter months occupancy is high, sometimes exceeding 100%. During the summer months a hospital usually has a low occupancy.

In 1948, at the time the Hill-Burton program was becoming operational, there were 3.4 beds per 1,000 population. There are currently 4.3 nonfederal general medical and surgical hospital beds per 1,000 population. The distribution over the country of hospital beds has become more nearly balanced. Mississippi, Alabama, Arkansas, Georgia, and Tennessee had the lowest bed/population ratios in 1948, but now are at the national average or above it. Some of the states with particularly high bed/population ratios in 1948 have actually experienced a decrease. Within states there is also improved balance in hospital facilities between the less affluent and more affluent areas. There has been a shift in recent years from construction and expansion to the modernization of existing hospitals and clinics.

While the number of community short-term hospital beds has been increased, there has been a sharp reduction in the number of other types of hospital beds. The number of federal hospital beds has dropped from 1.7 per 1,000 total population in 1946 to 0.7 beds per 1,000 total population in 1973. The number of nonfederal psychiatric and tuberculosis beds has also dropped, resulting in a reduction in the overall bed/population ratio from 10.3 to 7.3 per 1,000 population.

Only one-third of all general medical and surgical hospital beds are under governmental ownership, whereas most psychiatric beds are in hospitals owned by state and local governments. These differences are partly historical, partly economic.

Hospitals offering a full range of special, highly technological services have increased in number over the past decade. Such facilities as intensive care, open-heart surgery, radioisotope, and renal dialysis units have proliferated. This addition of special facilities to a hospital's service capacity has been one of the factors in the rising hospital costs and the general inflation of the medical care dollar.

The number of beds in nursing homes more than doubled between 1963 and 1973, from 569,000 to 1,328,000. This increase resulted in part from the coverage of the charges for certain types of nursing home care under the Medicare and Medicaid programs, as well as changes in family living arrangements and advances in medical technology. Some of the growth in nursing home use appears to be the result of placement in nursing homes of older patients who in earlier years would have been residents in state and county mental hospitals.

There are 451,000 beds in residential health facilities other than hospitals and nursing homes. These include facilities for the mentally retarded (217,000 beds), orphans and dependent children (49,000 beds), the emotionally disturbed (60,000 beds), alcohol and drug users (33,000 beds), the deaf and blind (24,000 beds), and the physically handicapped (5,000 beds).

Increases in hospital employees, including physicians, nurses, and other personnel, per patient in short-term hospitals have been one of the factors in the rising cost of hospital care. In 1950 there was a full-time equivalent of 1.78 employees per patient in a nonfederal short-term hospital. By 1973 the number had increased to 3.15 full-time equivalent employees per patient. (Full-time equivalents are calculated by counting two half-time employees as one full-time equivalent employee.)

The availability of home health services is often a factor in determining if a patient must be hospitalized or can remain at home. The number of home health agencies approved for participation in the Medicare program increased appreciably between 1966 and 1970,

the first 4 years of the program. Since then the number of approved agencies has remained stable at about 2,200. Most of these agencies are governmental health agencies or visiting nurse associations (VNAs).

Poison Control Centers in the country have almost tripled in number since 1960. There are now 594 centers providing emergency and other care for persons who have come in contact with poisonous substances. Other forms of emergency medical services and ambulatory (outpatient) health facilities in general are increasing in number and utilization.

COST OF PERSONAL HEALTH SERVICES

In the United States in 1976 total expenditure for medical care was $139 billion. Of this, 58% was private expenditure, and $59 billion, or 42%, was public. This would appear to be a monumental sum, but it should be considered in terms of total personal consumption expenditures. In 1976 total personal consumption expenditures in the United States were $615,840,000,000. Medical care expenses constituted but 7.8% of this total (Fig. 18-7), but this is a growing proportion of personal consumption and family budgets.

In 1976 the per capita national and private consumer expenditures for health and medical care were $638. Of this, $369 was private consumer expenditure. The consumer medical dollar was divided as shown in Fig. 18-8. Hospital costs will continue to rise, despite the decline in the average length of hospital stay resulting from advances in medication, surgery, and other procedures. Nursing homes and rest homes as adjuncts to the general hospital have reduced the cost of hospitalization during the period of convalescence. Patients who do not require extensive care of hospitals can recover as rapidly in these homes at a lower cost, and at even lower costs with good home health care services and self-care education.

What should be the compensation of the physician? Three years of premedical study, 4 years in medical school, and 3 years of in-

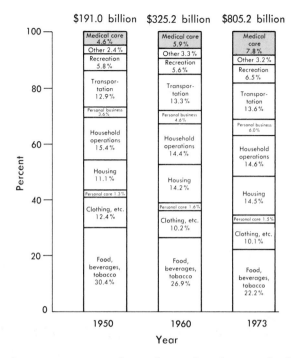

Fig. 18-7. Personal consumption expenditures by product shows medical care taking an increasing share from 1950 to 1960 and 1973. (From U.S. Department of Commerce, Bureau of the Census: Statistical abstract of the United States, 1974, Washington, D.C., 1974, U.S. Government Printing Office, Table 605; and U.S. Department of Commerce, Office of Business Economics: Survey of current business, vol. 54, no. 7, July 1974, Table 2-5)

ternship and residency add up to 10 years of lost earnings, in addition to the items of tuition, books, and other costs. Yet taxpayers also have an investment in the physician's education. They provide and maintain the colleges, the medical schools, and the hospitals where physicians receive their education. The average income of physicians today is more than $40,000 per year.

The medical profession has a virtual monopoly in the American economy, but physicians are sensitive of their image as a profession and exercise a supervision and discipline over all members of the profession. Instances of exorbitant medical charges have been substantiated. At the other extreme are the instances in which physicians have donated their professional services. It is not the extremes of overcharging or charity where the problem of the cost of medical care rests, but in the general inflation of prices in this

relatively uncontrolled sector of the economy.

The cost of dental care does not vary greatly from year to year for an individual or a family. In 1970 in the United States, consumers paid $8.6 billion for dental services, an average of about $120 per family. Because many Americans have never been in a dental office, the average of $120 does not express actual cost per year for those families who do use dental services.

But it is neither physician services nor dental services that account for the main increases in health expenditures. As shown in Figure 18-3, the proportion of national health expenditures taken by hospitals and nursing homes has increased while every other category of health expenditure has decreased in percentage. The economics of these trends are beyond the scope of this text, but three major causes and the national policy initiatives to remedy or check these

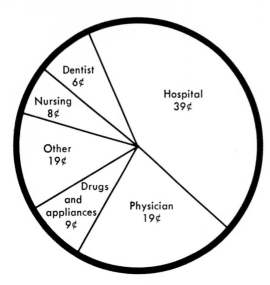

Fig. 18-8. Consumer medical dollar divided. Hospital care has become the major cost with cost of physician services becoming proportionately less. (From Social Security Administration, Office of Research and Statistics, Note No. 27, December 22, 1976)

sources of runaway hospital prices are central to community health (see box below).

ABILITY TO PAY FOR PERSONAL HEALTH SERVICES

Reports from the Department of Commerce, Bureau of the Census, indicate that a considerable proportion of families have an income too low to pay for all of their medical needs. The U.S. Census indicates that one-fifth of the families in the nation have an annual income of less than $6,000. How much can a family pay for medical care if it has an income of $6,000?

It was acknowledged in 1966 that a family with an annual income of less than $3,000 may be able to pay nothing for medical care. This family would find difficulty in paying monthly premiums on a hospital and medical insurance policy. A medical bill of $600 would be a financial hardship and even a disaster. This family was offered assistance from governmental agencies that began in 1967 to provide medical insurance or otherwise subsidize medical costs of families in low-income brackets. Families on public welfare increasingly have their medical needs provided by the government. The low-to average-income family not on welfare also needs assistance and protection against the increasing threat of hospital bills. Fig. 18-10 illustrates the increasing reliance on third-party payment mechanisms.

THE "CRISIS" OF MEDICAL CARE

This nation has the most technically prepared medical personnel among the finest medical care facilities to be found any-

Source of cost increases	Recommended policies
Physician salaries	Increasing use of paraprofessional, allied health, and "physician-extender" personnel
Unnecessary hospitalization, laboratory tests, length of stay, and elective surgery	Increased incentives for keeping patients out of hospitals by allowing physicians to share in the profits of prepaid medical plans and Health Maintenance Organizations; also, peer review of medical practice and utilization review of hospital practice
Increased utilization of medical services for conditions that might have been prevented and readmissions for chronic conditions not adequately controlled by patients	Increased emphasis on preventive medicine and health education, including occupational health, patient education, and self-care education

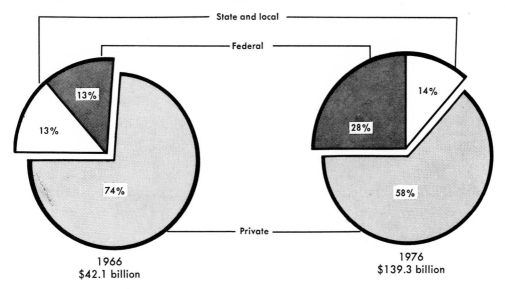

Fig. 18-9. Public funds pay 42¢ out of every medical dollar spent. The medical care dollar is financed both publicly and privately. The private share has always been by far the larger, but in recent years, with the addition of the new programs of Medicare and Medicaid, a shift to more public (especially federal) financing can be seen. (From Social Security Administration, Office of Research and Statistics, 1976)

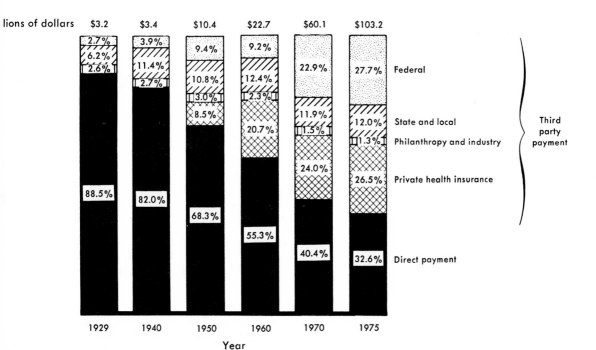

Fig. 18-10. Distribution of personal health care expenditures, by source of funds, selected fiscal years, 1929 to 1975. (From Social Security Administration, Office of Research and Statistics)

where. The problem is that of making accessible to every citizen the medical care he or she needs, which involves the economic interests of the public and the professional interests of the medical profession.

Access to essential services and freedom from the insecurity of catastrophic medical costs are the concern of communities and the public. Independence in medical practice is the concern of the medical profession.

Much of the current "national crisis in health care" is only a surfacing and recognition of conditions that have existed since the beginning of American concepts of *medical* care. Just as the recognition and redefinition of unacceptable conditions must be attributed largely to an increasingly educated and aware public, so too must their further analysis and solution be achieved through the participation of an informed public. No solution imposed on the public by technicians, politicians, or administrators will henceforth be acceptable without such participation in the planning process. We have reached that point in cultural evolution and public sophistication where autocratic, plutocratic, and technocratic solutions, at least in the area of health, are no longer sufficient. Decisions must be reached in close collaboration with informed consumers.

The issue of an educated public arises also in other contexts of the national health crisis. The proper utilization of good health services and health insurance mechanisms requires an informed and motivated public. If the *ideal* health care system for the United States were installed tomorrow, it would be highly subject to disuse, misuse, and abuse by an unprepared public operating under the control of habits, attitudes, and expectations inculcated by a lifetime of coping with the ancient fee-for-service system. Many of the failures or temporary breakdowns in the implementation of new programs in this and other countries have been traced to problems of communication, knowledge, attitudes, and habits. These

educational problems have been diagnosed in both the lay and professional communities.

A third context in which community health and health education is critical to consideration of the national medical crisis is in disease prevention or health maintenance. Given the available health care resources of the United States, any new plan that makes health care more accessible and more acceptable to more people (which should be the case) would place untenable pressure on those resources without a new orientation to prevention and health maintenance. A major criticism of the traditional fee-for-service structure of American medicine is that it provides no incentive for the providers of services to give attention to prevention, health maintenance, and health education. The rewards are tied almost entirely to treatment of the sick. When Americans speak of health care, they mean disease and medical care. There can be little doubt that the primary element in illness prevention and health maintenance is, and will increasingly become, health education.

A fourth area of community and educational concern, also related to the problem of resources, is the training and supervision of personnel in new categories of health service, as well as the continuing education of existing professionals in concepts of communication, group work, and other methods of patient and community education. The health manpower pool must be expanded and the existing pool of health professionals must become better trained to communicate effectively with patients and consumers. These training needs call for the deployment of advanced educational technology and will strain educational resources as much as the health resources themselves. Students too have become more informed consumers in higher education systems and have begun to redefine traditional teaching systems as "unacceptable," forcing yet another "crisis" in higher education and health professional training. Thus there is an educational crisis within the health crisis calling for expansion and upgrading of training programs for educators, educational administrators, and public health educators.

The educational and community health perspective on the national health crisis, then, focuses on problems of consumer participation in planning, problems of appropriate utilization of health care systems, problems of preventive health maintenance, problems of communication with patients, and problems of health manpower training and self-care. The remainder of this chapter comments specifically on national health plans, including those of other countries and some now before Congress for this nation. In view of the medical, economic, and political perspectives that have dominated the planning and debate surrounding most proposed and existing systems, this text will emphasize the community health and educational perspective outlined previously.

SOME SUGGESTED PRINCIPLES

As a guiding set of principles and goals for national action on the health crisis, the following recommendations of the American Assembly (The American Assembly, 1970) are helpful in assessing alternative plans and proposals:

1. Access to adequate health care for all in the United States must be recognized as a basic right. This requires commitment and incentive for local official and voluntary action.

2. The federal government should establish a Council of Health Advisors in the Executive Office of the President, required to make an annual report on the status of the nation's health and health system.

3. To correct the uncoordinated nature of the many federal health programs, immediate steps must be taken at the highest level of government to implement coordinated policy and program development.

4. The nation's health strategy must now emphasize health maintenance through preventive medicine, health education,

and environmental management, in addition to treatment.

5. It is an urgent national priority to fashion comprehensive health services systems available to all people. These systems must include:

   a. Identification of areas, by population or geography, but not necessarily by political boundaries, within which local responsibility for development and coordination of services can be promoted through appropriate consumer and provider participation in the policy-making processes of all health agencies in the area.

   b. Maximum utilization of local public and private agencies for organizational responsibility, through substantial federal incentives for action in the form of financial support and development of criteria and standards to implement such responsibility.

   c. Emphasis on provision of primary care through facilities for ambulatory patients readily available in their own localities. This must provide for professional supervision of a full continuum of services for individuals and families—a concern for the whole man in his environment and not just a part of the body or a category of disease.

   d. Emphasis should also be placed on restructuring the role of the hospital to assure that it plays a positive leadership role in the rationalization of community and regional health services. To this end, the criteria and machinery of voluntary area and regional health planning and of state health facilities licensing should be strengthened to include the concepts of community need and responsibility (usually referred to as franchising) for all hospitals and related facilities and services.

   e. Incentive to encourage more efficient arrangements as a way of containing costs. This should include continuing assessment of the cost and effectiveness of the services provided in each region, using nationally uniform data collection and evaluation criteria.

6. We further recommend an intensive effort

by medical schools and other interested agencies to recruit and train personnel for new categories of health service, such as physician assistants, to support this system. Modifications of licensing provisions and legal liability will be required to permit effective utilization of such personnel while assuring quality of services.

7. Rapid advances in medical knowledge requiring ever increasing specialization, and practical limitations precluding the training of enough doctors to maintain the family physician tradition, dictate the need for maximum utilization of the skills and talents of all health personnel currently available. Efficient delivery of comprehensive personal health services can be carried out most effectively through the vehicle of group practice, pooling a variety of specialized talents as contrasted with solo practice; and incentives for physicians and other health personnel to organize such group practices.

8. Federal payments for personal health services should encourage development by organizations offering comprehensive health care with a variety of reimbursement methods, particularly annual per capita payments. Alternatives to the individual fee-for-service method of reimbursement must be vigorously and promptly developed and implemented, and legal barriers to group practice prepayment should be eliminated.

9. The nation should commit itself to a universal financing system for comprehensive health care, with public-private participation, generally referred to as national health insurance. However, unless the delivery system is geared up and efficiently organized to provide comprehensive health care to all, the availability of more dollars for purchase of services not available will unduly raise costs further, frustrate expectations among many, and compound the chaos now existing in the delivery of personal health services. In preparation for national health insurance, the nation should begin to restructure the system, using already existing purchasing power to promote national organization and reward efficiency in the nation's competitive and pluralistic tradition.

10. Adult and child health education should be vigorously promoted. Particular attention must be given at appropriate levels of elementary, secondary, and higher education to assure fundamental knowledge of life processes for purposes of voluntary individual action for health protection and maintenance. This includes special emphasis on life-style, immunization, sex information, and effects of such hazards as smoking, drugs, and alcohol. We especially encourage the use of peer-group counseling in these matters where appropriate.

11. A national policy must be developed to determine procedures and criteria, with full disclosure, whereby society may decide who should receive specific life-saving services, such as kidney dialysis and organ transplants, not available to all—judgements which physicians should not have to make alone.

12. New knowledge is essential to improvement of the nation's health. Recent reduction in support for biomedical research is a policy leading to disaster, which must be reversed. Further, additional support must be provided for research in behavioral and social sciences related to health and delivery of health services.

NATIONALIZED MEDICAL SERVICES

A medical program is socialized when it is administered by the government. More than fifty nations have national medical service programs, and virtually all of these are socialized programs. For generations the United States has socialized various services—mail service, education, and police and fire protection. A city that sells water or electricity to its residents is engaged in the socialization of an economic enterprise.

National medical programs vary from one nation to the next, but three national medical programs in Europe have been of special interest to Americans. These programs have similarities and dissimilarities and represent three basic types of national medical programs.

Germany. The first national medical program was the German Sickness Insurance

Plan (Krankenkassen), which was launched in 1883. The Socialists in the Reichstag were planning to present a health and retirement program. To spike the guns of the Socialists, whom he despised, Chancellor von Bismarck instituted his own program. The Krankenkassen is nationalized but not socialized. Supervised by the government, the plan is administered by nonofficial societies or organizations. Practically all workers and their dependents are required to participate in the program. A worker's employer deducts the insurance premium from the worker's pay and adds half that amount as the employer's contribution. This amount is sent to an approved society of the worker's choice. The society may be a social organization, an athletic society, or other civilian organization that has been approved for participation by the central government. If workers or their dependents have any medical service, the attending physician's statement is sent to the worker's society for payment.

Each worker and dependents have a choice of physician, who is paid on a fee basis established by the government. All of the worker's dependents participate in the program, and practically all medical and hospital costs are paid by the insurance program. Fully 95% of Germans are in the program.

England and Wales. England has had a national health program since 1910, but the early plan was totally inadequate. It provided little more than a medical consultant service for workers and did not include dependents. The plan did not solve the problem of providing medical care for the public, and the cost of medical care that fell unevenly on the people became a burden from which the public demanded relief.

England and Wales instituted the present National Health Service in 1947. It is under the Ministry of Health, with executive councils and regional hospital boards. Approximately 97% of the population are included in the program, and about 98% of the practicing physicians participate. The weekly premium of a worker is about $0.35,

and the employer adds about $0.08. About 75% of the funds for the program come from the National Exchequer, and the premiums paid by the participants and employers provide about a fourth of the funds. About a fourth of national public expenditures goes to the health program.

Participating persons and their dependents have a choice of physician, who may accept or refuse a person as a patient. Each physician has a "list" of patients and is limited to 3,500 names. Physicians are paid on a per capita basis, regardless of how often they serve a patient or if the patient is served at all. Physicians receive about $3.00 per year for each name on their list. Physicians starting practice must have their location approved by the Ministry of Health in order to provide a uniform distribution of practitioners. Specialists are salaried and have higher incomes than general practitioners. General practitioners refer patients to the specialists.

All hospital and medical services are without cost to the patient. A minor charge is made for each prescription, spectacles, and filling or other dental treatment.

The British program has been considered successful, despite some shortcomings. Physicians complain that they are underpaid and overworked. Yet England and Wales are satisfied with their National Health Service and no political party would propose that it be terminated.

Sweden. Medical economists generally agree that Sweden has the best structured and administered national health program. Sweden's experience in pension programs, maternal and infant care programs, geriatrics programs, and welfare programs was an excellent preparation for establishing the System of Medical Care and Sickness Benefit insurance, which the Riksdag instituted on January 1, 1955.

All Swedish citizens 16 years of age or over must participate in the program. Children are insured as dependents. The program includes everyone except certain people in institutions. Employees pay a premium not to exceed 2% of their wages, employers pay a tax of 1.1% of their wage total, and the state subsidizes the remainder from general tax revenues.

Sweden's program is administered by the National Social Insurance Institute. On the local level each county has a central "Fund," elected by the local people responsible for local problems. A managing committee composed of a delegate from the Fund, a physician, and a supervisory official conducts necessary business between meetings of the Fund.

Physicians are in private practice and are not government employees. Clinical practice prevails in Sweden. Hospitals are operated by the government. All hospital and medical costs were paid when the program first started, but, because people took unfair advantage of the program, a change in policy was made. Today the program pays 75% of medical costs, based on fees established by the government. Physicians protest that the fees are too low. The program pays all hospital costs at public (four-bed) ward rates, limited to 730 days for each sickness. When better facilities are requested the patient pays the cost difference.

The Swedish program is very much like the hospital and medical insurance programs in America, except that in Sweden the government is the insurance company and sets physician and hospital fees. In Sweden consumers of medical and hospital services also have a voice in the policies and administration of the program.

AMERICAN PROGRAMS

Through the years, various plans to make medical care available have been developed in the United States. For decades industrial firms have provided medical and hospital services for all employees and their dependents. For generations the medical profession has used a sliding scale of fees based on the ability of the patient to pay. The practice is legal, although it has been questioned on ethical or moral grounds. Socialized medicine was in existence in the United States before the turn of the century. The federal government has provided medical and hospital care for members of the Armed Services and their dependents, war veterans, Indians on reservations, foreign service personnel, and various categories of government employees. The federal government, together with the state and local governments, has provided medical and hospital services for families on welfare.

Private health insurance

As shown in Fig. 18-10, America's need to make medical and hospital care available to all at prices people can afford has resulted in the development of extensive programs in medical and hospital insurance. Commercial insurance companies were reluctant to initiate health insurance but began with hospital insurance where actuarial data were available and costs were reasonably stable and predictable. Success with hospital insurance encouraged the companies to expand to medical insurance and, finally, insurance for physician visits. Voluntary, noncommercial organizations, notably the American Medical Association, developed insurance programs for both groups and individuals.

Insurance is a device that substitutes average costs for variable costs. It is not possible to predict the medical and hospital expenses for one person for the next year, but it is possible to predict total medical and hospital expenses for a million people. From such data, insurance premiums are determined and the medical and hospital costs are spread among many rather than falling heavily on a few.

In 1963 68% of all individuals had hospital insurance. In 1970 this figure had risen to 77%. About 74% of the population has surgical insurance. Hospital and surgical coverage increased with age, family size, education, and income. The surveys by the Public Health Service indicate that those who may have greatest need for hospital and surgical insurance coverage do not have such insurance.

Commercial insurance companies issue policies covering about 51.1% of the people with hospital insurance. Of these, about two-thirds had group insurance. Blue Cross–Blue Shield issued policies covering about 45.6% of the people with hospital insurance. The remaining 3.3% are covered by other programs.

Hospital insurance usually provides for full payment of a bed in a four-bed ward for a period of 70 days for a disability. The policy usually pays half of hospital costs for 5 months beyond the 70 days. Incidental hospital charges are also paid by the policy. Medical insurance policies are written to pay about 75% of all surgery and some of the extended treatment. Policies have a schedule of surgical fees, but the cost of surgery rises at a more rapid rate than the fee schedule. As a result, the policy rarely pays more than half the actual cost of surgery.

Policies to pay physician's services have not been popular. These policies pay $5 for each visit to a physician, beginning with the second visit. The problem for most people is not paying $5 for a visit to a physician. It is paying for major surgery and extended medical care.

Catastrophic insurance plans have considerable merit. These are usually group plans that cover both hospital and medical expenses and are designed to cover the major part of heavy hospital and medical costs. A base of $10,000 is usually established for the insured and his or her dependents. The policy pays 80% of medical and surgical expenses after the insured pays the first $50. The policy pays hospital charges for a bed in a four-bed ward. If, in a year, $4,000 is paid to the beneficiary, the basic fund is reduced to that amount; but each year thereafter, another $1,000 is added, until the basic fund is back to $10,000.

It must be recognized that premiums for any insurance policy are based on the benefits to be granted. No insurance firm could continue in business if it paid out more than it took in.

HEALTH MAINTENANCE ORGANIZATION (HMO)

Perhaps the most significant American advance in providing prepayment medical care has been the development of Health Maintenance Organizations, sometimes identified merely as prepaid group practice. In recent instances the programs have been subsidized, at least at the outset, but in the main, these have been self-sustaining enterprises. According to the Department of Health, Education and Welfare, four principles characterize a Health Maintenance Organization: It is (1) an *organized system* of health care that accepts the responsibility to provide or otherwise assure the delivery of (2) an agreed upon set of *comprehensive health maintenance and treatment services* for (3) a voluntarily *enrolled group* of people in a geographical area and (4) is reimbursed through a prenegotiated and fixed periodic payment made by or on behalf of each person or family enrolled in the plan. These four principles of HMO development are further defined and described by Congress in the HMO Assistance Act of 1973.

An *organized system* of health care is one that is capable of bringing together directly, or arranging for, the services of physicians and other health professionals with the services of inpatient and outpatient facilities for preventive, acute, and other care, as well as any other health services that a defined population might reasonably require. The system is organized in such a way as to assure for the enrollee the most efficient and effective entry into the health care system. It also promises continuity of care for the enrolled population through linkages between the components of organization.

Comprehensive health maintenance and treatment services means that the HMO is capable of providing or arranging for the provision of the health services that a population might require, including primary care, emergency care, acute inpatient hospital care, and inpatient and outpatient care and rehabilitation for chronic and disabling conditions. Primary care, one of the keystones of the HMO, emphasizes those services aimed at preventing the onset of illness or disability, at the maintenance of good health, and at the continuing evaluation and management of early complaints, symptoms, problems, and the chronic aspects of disease. It may be more graphically described as "personal physician care" or the entry point into the system, from which referrals to specialists are made.

An *agreed upon set* of services means that the consumers and the HMO will agree upon which services will be purchased from the HMO in return for the prepayment figure. Because some HMOs may have groups or enrollees paid for by Medicare, Medicaid, or employer-employee arrangements, the benefit schedule for population groups may differ.

Enrolled group means those people who voluntarily join the HMO through a contract arrangement in which the enrollee (or head of household) agrees to pay the fixed monthly or other periodic payment (or have it paid on his or her behalf) to the HMO. Enrollees agree to use the HMO as their principal source of health care if they become ill or need care.

The concept of health maintenance organizations grew from the success of a variety of medical foundations and prepaid group practice organizations in various parts of the United States that are now providing health care services for more than 7 million people.

The Kaiser Foundation Health Plan, for example, now cares for almost 2.8 million members, mainly at various locations in California, Oregon, Washington, and Hawaii. The Health Insurance Plan of Greater New York cares for three-quarters of a million people. The Group Health Cooperative of Puget Sound, of Seattle, Washington, the Group Health Association of Washington, D.C., and the San Joaquin Medical Care Foundation of California are other major prepaid plans.

These and the 180 other HMOs at the end of 1974 had been started and now operate under a variety of sponsors and financing mechanisms. Their continued effectiveness had led to the conviction that a much greater number of HMO organizations can be created through financial and technical assistance, and that thereby the health services delivery system in our country will be markedly improved.

An HMO can be organized and sponsored by a medical foundation (usually organized by physicians), by community groups who bring together various interested leaders or organizations, by labor unions, by a governmental unit, by a profit or nonprofit group allied with an insurance company or some other financing institution, or by some other arrangement. The HMO may be a hospital-based, medical school–based, or a freestanding outpatient facility.

The Health Maintenance Organization Act (PL 93-222) began offering federal support for HMO development in 1974 if medically underserved populations were enrolled. HMOs applying for federal grants and loans are required also to have provisions for quality assurance and grievance procedures, continuing education for their professional staff, home health services, and preventive services including health education, family planning, and preventive dental care. The most innovative and educationally sound programs with far-reaching implications for the future of medical and health care are those of the Group Health Cooperative of Puget Sound in Seattle and the Kaiser-Permanente Medical Care Program in Oakland, California.

Based on their long experience with prepayment medical care, the Kaiser-Permanente and Group Health Cooperative staffs are in a better position than most to anticipate some of the problems that medical centers will face if national health insurance is implemented. Dr. Sidney Garfield (1970) specifically describes the problem of overloading "sick-care" services with nonsick patients. He divides the anticipated "entry mix" of patients into five groups: the well, the worried well, the early sick, the chronically sick, and the acutely sick. Through the development of a health testing and referral service at the entry point of the system, using paramedical staff and automated history and test analyses, these five groups of patients can be channeled appropriately to one of three centers optimizing the utilization of specialized manpower and services. The well and worried well would be referred to a "health-care center" featuring health education, health exhibits, counseling, and special clinics on nutrition, adolescent problems, family planning, and prenatal and well-baby supervision. The acutely sick would be referred to the sick-care center, featuring integrated facilities of clinics and hospitals, special laboratories, radiotherapy, intensive care units, and extended care wards. The early and chronically sick would be referred either to the sick-care center or to a preventive-maintenance service, depending on their symptoms and prior experience. The preventive-maintenance service would have clinics on obesity, diabetes, hypertension, arthritis, back problems, mental health, geriatrics, and rehabilitation.

Patients would be referred from one center to another and in particular could be referred routinely to the health education service on exit from the system. Experience at Kaiser has shown that physicians in various departments are relieved from repetitive and, to them, boring educational tasks by being able to refer patients to health education and health exhibits by prescription. Hence the system proposed by Garfield provides for the efficient utilization of both clinical and social medicine resources.

The Kaiser program and other HMOs have demonstrated what can be done with organized prepayment medical services. Balanced use of services and facilities, together with efficient administration, is the key to HMO success.

MEDICARE

The United States launched its first widespread program of socialized medicine on July 1, 1966, when the Medicare program went into operation. It is a combination compulsory hospital and optional medical care program and is available to over 95% of people 65 years of age and older. The program is designed to give the elderly a certain degree of security against overburdening hospital and medical costs and to assure them the essential hospital and medical services. Medicare (PL 89-97) is three plans in one—the basic plan, the voluntary supplement plan, and the extension of the Kerr-Mills plan of medical assistance for the aged, now know as Title XIX or Medicaid.

The basic plan provides hospital care automatically for all people 65 years of age and older except certain federal employees and certain aliens. Whether persons are working or retired they are entitled to the benefits of the basic plan, which is financed by an increase in the Social Security tax but is not limited to those receiving other Social Security benefits.

The basic plan (Title XVIII, Part A) provides for hospitalization up to 90 days for each illness, although the patient must pay the first $92 of the hospital charges (deductible). Hospital care is provided for another 60 days, but the patient must pay a fixed amount (co-insurance) for each of the 40 days of additional hospitalization. Care covers all services usually provided by hospitals for inpatients, such as the following:

1. Semiprivate room and board (two- or four-bed ward) and private room when isolation is necessary
2. Regular duty nursing services
3. Use of operating and recovery rooms
4. Services of anesthesiologists, pathologists, and radiologists
5. Drugs and biologicals
6. Blood transfusions after the first 3 pints
7. Appliances and supplies such as wheelchairs and crutches

Medicare pays the entire cost of home care, up to 100 visits, and posthospital care for 20 days in an "extended care facility" for each illness, plus the additional 80 days for which the patient pays a fixed amount per day. "Extended care facilities" means a special convalescent wing in a hospital or a nursing home with registered nurses. At least 3 days' hospitalization is required before extended care facility services are provided. This last requirement may be dropped to discourage unnecessary hospitalization.

The voluntary supplemental plan (Part B) provides medical care and is subscribed to by over 95% of those covered by Part A. They paid a $6.70 per month premium beginning July 1, 1973. This amount is deducted from the Social Security monthly check if the enrollee is a Social Security recipient. Others are billed for the 3-month premium. The federal government matches this premium, and these are the sources of funds for the medical assistance plan.

Each year the enrollee pays the first $60 of his or her medical expenses (deductible). Thereafter the plan pays 80% of the remaining expenses. Services of a doctor of medicine or a doctor of osteopathy are provided for in the plan. This includes office calls, home calls, consultation, diagnostic tests, surgery, certain types of dental surgery, splints, rental facilities such as oxygen tents, and ambulance services. On a limited basis, treatment outside the hospital for mental disorders is paid up to $250 per year or half of the expenses, whichever is less.

Not covered by the medical plan are such things as eye examinations, eyeglasses, chiropractor services, podiatrist services, private duty nurse service, routine health examinations, drugs and biologicals, and dental services. The government is now considering adding certain preventive services in the hope of controlling costs in the long run.

Commercial insurance companies serve as agents for the Medicare program. Claimants under the program fill out a form and mail it to the designated insurance company serving as agent for the government. Receipts of payments made are attached to the form by the claimant.

The Medicare law specifically prohibits federal interference in the physician-patient relationship, to pacify the medical establishment, but this also precludes monitoring of quality. Freedom of choice is guaranteed—there is no closed panel or prescribed groups of physicians. The use of third-party insurance carriers is a further concession to the private sector.

The $92 deductible would seem to save the government from dealing with petty accounts, but it only adds to the administrative complexity of the financing. Premiums have had to be raised since the program began in order to cover deficits. The payment system has discriminated against federal providers by disallowing payment to certain categories of providers.

The relative isolation of the aged and the lack of an adequate educational program accompanying the introduction of Medicare resulted in low utilization of benefits during the initial years, but also in the delay of preventive care that might have reduced later utilization. The Senate Committee on Finance asked the Secretary of Health, Education and Welfare to submit to Congress by January 1, 1969, a report on "the possible coverage under Medicare of the cost of comprehensive health screening devices and preventive services designed to contribute to the early detection and prevention of diseases in old age and the feasibility of instituting informational or educational programs designed to reduce illness among Medicare beneficiaries and to aid them in obtaining needed treatment."

The Secretary's Report to Congress (Feasibility Study on Preventive Services and Health Education for Medicare Recipients, December, 1968) recommended that the federal government act to strengthen local community educational activities to reduce illness among Medicare beneficiaries. The Staff and Advisory Committee report submitted to the Secretary of Health, Education and Welfare originally recommended amending "the conditions for participation in Medicare to require that hospitals, extended care facilities, and home health agencies include qualified educational specialists on their staffs or use qualified consultants to help insure that educational components of their services are soundly developed." This was apparently too close to "federal interference" from the point of view of the Secretary's office. The Secretary's official report recommended "a national, cooperative, voluntary effort directed at health education for the aged" to be *initiated* by Health, Education and Welfare "in cooperation with medical societies, women's auxiliaries, voluntary agencies, advertising groups, consumer groups, senior citizen's organizations, community hospitals and other providers of services, public health agencies, insurance companies, news media and other groups interested in and capable of providing local leadership, initiative and effective action." To implement this recommendation, the Secretary went on to recommend Congressional appropriations and the establishment of a "focal point for coordination of health education efforts in the Office of the Assistant Secretary for Health and Scientific Affairs." Thus, in effect, the Secretary's recommendation differed from the original in that it placed the responsibility for local educational efforts on a wide range of lay and professional resources at the community level, with consultation and assistance rather than enforcement at the federal level.

This represents a "community organization" and participatory approach to community health and health education and is one that is needed for Medicare as well as for other national health insurance and health care programs. Unfortunately, as in many federal agencies, there has been a decline in the number of professionally qualified public health educators in the Medicare offices, and there has been no appointment of a public health educator in the office of the Assistant Secretary for Health and Scientific Affairs, as recommended in the Secretary's report to Congress. And there is but one professionally qualified public health educator in the entire Social Security Administration (consulting on industrial hygiene programs with little relationship to Medicare). The information offices of the Social Security Administration and most other agencies of Health, Education and Welfare are more concerned with public image and public compliance with regulations than with health education. One must therefore question pronounced federal commitments to the concept of health education for the aged, either as a rightful component of health care for Medicare beneficiaries or as a means to reducing Medicare costs.

MEDICAID

Title XIX or the Kerr-Mills medical assistance plan (Medicaid) provides medical care not only for indigents 65 years of age and older but for those of any age who were defined medically indigent. This program is a joint enterprise of the federal and state governments, which subsidize all of the costs. In 1977 every state except Arizona participated.

Like Medicare, the Medicaid "Grants to States for Medical Assistance Programs" was addressed exclusively to the problem of purchasing power and made little or no effort to deviate from "usual and customary fees" to hospitals and physicians or from the prevailing organization of delivery systems. Both programs under Public Law 89-97 were established on the assumption that the existing delivery systems would respond to the needs and demands of the population if sufficient fees for services were provided. The only thing that seems to have responded is prices. Together the costs of the two programs rose from $5 billion in its initial year to nearly $28 billion in 1975. The growth and distribution of these costs are shown in Figs. 18-11 and 18-12.

The purpose of Medicaid was to provide medical assistance for the "medically indigent" families with dependent children, the aged, the blind, and the disabled. The law extended to rehabilitation and other services to help such families attain independence and self-care. The distinguishing mechanism of this plan is that it authorizes appropriations on a fiscal year basis for payments to states that submit approved plans. The act requires that state plans must (1)

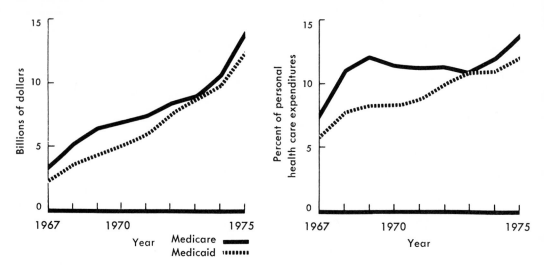

Fig. 18-11. Growth of Medicare and Medicaid funding in dollars and percent of personal health care expenditure, fiscal years 1967 to 1975. (From Social Security Administration, Office of Research and Statistics)

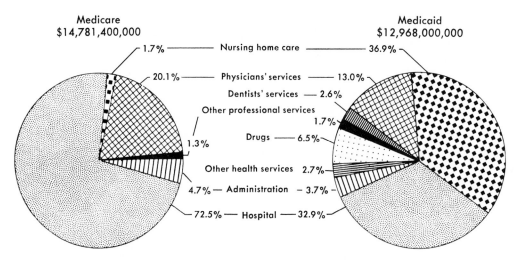

Fig. 18-12. Medicare and Medicaid payments by type of service, 1975. (From Social Security Administration, Office of Research and Statistics)

cover the entire state, (2) contribute at least 40% of the nonfederal share, (3) provide for a fair hearing to any individual whose claim is denied or delayed, (4) provide for administration of the state program or supervision of locally administered plans, (5) designate a single state agency for administration or supervision of the plan, (6) provide reports to the Secretary of Health, Education and Welfare, (7) provide safeguards for confidentiality of records, (8) provide that all individuals wishing to make application for medical assistance under the plan have an opportunity to do so, and (9) designate an authority for establishing and maintaining standards for participating institutions.

Consider some of the implications of these nine requirements. Numbers 1 and 2 clearly distinguish Medicaid from Medicare as a *state* plan. Number 3 places emphasis on repairing damage that should be prevented by requirements 8 and 9. If number 8 is viewed from the educational perspective, it would require states to include coordinated programs to assure that all eligible beneficiaries know of their eligibility and that all applicants know of and have access to sources of assistance in maneuvering the application process. According to a survey in California, 95% of the potential beneficiaries and many of the community workers interviewed confused Medi-Cal (The California name for Medicaid) with welfare and with Medicare. (Some thought it was a soft drink.) Even among those using the program, 90% thought it was the same as welfare. The welfare stigma was found to be highly unsettling for most users, a cause of misuse, and a clear deterent to utilization by potential beneficiaries (Berger, 1969).

Requirements 10 and 11 for state plans specify the relationships with welfare. Number 10 requires the state to provide medical assistance to all individuals under their existing welfare categories *plus* coverage of the "medically indigent" with services of the same scope (no less than services provided under any other state plan). Number 11 then requires cooperative arrangements with health agencies, thus allowing Welfare to be the coordinating agency but suggesting that the state health department should assume responsibility for the health aspects of the program. In view of the California study and experience in other states that have placed the Medicaid administration in welfare departments, the administration *at least* of the part of the program dealing with non-welfare medically indigent patients should be delegated to health departments. Along with this transfer, health educators should replace welfare workers as planners of community organization, information, and education programs. Emphasis then might be placed more on prevention of illnesses and their recurrence, appropriate utilization of health resources, anticipation of problems in negotiating the health care system, preparing unsophisticated patients to get the most out

of their brief encounters with physicians (what questions to ask, what rights to demand, etc.), and related problems that health educators could presumably deal with more adequately than welfare workers. But most important is the removal of Medicaid from identification with welfare (Bernstein, 1970).

These needs are underscored by the "Report of the Task force on Medicaid and Related Programs" submitted to the Secretary of Health, Education and Welfare in 1970:

Programs of health education, provided they meet adequate standards set by the Federal Government, should be considered integral components of any health care service, and therefore, included in the budget of such service. All agencies and institutions providing health services that receive Federal support must provide continuing programs of health education to their consumers.

The report continues:

State Medicaid Programs should be required to undertake educational efforts designed to: improve recipients' use of the Medicaid program; improve the health of Medicaid recipients through preventive education; improve providers' use of the program; and provide for greater participation by provider and consumer in the planning, implementation, and evaluation of the program.

In order to assist State Medicaid Programs in developing effective educational and informational programs, guidelines, materials, consultation and technical assistance should be provided by Health, Education and Welfare. "Model educational programs" should be developed in consultation with the States. The approach used should also include "outreach" education utilizing potential Medicaid beneficiaries. Efforts should be made to involve voluntary health agencies, consumer organizations and professional organizations, many of which have substantial and successful health education experience.

This last recommendation relates to the need for coordinating existing community health resources and planning for health on a more comprehensive basis. Medicare and Medicaid must be regarded as failures if they were expected to achieve this kind of coordinated and comprehensive approach to community health planning. The real potential for such an approach was intended to be provided by legislation passed the following year as Public Law 89-749.

Comprehensive Health Planning Act of 1966. This Act (PL 89-749) declared as its purpose (1) "promoting and assuring the highest level of health attainable for every person" (2) through "an effective partnership, involving close intergovernmental collaboration, official and voluntary efforts, and participation of individuals and organizations" (3) with federal financial assistance "to support the marshalling of all health resources—national, State, and local—to assure comprehensive health services of high quality for every person," (4) "but without interference with existing patterns of private professional practice of medicine, dentistry, and related healing arts," therefore requiring (5) "comprehensive planning for health services, health manpower, and health facilities . . . at every level of government," (6) "strengthening the leadership and capacities of State health agencies," and (7) "support of health services provided people in their communities should be broadened and made more flexible."

This law has since been replaced (superceded) by the National Health Planning and Resource Development Act of 1974 (PL 93-641), which will be discussed in Chapter 20, but some important insights into national health policy, politics, and trends can be gained by examining the wording of the original preamble. "Assuring the highest level of health attainable for every person" was little more than a platitude in this context. It did not represent a commitment of the federal government, but rather the ultimate goal toward which specific provision of the act might contribute with some federal assistance. The term "partnership" in part 2 clearly exempted the federal government from ultimate responsibility. Note also in part 3 that federal *financial assistance to support the marshalling* of resources was consciously different from *providing resources.*

The ultimate concession to the medical establishment is found once again in part 4. Not to interfere with "existing patterns of private professional practice" virtually nullified the community potential of the Act. The main emphasis of the law became the development and support of planning capacities, especially at the state health department level (see Chapter 20). One section of the Act provided for Project Grants for Areawide Health Planning.

The appointment of community planning councils was required to have consumers in a majority of the councils. How to define "consumers of health services" and how to obtain "representatives" of such consumers became one of the most controversial aspects of this Act's implementation. Some communities merely relabeled selected professionals and agency representatives as "consumers." The interaction of health professionals and lay consumers working together on planning councils has been an exciting and at times difficult process. Professionals tend to be threatened by and resistant to the challenge to their traditional roles. Consumers are sometimes intimidated by their lack of technical knowledge, but because they usually are placed on these councils as representatives of special interest groups rather than as representatives-at-large or homemakers, they have usually acted as advocates for specific groups rather than consumers in general. The successful conduct of planning meetings bringing together such diverse interests and skills calls for training and experience in group process and discussion leadership. These and other planning skills are in relatively short supply.

The availability of planners with such skills was recognized as a problem and has been addressed by manpower legislation. Unfortunately, the Planning Agencies and Councils had to be set up before training programs could turn out skilled planners. One of the reasons that health educators have disappeared from other programs (Medicare and community health department programs) is that their general skills in planning, community organization, training, and group process were suddenly in great demand with the enactment of Public Law 89-749 and many became reclassified as "administrators," "planners," and "directors" in Comprehensive Health Planning Agencies.

SUMMARY OF EXISTING AND PROPOSED NATIONAL HEALTH POLICIES

We have ranged rather superficially over the history and current status of health legislation already enacted by Congress. We have identified some major gaps and weaknesses in these acts, especially as related to their failure to take adequately into account the knowledge, attitudes, behavior, resources, and health needs of consumers and communities and thereby to challenge the existing medical establishment to make significant changes in the structure and form of personal health care delivery systems. The tacit assumption underlying these acts is that given more resources and better coordination of existing resources, the existing system (or nonsystem) can be strengthened to meet the needs and demands of the population.

The Comprehensive Health Planning Act and the National Health Planning and Resources Development Act come closest to challenging the existing order through participation of professionals and consumers in decentralized decision making, but the financial support and the power to implement the decisions still are lacking at the community level.

Proposed national medical care programs. A growing nationwide realization that the existing national program for providing medical and hospital care is not adequate has motivated groups in and out of government to propose national health care or health security programs. These proposals differ both in philosophy and in their basic forms, yet their differences are not irreconcilable. Any final program doubtless will contain elements of these various proposals. For purposes here, two types of proposals will be presented for contrast: that of the American Medical Association and that of Senators Edward M. Kennedy, Martha Griffiths, and twenty-four other senators.

The United States has not suddenly decided to follow the example of other countries. Although the seventeen countries that rank higher than the United States in life expectancy statistics all have a national health program (either financing or providing services) and all have lower per capita costs for health care than the United States, these experiences only lend support to a movement for national health insurance in this country that began with the 1912 presidential campaign of Theodore Roosevelt. Franklin Roosevelt's report to Congress in 1935, which formed the basis of the Social Security Act, endorsed the principle of compulsory national health insurance but made no specific program recommendation.

President Truman also proposed a comprehensive, prepaid medical insurance plan in 1945 and again in 1947, 1949, and 1950, which led ultimately to OASI, which in turn led to the Kerr-Mills bill (Medicare) in 1965.

Numerous proposals on restructuring the health care system have been introduced recently by public and private groups recognizing the inadequacy of the Social Security Amendments on Medicare and Medicaid to provide health insurance for the elderly and the medically indigent. The major proposals now before Congress for national health insurance plans place major emphasis on insurance protection. The National Health Insurance Plan, proposed by the Committee of 100 and first introduced by Senator Edward Kennedy, is probably the most comprehensive of all and strongly emphasizes preventive care and manpower training. Even this relatively "liberal" proposal, however, exempts the government from managing direct care services.

All of the proposals offer protections to the pocketbooks and assets of both consumers and providers. All involve some use of federal tax devices, and at least one proposal makes further use of state taxes. The American

Medical Association proposal, of course, would interfere least with the existing organization and delivery of medical care. It involves federal income tax credits for individuals who purchase health insurance; voluntary free choice of benefit packages that include all physician services; some method of pooling of risks among insuring agencies; and control of quality, use, and efficiency by providers only. An approach that minimizes the possibility of change in the health care delivery system and the participation of consumers may fall short of national needs.

There is increasing general agreement that some form of universal coverage is essential through federal legislation. Nevertheless, there are substantial disagreements over the approach that should be taken. Principally, there is the contention that a mandate for payment for a national health insurance program would inflate the cost of medical services because of deficiencies in organization, facilities, and manpower available to furnish medical care under the uncoordinated schemes that we now operate. Medicare and Medicaid are prime examples of the inflationary results of pumping large sums of federal financial resources into the present health complex. Billions of dollars placed in the hands of health services consumers, pressing against a system incapable of providing these services on an adequate scale, would produce further inflation of the cost of medical care unless specific resources are developed and the system restructured.

Some form of universal health insurance is foreseeable in the near future. National health insurance seems to be the most politically feasible first step toward the development of a broad-spectrum universal financing mechanism that will provide incentives for improving the health care delivery system. Underlying the promotion of any national health insurance program is the recognition that there is little point in pouring vast federal sums into health insurance without a concomitant commitment to reorganize the delivery system, to continue developing manpower resources, to place emphasis on prevention, and to involve consumers in decisions regarding the delivery of services at the local level.

The American Medical Association has advanced what has been termed the "Medicredit" plan. The protection may be in the form of a health insurance policy from a company; membership in a prepayment plan such as Blue Cross–Blue Shield; or membership in a prepaid group practice plan. Choice of the kind of protection desired is made by the individual or the family. Medicredit will be approved by the respective states to assure that benefits meet national standards. Medicredit does not obligate the government to pay for the care of people who can afford to provide most of the payment for their medical problems themselves.

There are two forms of protection offered under the plan: basic coverage, and catastrophic coverage. Basic coverage provides for the payment of expenses for services such as inpatient care in a hospital or extended day facility for 60 days during a 12-month policy period, in a semi-private room. Within the 60 day limit, 2 days in an extended care facility count as only 1 day. Inpatient hospital services cover all care customarily provided in a hospital including nursing services, drugs, oxygen, blood and plasma (after the first 3 pints), biologicals, appliances, surgery, delivery or recovery room, intensive care or coronary care unit, rehabilitation unit, and other customary provisions. Extended care facility services cover all care customarily provided in an extended care facility. Outpatient emergency care covers diagnostic services: x-rays, laboratory tests, electrocardiograms, and other diagnostic tests.

Medical services—preventive, diagnostic, or therapeutic—provided or ordered by a doctor of medicine or doctor of osteopathy, wherever provided, are covered. This includes dental or oral surgery, and ambulance service, but does not include cosmetic (plastic) surgery unless related to birth defects or burns or scars caused by injury or illness.

Catastrophic coverage would pay for an additional 30 days in a hospital or extended care facility. Since medical care services continue without limit under basic coverage, no additional medical services are necessary.

Who pays for what? Medicredit is designed to give maximum help to those who need it most, and minimum help to those who are best able to pay their own way. Financial condition is determined solely by the amount of federal income tax a person or family pays whether by withholding or direct payment by individuals when they file their tax return. A person or family paying no federal income tax has all basic and catastrophic coverage paid by the federal government. For a person or family who pays federal income tax, the federal government pays for the catastrophic coverage. The cost of the basic plan is prorated on the basis of federal income tax paid.

What is covered? Under basic coverage, the patient would pay:

1. $50 per stay in the hospital as an inpatient
2. 20% of the first $500 of expenses for outpatient or emergency care (maximum of $100) in a 12-month period
3. 20% of the first $500 of expenses for medical care services (maximum of $100) in a 12-month period

Medicredit was designed to solve the most immediate problem relating to medical and health care. Companion programs are being proposed by the AMA to solve the various problems inherent in providing medical and hospital services for all citizens.

The Health Security Act was introduced in the United States Senate by Senator Edward M. Kennedy and is a national health insurance plan to be administered by the federal government, covering all United States citizens and certain aliens. It would repeal Medicare but would continue Medicaid as a supplemental program.

The plan provides for comprehensive health benefits, including physicians services, inpatient and outpatient hospital care, home health services, supporting services such as optometry, podiatry, devices, and appliances subject to the following exclusions:

1. Dental care initially limited to children under 15; covered age group is to be extended in each of the succeeding 5 years until all under age 25 are covered
2. Drug benefit limited to inpatient drugs, specified drugs necessary for chronic conditions, drugs provided through group practice systems
3. Skilled nursing home care initially limited to 120 days with provision for expansion when feasible
4. Mental hospital care limited to 45 days per year active treatment; limit of twenty consultations per year for outpatient psychiatric care if provided by solo practitioner

Benefits are covered in full with no deductibles, co-insurance, waiting periods, maximums, or cutoffs other than as previously indicated.

Hospitals, homes with skilled nursing, and home health agencies would be paid on a schedule of reasonable costs. Health maintenance organizations or professional foundations will be paid on a per capita basis or approved budget. Independent physicians and dentists may be paid on fee-for-service basis or per capita. Supplemental stipends may be paid to practitioners located in remote or deprived areas. Practitioners may be reimbursed for costs of continuing education.

Administration of the program is to be by means of a five-member Health Security Board within the Department of Health, Education and Welfare. A National Health Security Council, representing consumers, providers of care, health organizations, and others would advise the Board on program operation. Regional authorities would be given strong discretionary powers. The program would substantially supplant private health insurance.

The program is to be financed by a 3.5% tax on employer's payrolls (36% of costs); 1.0% tax on employees (12% of costs); 2.5% tax on self-employed (2% of costs); and the balance (50%) from general tax revenues.

The Act also provides $600 million for a Health Resources Development Fund to be used in 2 years preceding program operations for development of health manpower.

Some general principles under which the Kennedy-type of proposal would operate are the following:

1. The national health insurance program should be an integral part of the national social insurance system financed by employer-employee and federal tax revenues.
2. The spectrum of program benefits should include preventive, curative, and rehabilitative services.
3. Payments for the services provided as benefits should assure full financial protection for the consumers and should be fair to the providers of services.
4. There should be provisions within the program design to safeguard quantity, quality, effectiveness, continuity, and economy of the family health care services it finances.
5. Organization of auxiliary and professional health personnel into health teams should be supported, financed, and trained.
6. There should be public control of the basic policies governing the program through consumer participation and full public accountability for its financial and operational activities.
7. National development of adequate manpower, facilities, and organizations needed for effective delivery of health care services should be an integral part of the program design.
8. Although primarily directed to the development of comprehensive personal health care services, the national health insurance program should have concern for the development of effective community health and welfare programs at the national, state, regional, and local levels through comprehensive health planning.
9. There should be advocation of reform and realignment of federal agencies concerned with health programs into a coordinated entity that will provide common objectives and common action toward developing integrated health systems.

One of the most positive aspects of this bill from the point of view of political develop-ment and participation is the broad base of support and input that has been included in its formulation. The Committee for National Health Insurance or "Committee of 100" was originally formed by the late Walter Reuther in 1968. Three of the 100 members, along with twelve other Senators, first sponsored the bill in August, 1970. It was later merged with a similar bill sponsored by Congresswoman Martha Griffiths and the AFL-CIO. Unlike the other plans with their emphasis on the private sector, this bill convincingly proposes "a working partnership between the public and private sectors." Although the bill clearly disavows any intention of government-owned or government-managed facilities, it does set down a variety of provisions for consumer and community participation. For example, consumer organizations will be encouraged to give health care a high priority in their overall activities and to sponsor and develop comprehensive, community-wide health care organizations. Along with comprehensive health care programs to be developed by hospitals, physician groups, and combinations of professionals, the consumer-sponsored organizations will be supported and recognized by Health Security.

Effective participation by consumers at all levels of policy formulation and program development of Health Security will be assured on the Board, on the National Advisory Council assisting in its continuing public administration, and on regional and local advisory councils. There will be public control of the basic policies governing the program, and full public accountability for its financial and operational activities.

There are also major provisions for and commitments to preventive health in this bill, along with concomitant concerns for the development of health manpower and support for the location of needed health personnel in urban and rural poverty areas. Health education is specifically cited as an essential component of the program.

Appraisal. All of the proposed national

health program proposals have certain merits. Doubtless any final program accepted and put into operation will incorporate certain features of each of the proposals. When such a national program will be instituted in the United States depends on a combination of circumstances. An economic recession would dramatize the need for some type of program, but it is to be hoped that the architects of any program will not work under the pressure of an emergency. In addition, the voices of the health professions must be heard in an atmosphere of deliberation and consideration. To convert to a national health program is no small task for a nation as large, dynamic, and varied as the United States.

The inability of private health insurance to meet the medical and other health needs of the United States population fully has been demonstrated. The commercial plans have taken away most of the low-risk, high-income consumers, leaving the nonprofit Blue Cross and Blue Shield plans with the necessity of raising premium rates on their poorer customers. As Senator Kennedy pointed out in his speech introducing the Health Security Act (Congressional Record, 5.4297, August 27, 1970), private insurance in 1968 met only one-third of the private costs of health care and much of that was where it was needed least:

20% of all Americans under 65 had no hospital insurance

22% had no surgical insurance

34% had no inpatient medical insurance

50% had no outpatient x-ray and laboratory insurance

57% had no insurance for office visits or home visits

61% had no insurance against the cost of prescription drugs

97% had no dental care insurance

Moreover, Kennedy continued, private health insurance is not sufficiently prevention-oriented, it is *sickness* rather than *health* insurance. It gives partial rather than comprehensive benefits. It fails to control either costs or quality. "Health insurance coverage in America today is more loophole than protection," he said.

The health insurance industry itself has acknowledged the problem and has developed a series of "new objectives" for which a program has been proposed for federal action.

1. Health care delivery systems should be *responsive and relevant* to the continuing health needs of people rather than only to their episodic medical needs. Systems should be oriented to the whole person and his needs for disease prevention and health maintenance, rather than primarily to medical treatment and management of disabling conditions.

2. Health care delivery systems should *integrate and interact* with other social and environmental systems that serve in the public interest, including employment, education, housing, transportation, communications, recreation, etc.

3. Health care delivery systems should be *reflective of consumer and professional interests*, operating not only to provide the quality of care needed and desired by the citizen-consumer, but to assure that the means of delivering services are in keeping with the professional concepts and standards of the providers of service.

4. Health care delivery systems should be adaptively structured and interrelated so as to *provide access to quality health care by all residents* regardless of such factors as geographic location, economic resources or cultural or social variables.

The personal health system for the future as envisioned by the Health Insurance Association of America would have the following characteristics:

5. Multiple and organized systems providing relatively comprehensive services and continuity of care, with the needs of the individual taking precedence over institutional requirements, and with extensive utilization of group practice and team methods of delivering personal health care services.

6. Access to personal health care reasonably near to those being served, with more care provided on an ambulatory basis, and limited in-patient care adapted to the needs of

the patient and economy and effectiveness of service.

7. Emphasis on preventive services, health maintenance procedures, and health education concerning individual and family health behavior and the use of health services.
8. Active involvement of "consumers"—including those of low income, of minority and ethnic groups, and of the areas being served, as well as middle and upper income people—in planning, development, and management of services and facilities, and in determination of priorities.
9. Many different efforts separately and jointly by governments, professions, and private industry to try out new ways and means of delivering health care services and similar pluralistic approaches to financing—including strong reliance on insurance and other forms of prepayment as well as governmental subsidies (Gulick, 1970).

The United States will someday have a national health insurance program, but when and how is still a matter of conjecture. To duplicate Sweden's program would be a formidable and questionable task. What works effectively in Sweden, a nation of about 8 million people, may not fit at all for a nation of more than 25 times that population. The medical profession, with much at stake, will have its voice heard in any proposal for a nationalized program. Other professional and consumer groups less well organized will need to combine forces to be heard as clearly.

QUESTIONS AND EXERCISES

1. Why do we say that it is paradoxical that the United States does not have the highest level of health nor the greatest life expectancy?
2. Why is health education of the poor an urgent need in the United States?
3. Why does quackery tend to flourish in the United States?
4. Why has the Administrator of the Federal Food and Drug Administration proposed that most patent medicines be banned from sale?
5. Name some patent medicines you think should be banned from sale and indicate the reasons.
6. Why will an adult citizen in the United States wear a charm around his neck to keep sickness away?
7. What should the communications media do to protect the public from quackery?
8. Is the United States general and special hospital

admissions rate of 146 per 1,000 population too high or too low? Why?

9. What is the ratio of physicians to population in your county and what is your appraisal of the situation?
10. How does your county measure up to the standard of four and one-half beds per 1,000 people?
11. Why is the average length of stay in a hospital of limited value in the analysis of medical and hospital costs to citizens?
12. To what extent should nursing homes and personal care homes be increased in the next 10 years in your community?
13. Why are medical and hospital costs increasing faster than the cost of living index?
14. What is your proposal for paying for hospital and medical care for the low-income families not on welfare?
15. Why are people slow in paying their medical and hospital bills?
16. What is the case for and against the federal government totally subsidizing education in the medical, dental, and other health professions?
17. Why should the consumer of medical service have a voice in how medical service is to be paid?
18. What evidence have you that the public seeks to control medical practice?
19. Make a survey among 100 adult acquaintances under age 65 to determine the percentage carrying hospital and medical insurance and compare it with national figures.
20. Propose a National Hospital and Medical Service Program for the United States.

REFERENCES

The American Assembly: The health of Americans, New York, 1970, Columbia University Press.

Andersen, R., Smedby, B. J., and Anderson, O. W.: Medical care use in Sweden and the United States—a comparative analysis of systems and behavior, Chicago, 1970, University of Chicago Press.

Anderson, O. W.: Health care: can there be equity? The United States, Sweden, and England, New York, 1973, John Wiley & Sons, Inc.

Becker, M. H., editor: Personal health behavior and the health belief model, Health Education Monographs **2:**324-473, 1974.

Bennett, A. E.: Communication between doctors and patients, London, 1976, Oxford University Press for the Nuffield Provincial Hospitals Trust.

Berger, J.: A study of information needs in the community on the Medi-Cal program, Berkeley, Calif., 1969, Bureau of Health Education, California State Department of Public Health.

Bernstein, B. J.: Public health—inside or outside the mainstream of the political process? Lessons from the passage of Medicaid, American Journal of Public Health **60:**1690-1700, September, 1970.

Blum, H. L.: Expanding health care horizons: from a general systems concept of health to a national health policy, Oakland, 1976, Third Party Associates.

Brenner, M. H.: Estimating the social costs of national economic policy, Washington, D.C., 1976, U.S. Government Printing Office.

Cambridge Research Institute: Trends affecting the U.S. health care system, Rockville, Bureau of Health Planning and Resources Development, DHEW Publication No. (HRA) 76-14503, 1976.

Chapman, J. E., and Chapman, H. H.: Behavior and health care: a humanistic helping process, St. Louis, 1975, The C. V. Mosby Co.

Crowley, A., editor: Medical education in the United States, 1973-1974, Journal of the American Medical Association, Supplement, January, 1975.

Editors of Consumer Reports: The medicine show, Mount Vernon, N.Y., rev. ed. 1974, Consumers Union.

Forward Plan for Health, FY 1978-82, Washington, D.C., 1976, Public Health Service, DHEW Publication No. (05) 76-50046.

Fuchs, V. R.: Who shall live? Health, economics and social choice, New York, 1974, Basic Books, Inc., Publishers.

Garb, S.: Abbreviations and acronyms in medicine and nursing, New York, 1976, Springer Publishing Co., Inc.

Garfield, S. R.: The delivery of medical care, Scientific American 222:15-23, April, 1970.

Golden, A. S.: An inventory of primary health care practice, Cambridge, Mass., 1976, Ballinger Publishing Co.

Goodrich, C. H., and associates: Welfare medical care, an experiment, Cambridge, Mass., 1970, Harvard University Press.

Gulick, M. A.: The health care crisis, The Conference Board Record 7:50-51, 1970.

Health, United States, 1975, Rockville, Md., 1976, Health Resources Administration, National Center for Health Statistics, DHEW Publication No. (HRA) 76-1232.

Health Resources Statistics, 1974, Rockville, National Center for Health Statistics, DHEW Publication No. (HRA) 75-1509.

Hepner, J. O., and Hepner, D. M.: The health strategy game: a challenge for reorganization and management, St. Louis, 1973, The C. V. Mosby Co.

Hiatt, H. H.: The politics of health care: nine case studies of innovative planning in New York City, New York, 1973, Praeger Publishers, Inc.

Kennedy, E. M.: In critical condition: the crisis in America's health care, New York, 1972, Simon & Schuster, Inc.

Lalonde, M.: A new perspective on the health of Canadians: a working document, Ottawa, 1974, Ministry of National Health and Welfare, Government of Canada.

Levin, L. S.: Self-care: new initiatives in health, New York, 1976, Neale Watson Academic Publications, Inc.

Lewis, C. E., Fein, R., and Mechanic, D.: A right to health: the problem of access to primary medical care, New York, 1976, John Wiley & Sons, Inc.

Marmor, T. R.: Politics of medicare, Chicago, 1970, Aldine-Atherton, Inc.

McKinlay, J. B., editor: Economic aspects of health care, New York, 1973, Prodist.

Munts, R.: Bargaining for health: labor unions, health insurance and medical care, Madison, 1967, University of Wisconsin Press.

Myers, E. S.: Insurance coverage for mental illness: present status and future prospects, American Journal of Public Health 60:1921, 1970.

National Center for Health Statistics: The nations' use of health resources, 1976 edition, Rockville, Md., 1977, Health Resources Administration, Public Health Service, DHEW Publication No. (HRA) 77-1240.

National Commission on Community Health Services, Report of the Task Force on Health Care Facilities: Community health facilities: the community bridge to effective health services, Washington, D.C., 1967, Public Affairs Press.

Navarro, V.: Medicine under capitalism, New York, 1976, Prodist.

Norman, J. C.: Medicine in the ghetto, New York, 1969, Appleton-Century-Crofts.

Otten, A.: Doctor's helpers, Wall Street Journal, April 4, 1974.

Preventive Medicine USA: Theory, practice and application of prevention in personal health services and quality control and evaluation of preventive health services, New York, 1976, Prodist.

Reynolds, F. W., and Barsam, P. C.: Adult health services for the chronically ill and aged, New York, 1967, The Macmillan Co.

Richardson, J. T.: Origin and development of group hospitalization in the United States, 1890-1940, Columbia, 1945, University of Missouri Press.

Roemer, M. I.: Organization of medical care under Social Security, Washington, D.C., 1971, International Labour Office.

Roemer, M. I.: Rural health care, St. Louis, 1976, The C. V. Mosby Co.

Sackett, D. M., and Haynes, B.: Compliance with therapeutic regimes, Baltimore, 1976, The Johns Hopkins University Press.

Shonick, W.: Elements of planning for area-wide personal health services, St. Louis, 1976, The C. V. Mosby Co.

Social Security Administration, Office of Research and Statistics: National health expenditure highlights, fiscal year 1976, Research and Statistics Note No. 27, December 22, 1976.

Stimmel, B.: The Congress and health manpower: a legislative morass, New England Journal of Medicine 293:68-74, July 10, 1975.

U.S. National Center for Health Services Research: Changes in the costs of treatment of selected illnesses 1951-1964-1971, Rockville, Md., 1976, DHEW Publication No. (HRA) 77-3161.

U.S. National Center for Health Statistics: Hospital discharges and length of stay; short-stay hospitals, United States—1972, Rockville, Md., 1976, DHEW Publication No. (HRA) 77-1534.

Weaver, J. L.: National health policy and the underserved, St. Louis, 1976, The C. V. Mosby Co.

White, K. L.: Epidemiology as a fundamental science—its uses in health services planning, administration, and evaluation, New York, 1976, Oxford University Press, Inc.

Wing, K.: The law and the public's health, St. Louis, 1976, The C. V. Mosby Co.

19 ▪ COMMUNITY HEALTH SERVICES

The public must and will be served.

William Penn

A community recognizes there are some things important in the promotion of health that individuals cannot do for themselves and that must be done through collective action. There are also some things that the individual can do but that can be done better on a community or cooperative basis. In the complex society of today, no one is totally self-sufficient in dealing with all threats to health. To facilitate and supplement what the individual does in health promotion, official and voluntary health organizations have been established on local, state, national, and international levels. Operating both cooperatively and independently, these organizations protect and promote the health of the community.

COMMUNITY RESPONSIBILITY

Need, demand, custom, and gradual development have led society to accept as a community responsibility certain health services on behalf of all citizens. As the population increases and tends to concentrate in urban centers, some new health problems develop, but most of the health problems that have long been with communities become more complex and more difficult to manage. If community health problems of today are more complex, society has advanced its technology in dealing with some of them.

Most community health services directly or indirectly will be of value to all citizens but of greater value to lower income groups than to higher economic groups. As an example, community immunization services will have a greater protective impact on lower income groups but will have some value, direct or indirect, for people on all income levels.

Health services and functions accepted as community responsibility include safe, ample water supply, safe milk supply, regulation of food establishments, waste disposal, control of air pollution, insect control, rat control, nuisance elimination, screening and referral for detection of chronic diseases, collection and recording of vital statistics, communicable disease control, infant, maternal, child, adult, and senior citizen health promotion, mental health, nutrition education, health education, laboratory service, and other services specific for certain communities.

PROFESSIONAL PERSONNEL

In the previous chapter the supply and demand for physicians, nurses, dentists, and other providers of personal health services were reviewed. These personnel provide the base for community health services as well, but an additional cadre of professionally qualified community health specialists is needed to plan, organize, administer, and evaluate community health programs. Of the 780,000 employed nurses in 1972, for example, only 54,800 (7%) were employed in public health agencies and schools, compared with 74% in hospitals and nursing homes (Health resources statistics, 1974). Less than 5% of these nurses employed in schools and public health agencies have master's level

299

training in public health (Hall and associates, 1973).

Table 19-1 presents the developing manpower picture in the current decade, using estimates from a variety of sources to compare the 1970 supply with the 1980 projected requirements. The "school output" includes the graduates of schools of public health as well as those receiving similar advanced degrees in community health education from schools of education, community health nursing from schools of nursing, health services administration from schools of business, and environmental health from schools of engineering. These figures were verified and endorsed by the Milbank Memorial Fund Commission on Higher Education for Public Health (Sheps, 1976), which concluded, " . . . the greatest relative increases in public health manpower requirements will occur in mental health, health education, and health services administration."

Health education manpower requirements are expected to triple because of new programs in smoking, alcohol, diabetes, hypertension, and cancer control, which will depend heavily on health education as the main approach to behavioral change. Currently, fourteen of the nineteen accredited schools of public health have active graduate pro-

Table 19-1 ■ Estimated supply of and requirements for selected categories of professional health manpower for community health services

Occupational category	Professionals with master's level training or higher*			
	Base year supply (1970 unless specified)	1980 supply, assuming		Possible 1980 requirements‡
		Constant school output†	Reduced school output†	
Environmental health	2,200	4,300	3,800	5,000
Epidemiology	1,000	1,800	1,500	2,000
Health education	2,000	3,600	3,100	6,000
Health services administration	8,500	18,200	15,300	25,200
Health statistics	1,100 (1971)	1,700	1,500	2,500
Maternal health, family planning, and child health	800	1,800	1,500	2,000
Mental health	200	400	350	1,100
Public health dentistry	300	550	500	550
Public health nursing	2,500 (1968)	5,200	4,500	5,700
Public health nutrition	1,000	1,800	1,500	2,600
Public health veterinary medicine	200	350	300	550

Adapted from Hall, T., and associates: Professional health manpower for community health programs, Chapel Hill, 1973, University of North Carolina School of Public Health.

*Numbers over 1,000 are rounded to nearest 100; below 1,000, to nearest 50.

†"Constant school output" is based on the size of the average graduating class in the early 1970s. "Reduced school output" assumes that the Administration's fiscal year 1974 budget, resulting in a 35% reduction in the combined school output from the 1973/1974 academic year, is not replaced.

‡The projected requirements do not take into consideration the continuing demands being made on American schools of public health to train foreign students in connection with the U.S. foreign assistance program and the requirements of the World Health Organization. Foreign student enrollments have averaged over 15% in recent years.

grams conferring some 250 master's degrees per year in community health education (University of California at Berkeley, UCLA, Columbia University, Harvard University, University of Hawaii, University of Illinois, The Johns Hopkins University, Loma Linda University, University of Massachusetts, The University of Michigan, The University of Minnesota, The University of North Carolina, University of Puerto Rico, and Yale University). Another seven programs in other educational units have master's level programs accredited by the Council on Education for Public Health (California State University at Northridge and San Jose, Columbia Teachers College, Hunter College, University of Missouri at Columbia School of Medicine, New York University, and the University of Tennessee). An estimated twenty other programs are applying or soon will be qualified to apply for accreditation, indicating the rapid growth of this field. These programs admit graduates of nursing and clinical programs, health education, social and biological sciences, and others with at least 1 year of community health experience.

Mental health specialists with graduate preparation in public health are in increasing demand because of the growth of community mental health centers and other programs related to mental health in community agencies. There were only 197 graduates of schools of public health with a major in mental health between 1960 and 1970, less than 2% of the 11,851 graduates during that period (Richardson, 1973). Most of those receiving master's degrees in mental health from schools of public health had prior graduate degrees in medicine, psychiatric nursing, psychology, or social work.

Health services administration has seen a growth pattern similar to that of community health education, but on a larger scale. The number of new graduate programs more than doubled between 1960 and 1972, and many new programs are now applying for accreditation to add to the 650 master's level graduates per year (Sheps, 1976). Most of the new programs have grown out of hospital administration programs in the same way that new community health education programs are growing out of school health education programs outside schools of public health. Another trend that may partially offset the shortages in other specialties for community health is the development of specialty tracks within graduate programs of health services and public health administration, such as mental health, emergency health services, health maintenance organizations, family planning services, long-term care, and ambulatory care services.

SOURCES OF PUBLIC HEALTH LAW

Woodrow Wilson defined law as "that portion of the established thought and habit which has gained distinct and formal recognition in the shape of uniform rules backed by the authority and power of government." A more concise definition is: law is crystallized public opinion. Public health law is that branch of jurisprudence that applies common and statutory law to the principles of hygiene.

Public health law in the United States is derived from several sources discussed in the following paragraphs. All sources of public health law have some impact on health, but the closer to a community the source of a public health law, the greater will be its impact on and value to the community.

The Federal Constitution. The Constitution is a grant of authority by the states to the federal government but with reservations as expressed in the Tenth Amendment. "The powers not delegated to the United States by the Constitution, nor prohibited by it to the States, are reserved to the States respectively, or to the people." The word *health* is not used in the Constitution and nowhere in the Constitution is there any reference to public health. The States did not surrender their control over health and they retain it today under the "police power." While the control of public health is primarily a state function, the Federal Constitution contains many broad provisions that affect the control of health and spell out the general responsibilities of the federal government in promoting the public well-being. These are described in Chapter 21.

State constitution and legislation. Fundamentally, promotion of public health is the function of the state. Governments have long recognized health as a basic essential that government has an inherent obligation, right, and power to protect and promote. From colonial times, states have taken whatever measures are necessary to safeguard and promote the health of their citizens. This authority is vested in the *police power*, which is recognized by the courts as well as by the federal government.

County and municipal ordinances and regulations. The state legislature has the authority to delegate the police power to counties and cities to exercise within their own territorial boundaries. This is done through the delegation of "home rule" to counties and municipalities. A city thus may present a proposed city charter to the state legislature for consideration. If the legislature approves, it grants this charter and home rule to the city. In health matters, counties and cities may pass health ordinances and regulations to be effective within their own geographical boundaries. Community standards may be higher than state standards, but not lower. Generally, counties and cities adopt the same health standards and regulations found in the state sanitary code.

Common law. A heritage from Great Britain, the common law is distinguished from civil law and from ecclesiastical law. It is unwritten law and is based on custom or court decision as distinguished from statutory laws. Based on practice and experience, the common law is founded on court interpretation of a present situation in terms of court decisions of the past. Some health problems or controversies may be adjudicated on the basis of custom or past practice. To this extent, the common law represents a source of public health law.

Police power

Police power is the authority of the people, vested in the state government, to enact laws, within constitutional limits, to promote the health, comfort, safety, order, morality, and general welfare of the people. This means the authority to promote the welfare of the public, although it may mean regulating and restraining the use of freedom and property. The police power is based on the greatest good for the greatest number and may operate to the inconvenience and even distress of certain individuals. All persons, business firms, and corporations must regulate their conduct subject to the police power.

Any *reasonable* act done under the shield of police power will tend to be upheld unless contrary to constitutional provisions. Amendments 1, 4, 6, and 14 of the Bill of Rights safeguard the personal rights of the citizen. Although the Constitution guarantees freedom of religious belief, such a guarantee does not invalidate a school board regulation requiring students to have a health examination for admission to school. Likewise, it is a valid exercise of the police power for a state law to require marriage license applicants to have a physician's statement showing they are free from venereal diseases.

Jurisdiction of any official health department extends over all persons and things within its boundaries. A state law may extend the jurisdiction of a county or city health department beyond the county or city boundaries. Even in the absence of such law, a local health department may take action to abate a nuisance outside of its territory if its own citizens are affected. The state health department can assume jurisdiction in a health dispute or health problem involving two or more cities or two or more counties.

Nuisance. Blackstone defined nuisance as "anything which worketh hurt, injury, or damage." A public health nuisance is one detrimental to the physical or mental health of one person or a large number of people. Most nuisances are not health nuisances.

Some health nuisances are of major importance, and others are of minor significance.

Health departments take all possible action to prevent nuisances by passing regulations declaring certain conditions to be a nuisance. Such action is taken by state boards of health and local boards of health. The following conditions, which are nuisances, are of importance in terms of their threat to human health: pollution of water, improper sewage disposal, air pollution, contaminated milk, contaminated food other than milk, lead paint in housing, rat infestation, stagnant water providing for insect breeding, and excessive noise (see Chapter 17). Some conditions declared to be health nuisances are actually of minor health significance. Yet the public regards these factors as threats to health. Further, even though these conditions may have a minor effect on health they can interfere with the enjoyment of life. Such things as the following, which have been declared to be nuisances, have slight health significance—rubbish, untidy back yards, odors, pig styes, stables, dead animals, garbage, and dumps. Well-defined legislation or regulations that make it an offense to cause or maintain objectionable conditions can be the basis on which health officials can proceed to correct offensive conditions. In dealing with a nuisance, even when a condition has been defined as a nuisance by law or regulation, diplomacy and tact are still important. It is an indication of competence in health administration when undesirable conditions can be corrected without resorting to extreme measures. Education and diplomacy are sometimes not enough, and court action may be necessary. In the absence of a regulation covering the situation, the board of health may cite a person to appear before it to answer charges of maintaining a nuisance. The following recognized principles of responsibility apply to a nuisance:

1. Motive is not a consideration.
2. Time is not a consideration.
3. Possession of a license to conduct a business does not excuse a nuisance.
4. Negligence is not an excuse.
5. Lack of financial means to correct the condition is not a valid excuse.
6. Municipalities are not responsible for a nuisance in connection with a governmental function but are responsible in connection with a proprietary function.
7. A nuisance is a basis for the revocation of a license.

Courts recognize three classes of nuisances—private, public, and mixed. If the nuisance cannot be corrected by negotiation, action to abate any one of these may be taken by a private citizen or a public health official.

Private nuisance is one that affects, injures, or damages only one individual or relatively few people. Sewage from a septic tank from one house flowing on to neighboring property may be declared to be a nuisance if the offended citizen takes court action. Abatement of a private nuisance is to be found in a suit for damages.

Public nuisance is one that injures a considerable number of people. An industrial plant emitting objectionable fumes affecting a neighborhood could be considered a public nuisance. A group of citizens may themselves file court action or may request local health officials to take action in a court of equity. Plaintiffs ask the court to issue an injunction forbidding the continuance of the condition, or the court may order the defendant to reduce the degree of offensiveness.

Mixed nuisance is one that affects both an individual and a considerable number of persons. Smoke from a factory may affect one person and a whole neighborhood. Remedy could be a suit for damages or a suit in equity, asking that an injunction be issued restraining the responsible party from continuing the condition.

Immediate action is sometimes necessary, and there is not always sufficient time to resort to court action. In this event, summary abatement is the remedy. However, before any action is taken, notice should be given to the person responsible for the condition to permit correction of the condition. If action is not taken, summary abatement is necessary. Persons correcting the nuisance must proceed with caution because they are personally liable for their acts. Courts have held that summary action must be reasonable. If the person responsible for the condition should elect to sue the individual who undertook the summary abatement, the disposition of the case would depend on whether the action taken was reasonable.

CITY HEALTH DEPARTMENT

In the early development of official health agencies, it was the city health department that was most in evidence. Baltimore established the first city health department in 1798. Virtually all cities by the mid-twentieth century had a health department of some description. In the smaller towns the department consisted of a part-time health officer, a quarantine officer, a sanitarian, and a clerk. Activities consisted largely in enforcing isolation and quarantine in communicable disease control and in the inspection of unsanitary conditions. Some small communities still have part-time health officers who are not trained in public health, who are political appointees, and who regard their health duties as a sideline to their medical practice. They have neither the time nor the inclination to carry out the many necessary health duties, and they sometimes use their official position to promote their private practice. Fortunately, this is being phased out in America and is giving way to complete, professionally staffed health departments.

Large cities maintain well-qualified health staffs with a director, nurses, sanitarians, sanitary engineers, laboratory technicians, health educators, and other highly specialized personnel, such as experts in air quality control. The Washington, D.C., health agency is equivalent to a city as well as state health department. In many situations city health departments are giving way to county health departments. A city of 30,000 people in a county of 70,000 would be wise to depend on a county health department rather than have its own separate department. Yet many cities still retain their health departments, which have programs similar to those of the county departments. Baltimore still has its city health department because the surrounding county is politically separate and does not include the city. What will be said later about the program and services of county health departments applies equally to full-time, professionally staffed city health departments.

COUNTY BOARD OF HEALTH

Authority to establish a board of health and a health program is delegated by the state legislature to the legislation body of the county or parish, the county board of supervisors, county board of commissioners, or other title. State statutes may specify how the county health board is to be chosen and the number of people to be on the board. The county board of supervisors (or commissioners) usually appoints the county board of health. In some instances a county supervisor or commissioner may be appointed to the county board of health. This arrangement can provide a coordination between the board of supervisors and the board of health. In other states the members of the county board of health must be from outside the membership of the supervisors.

A county board of health may be composed of five, seven, nine, or any other number of members. Too small a membership may not provide adequate representation of the diverse public interests, and too large a number of members may create a debating assembly. Length of term of office varies from 3 to 6 years, and terms are staggered to provide for continuity as well as replacement. Many segments of the population are represented on the board so that a cross-section of the population is represented. At least one physician should be on the board, but no one profession should dominate the membership. A chairman is elected by the board from among its own members.

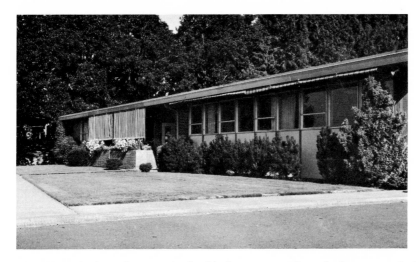

Fig. 19-1. Modern facilities for a county health department. These facilities provide for the sixty staff members of the health department of a county of 150,000 people.

Board responsibilities. Health authority in the county is vested in the county board of health. In many instances this authority will not extend over cities in the county that have their own full-time professional health department. The board has administrative, legislative, and quasi-judicial functions.

The board appoints a director of the county health department, a "health officer," to whom most *administrative* functions are delegated, including the recommendation of professional staff for board approval. The director is usually a medical doctor with professional preparation in public health. Increasingly, nonmedical directors are being appointed. The board also passes on the budget, as recommended by the director, and then sends the budget to the board of supervisors for approval. The board of supervisors has responsibility for the entire county budget, including that portion relating to health.

Legislative functions of the county board of health begin with the adoption of a county sanitary code. This code is the recommendation of the professional staff and is usually the state sanitary code modified to fit the county situation. The county can have more rigid standards than the state, but not less rigid. This county code has the effect of law and will be amended by the board from time to time as conditions require.

Quasi-judicial powers of the county board of health are inherent in the authority of the board to hold hearings preliminary to granting or revoking a license. The board has the authority to summon people to appear before it in cases where health regulations have been violated. Any decision by the board may be appealed to the courts by any citizen who believes that the decision was unjust.

Staff and finances. The health program of the county is carried on by salaried professional personnel. Size of the staff depends on the territorial area of the county, the population, special health problems, resources of the county, and the public's view of the importance of the work of the health department. No rule of thumb exists, but a general guide for professional staff can be represented somewhat as follows:

One health director	per 50,000 people
One public health nurse	per 6,000 people
One psychiatrist	per 50,000 people
One psychologist	per 50,000 people
One psychiatric social worker	per 50,000 people
One public health sanitarian	per 15,000 people
One public health educator	per 50,000 people
One laboratory technician	per 40,000 people
One public health dentist	per 100,000 people

Employment of an administrative assistant is economically sound because it relieves the director of many routine, time-consuming tasks. This action would increase the number of people the director could serve from 50,000 to 75,000.

For economic reasons, a population of 50,000 is regarded as the minimum unit for which a health department should be established. Smaller counties either contract for services from the state or unite two or more sparsely populated counties into a district health unit to have a population in the order of 50,000. Using a minimum of $5.00 per capita per annum and a population of 50,000, a minimum staff and budget could be proposed.

Personnel	Salary	Expense	Total
One director	40,000	3,000	
Eight nurses	92,000	14,000	
One laboratory technician	12,000	1,000	
Two sanitarians	24,000	6,000	
One health educa-tor-nutritionist	16,000	3,000	
Two clerks	14,000		
Office		12,000	
Quarters		8,000	
Miscellaneous		5,000	
			250,000

This budget is in line with the suggested minimum per capita appropriation. While acceptable and perhaps adequate, it is hardly a generous budget.

Staff functions

Direct health services to the people of the community are provided by the full-time professional staff. General and specific services vary greatly from county to county within a state and in counties from one state to another. State legislatures may require county health officials to perform certain special services. For example, one state requires county health directors to make medical investigations of deaths and to make investigations of the "battered child" cases. In many instances two county health depart-

ments will be giving the same service but under two different titles. One health department may give family health service and another health department may be giving the same service as maternal and child health service.

To cite all types of services given by county health departments would be to make an interminable list of unusual, rare, and minor services, as well as essential services. Services listed here are those that are quite generally accepted as the core of county health services. While each county health department has its own particular program, virtually all full-time county health departments carry on the following essential, highly important health services: (1) vital statistics, (2) communicable disease control, (3) promotion of maternal and child health, (4) promotion of dental health, (5) chronic disease control, (6) mental health promotion, (7) environmental health promotion, (8) laboratory service, and (9) health education.

Vital statistics. Biostatistics, public health statistics, human biometrics, and other terms are used to designate public health bookkeeping. Vital statistics consists of the application of statistical methods to the vital facts of human existence. For the health staff, vital statistics points out the health needs of the city or county as well as the strengths and weaknesses of the health program. Health data are obtained by registration and enumeration.

Registration of certain health information is required by law and health regulations. Physicians must report to the health department cases of certain communicable diseases. To make reporting easy, health departments provide all physicians with a simple form on which the physician can quickly record pertinent data and mail postage-free to the health department. Birth and death records usually come to the county health department from the county clerk.

Enumeration of health data usually requires that the health staff actually collect information. Health examinations, dental ex-

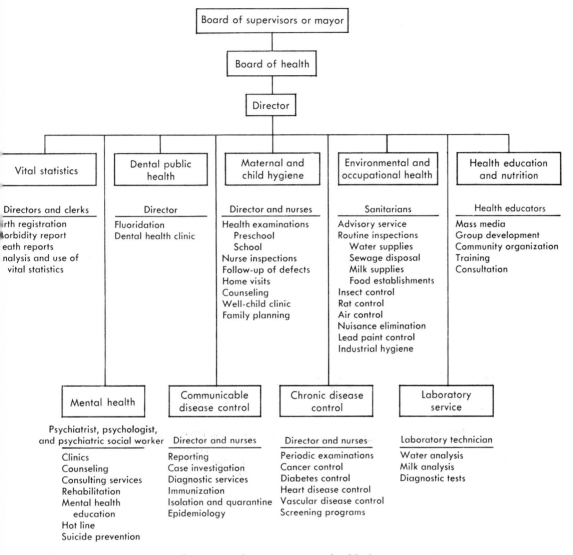

Fig. 19-2. Organization and services of a city or county health department. Many variations in health department organization exist and services vary from one health department to another, but the services listed in this chart represent the core of local health department activities.

aminations, and water samples provide important information. Special surveys and studies also provide information regarded as important by the health staff.

Health statistics are not an end in themselves but are a means to an end. They can picture health conditions, health levels, health needs, and health problems. Certain rates per year are of particular health significance.

1. Birthrate is the number of live births per 1,000 of the population.

$$\frac{\text{Number of live births}}{\text{Population}} \times 1,000 = \text{Birthrate}$$

2. General, or crude, death rate is the number of deaths per 1,000 of the population.

$$\frac{\text{Number of deaths}}{\text{Population}} \times 1,000 = \text{Death rate}$$

3. Infant mortality rate is the number of deaths under 1 year of age per 1,000 live births.

$$\frac{\text{Number of deaths under 1 year}}{\text{Number of live births}} \times 1,000 =$$

$$\text{Infant mortality rate}$$

4. Maternal mortality rate is the number of deaths of mothers from childbirth per 10,000 live births.

$$\frac{\text{Number of deaths of mothers (from childbirth)}}{\text{Number of live births}} \times$$

$$10,000 = \text{Maternal mortality rate}$$

5. Specific mortality rate is the number of deaths for a specific cause (or age group) per 100,000 population.

$$\frac{\text{Number of deaths (specific cause)}}{\text{Population}} \times$$

$$100,000 = \text{Specific death rate}$$

6. Case fatality rate is the number of deaths from a specific cause to the number of cases and is always expressed as a percent.

$$\frac{\text{Number of deaths from a specific cause}}{\text{Number of cases of the cause}} \times$$

$$100 = \text{Case fatality rate (\%)}$$

Other rates are also calculated to obtain an accurate picture of vital facts of health significance, such as marriage rates and divorce rates. Net and gross reproduction rates can be meaningful in terms of population directions. Within populations, rates for selected factors and for specific age, sex, and racial groups may have significance.

Rates will be affected by many variables that must be considered in interpreting the significance of a particular rate. For example, a particular "retirement" county in Florida had a low birthrate and a high death rate, understandable when one studies the age distribution of the population and finds a disproportionate concentration of older age people.

Communicable disease control. Constant vigilance is necessary to hold communicable diseases to a minimum. Programs can be planned and effectively administered so that epidemics do not occur and the number of outbreaks of communicable disease is held to a minimum. Such a program requires certain preventive measures: (1) immunization, (2) public health education, (3) protection of water, milk, and other food supplies, (4) promotion of sanitation, and (5) control of carriers. Control measures must concentrate on infected persons and their environment: (1) recognition of the disease, (2) prompt reporting of all cases, (3) isolation procedures, (4) quarantine when warranted, and (5) decontamination. Most city and county health departments provide immunization service. Others at least provide biologicals to be administered by private practitioners.

Promotion of maternal and child health. A public health nurse is a family health counselor. In some community health departments the nurse is given this title. The public health nurse does no bedside or hospital nursing except as a demonstration for the instruction of some member of the family or in an emergency. The health nurse is the key person in maternal and infant health.

In maternal health promotion, certain *direct* means are taken in behalf of the health of expectant mothers.

1. Promotion of prenatal care through early medical examination, prevention and correction of impairments, proper rest, proper nutrition, moderate exercise, sunshine, and avoidance of fatigue, smoking, drugs, and infection
2. Adequate delivery facilities in a hospital or home
3. Obstetrical and nurse-midwifery services
4. Postnatal care

Similarly, there are certain *indirect* means for promoting maternal health.

1. Public education and health education for other family members
2. Laws governing employment of women
3. Medical and hospital insurance with maternity benefits
4. Improvement of socioeconomic and environmental conditions

Infant health must begin with the education of the parents in the importance of considering all factors affecting infant well-being. In addition the public health nurse must assist parents in understanding the particular health needs and health problems of the infant, encourage the parents to have the infant examined at regular intervals by a physician, help secure medical diagnosis and treatment for the infant when such needs are indicated, and teach the mother care of the infant, including good nutrition, feeding, and parenting practices. The public health nurse can serve as a liaison between the family and the pediatrician or well-child clinic of the health department.

Many agencies, including the school, contribute to child health, and the county health department has an obligation to cooperate with all recognized agencies contributing to child health. This is in the best interests of the child. The health department contributes more directly to child health through the following activities of the public health nurse:

1. Counseling parents on health matters relating to children.
2. Assisting parents in understanding the health needs and conditions of their children.
3. Urging parents to have children receive a health examination at regular intervals and to complete their immunization series.
4. Helping parents in securing medical services for diagnosis and treatment of illness in the family.
5. Helping families to carry out essential sanitary and other health measures.
6. Teaching home nursing and parenting skills to members of the family.
7. Supervising family members who care for the ill children in the home.
8. Assisting in improving social conditions that affect health.
9. Recognizing and reporting signs of child abuse.

Family planning. As an example of guidelines for a specific, high-priority, program area, the recommendations of the Planned Parenthood Federation for family planning programs are more generally instructive:

1. Expand family planning services—through hospitals, health departments, private physicians, welfare agencies, Planned Parenthood and other voluntary agencies, and anti-poverty groups—to reach seven out of eight poor American women still denied these services.
2. Direct priority attention to incorporating effective services in existing big city health facilities and adding satellite clinics to serve outlying neighborhoods. Programs should also be initiated to deliver services in rural areas.
3. Priority should be given to development of convenient, familiar, and accessible services in or near officially designated "poverty" neighborhoods.
4. Services should not be directed exclusively to black areas. Emphasis on services for blacks alone will fail to reach the bulk of the population in need and may feed the suspicion that family planning advocates seek to reduce the number of blacks rather than to meet essential health needs.
5. Welfare referral and reimbursement programs and even Medicaid programs can meet only a small proportion of the need. Overemphasis on such programs diverts attention from needed changes in the health system to make family planning available to all of the poor.
6. Family planning clinics should be open evenings and weekends to serve working women. Adequate transportation and baby-sitting are needed for mothers who must remain home to care for young children.
7. Some of the women in need can be reached through newspapers, magazines, television, radio, and other traditional media, with information on the safety, effectiveness, and convenience of modern contraception,

and where they can get help. More personalized educational methods must be emphasized for some.

8. Humiliating marital status restrictions on provision of services will fail to meet the needs of a significant number of women who are separated, widowed, divorced, or single.

9. Good follow-up procedures are feasible and will have long-term benefits for the families in need of help.

10. Family planning programs should emphasize child spacing. By delaying and spacing pregnancies, couples will have a better chance to get more education and increase family income as well as to enjoy better health. Thus family planning services should seek to reach poor couples in their early twenties or even their teens.

These recommendations illustrate the general approach to preventive health delivery that should characterize all components of community health services. Similar recommendations would apply to other program areas such as mental health, diabetes, hypertension, maternal and infant care, and others.

Chronic disease control. Many if not most of the organic diseases of the late years had their genesis in middle age. Accordingly, adult health promotion gives emphasis to the

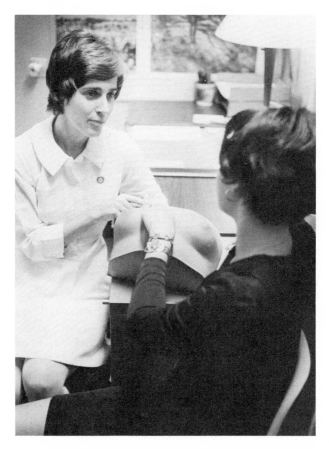

Fig. 19-3. Breast self-examination is a major strategy of the American Cancer Society and local health departments to detect early signs of breast cancer and to reduce delay in treatment. Breast self-examination is taught in clinics, classes, and women's self-help groups. (Courtesy Johns Hopkins Medical Institutions)

middle years of life as well as to the elderly years. Indeed, preventive efforts directed toward the younger years of age can yield the most productive dividends. A constructive adult health promotional program concentrates on the following three factors:

1. Periodic screening examination
2. Correction of all remediable disorders
3. Health education that emphasizes moderation and regularity in living, avoiding infection, treating infection immediately when it occurs, avoiding undue fatigue, exercise, proper diet, and checking with a physician when any abnormal condition persists

Community organization on the part of the health department is called for in getting adults examined. This is particularly true in getting men examined and assuring proper follow-up of those screened. Cooperation with the medical society, industry, labor unions, and service organizations backed by a good promotional program through various media is required.

Mental health promotion. Major emphasis in mental health promotion is placed on the mental health of the normal individual. The modern mental health program offers counseling, seminars, institutes, hot lines, demonstrations, lectures, and other services. Psychiatric, psychological, and social work services are available to normal individuals, people with minor disturbances, delinquents, people with serious emotional problems, the disordered, people in the process of rehabilitation, and to groups. The mere fact that the city or county health department provides a mental health center where a person may go for consultation is extemely significant for citizens in the community. It takes experience with this service before the public uses it effectively. It will take a few more years before mental health service is accepted as a phase of community health the way immunization has been accepted as an inherent service of the health department.

Environmental health promotion. Sanitarians are primarily occupied with public sanitation but provide consulting services when requested by householders. Home sanitation is encouraged through continuous

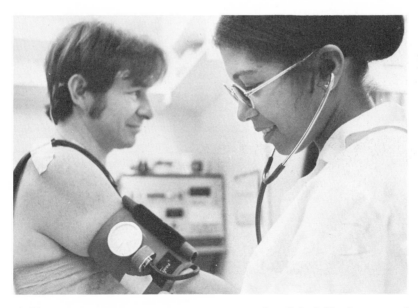

Fig. 19-4. Hypertension screening programs attempt to identify high blood pressure through special clinics and readings taken at fairs, work sites, and home visits. Only about 50% of the detected cases are followed up in treatment. (Courtesy Johns Hopkins Medical Institutions)

education measures. Most of the sanitarian's time and attention is directed to the inspection and appraisal of public water supplies, milk and milk products, sewage disposal, public buildings, swimming pools, bathing beaches, insect infestation, industrial operations, and nuisances. Preventing disease is the primary goal of the sanitation program, but promotion of an esthetic environment is usually a secondary benefit.

Laboratory service. Most health departments in low-census counties do not have their own laboratories but depend on the centralized laboratory of the state health department or a local laboratory in a hospital or a clinic. Water plant operators are usually competent to run bacteriological examinations of water. Even without its own laboratory a county health department can improvise sufficiently to provide limited laboratory service.

Having a county health department laboratory has many advantages in convenience and reduced time for running laboratory tests. Communicable disease control by means of laboratory tests requires promptness. Diagnostic tests, water and milk examinations, and food contamination tests can be done promptly in the county health department laboratory. When the health department supplies immunizations, the laboratory technicians keep the biologicals in stock and assume responsibility for dispensing them.

Health education. The base of the pyramid called community health is public health education, and the breadth and stability of the base largely determines the height to which the pyramid can rise. Health education is effective to the extent that it constructively affects people's health knowledge, health attitudes, and health practices. To be effective, public health education must get

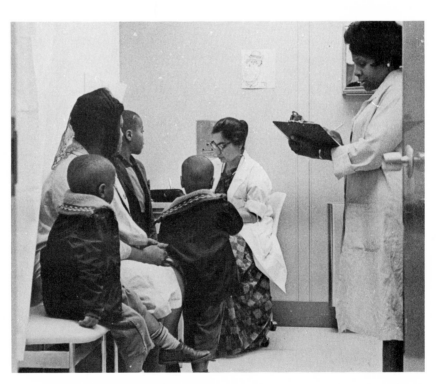

Fig. 19-5. Ambulatory care, primary care, and health maintenance through maternal and child health, children and youth, family health, and related clinical services are central to community health. (Courtesy Johns Hopkins Medical Institutions)

public *acceptance* of a program or practice, arouse a *desire* in people to benefit by it, and obtain *involvement* of the people.

Effective public health education is directed to different segments of the population for different purposes. Communications directly with those whose health behavior places them at risk are designed to gain their acceptance of a program or practice and to increase their motivation to benefit by it. Communications indirectly through parents, teachers, officials, employers, and peers are designed to provide a supportive social environment and reinforcement for the behavior. Communications directed to organizations, such as parent-teacher associations, service clubs, church groups, labor unions, health agencies, insurance companies, child study organizations, parent groups, and neighborhood organizations are designed to facilitate the behavior by organizing community resources that enable the health behavior to occur.

Public health education is beset with many obstacles, particularly false advertising, quackery, cultism, attitude toward health, superstition, professional indifference, and the human tendency to seek the easiest solution to every health problem. Yet a well-organized and effectively administered community health education program can be highly effective and can make an impact on the community's health.

The head of the community health education program is a professionally prepared community health educator. This person

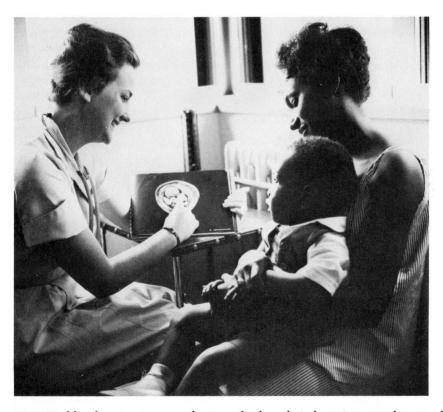

Fig. 19-6. Health education in prenatal care and other clinical services complements the home visits of public health nurses and the community organization and mass communications efforts coordinated by the community health educator. (Courtesy Johns Hopkins Medical Institutions)

supervises a number of organized units and individuals who have contributions to make. All members of the local health department staff properly are engaged in health education as a phase of their professional activities. The health educator coordinates the education efforts of the staff, provides consultation, and initiates action that will involve other staff members of the department as well as other agencies in the community.

In addition to the health department, the voluntary health agencies, child health councils, schools, medical society, dental society, and a number of other organizations in the city or county have contributions to make to health education. It requires imaginative, sensitive, and persistent leadership to get all of these organizations and individuals contributing in a coordinated way so that the health education program is effective and consistent.

Numerous services and materials constitute the methods used in community health education. Each medium makes its own contribution, but it is the composite effect of a coordinated program that achieves the goal of a health-educated public.

Services

Speaker's bureau (including others in addition to the health department staff)
Lecture series
Demonstrations
Seminars
Conferences
Health councils
Exhibits
Inservice education for teachers and others
Community organization
Consultation to health practitioners
Self-care discussion groups
Telephone hot lines and "dial-a-message" services
Smoking cessation groups
Weight control groups
Prenatal and parenting groups

Materials

Bulletins
Pamphlets
Newsletters
Films
Individual letters
Newspaper articles
Radio programs
Television interviews
Special reports for the media
Annual reports

Not indiscriminate use of every conceivable gimmick or device, but the considered use of the most effective means for obtaining specific health objectives is the scientific and professional discipline of health education.

Health education of the public is a continuous process. While some circumstances occasion a justifiable "blitz" program, these are of value only as they are part of the overall, year-round, continuing public health education program.

Other county health department services. Either through legislative requirement, local pressure, custom, or even coincidence, a county health department may be engaged in one or more unique services not included in the usual list of responsibilities. Some county health departments are responsible for the medical investigation of deaths of unknown cause. "Battered child" cases may be referred to the health department. Inspection of foster care homes is an activity of some county health departments. Speech therapy, occupational and physical therapy, rehabilitation, and medical questions relating to commitment to mental hospitals are but some of the unique activities of different county health departments. Someone must perform these services, but if these activities interfere with the effective performance of the basic public health functions of the department the public may lose more in health protection than it gains in social services.

Community health council

On the county level, health councils have been valuable in coordinating the health services of various agencies and individuals. Health councils are usually not official organizations but are voluntary and composed of representatives from various organizations and groups having special health interests or needs. Councils may vary from ten to thirty in membership, with representatives from such groups as voluntary health agencies, medical profession, dental profession, parent-teacher organizations, labor unions, chambers of commerce, women's clubs, church groups, social agencies, and various other groups. The council usually represents a cross-section of the population and can make known the health needs of the people. It can make recommendations to the county health department and can be called on to support certain activities of the department.

A community health council can provide a valuable community service so long as it considers the overall health needs of the county and strives to assist, support, and supplement the health department. It serves as a health-promoting force in the community and provides for citizen involvement in public health.

FEDERAL SUPPORT FOR COMMUNITY HEALTH SERVICES

Following the early stage of grants-in-aid to states for maternal and child health programs and to state and local governments for the establishment and development of health departments (Titles V and VI of the 1935 Social Security Act) came the "decades of investment." The Hill-Burton Hospital Survey and Construction Act of 1946 assisted more than 3,800 communities to build hospitals, extended-care and rehabilitation facilities, and public health centers. The National Institutes of Health was also developed during this post-war period of federal investment, contributing over $14 billion toward the development and support of biomedical and health-related research. Support for health manpower development also began during this period, providing traineeships for public health specialists, most of whom were already employed in community health agencies but without formal training in public health.

By the early 1960s there was considerable disillusionment with the results of these massive investments in the three major areas of national health resources—facilities, knowledge, and manpower. We had reached the highest level of per capita expenditures for health in the world, but our health services and our health statistics rated poorly among developed nations—thirteenth among industrial countries in death of infants during the first year of life; seventh in the percentage of mothers who die in childbirth; eighteenth in the life expectancy of males and eleventh for females; and sixteenth in the death rate of males in their middle years.

It was apparent that the investment period had succeeded in building a massive health and medical care complex, but this complex had failed to adjust its structure appropriately to trends in the distribution of illness, demands for services, specialization of practitioners and medical equipment, and demands among office and hospital personnel for competitive wages. Physicians and hospitals clung tenaciously to traditions of individualism, endeavoring to be all things to their patients despite the obvious need to pool specialized facilities and services. Rural areas most notably were still without community health services. We faced what is now referred to as the "national crisis in health care." By the mid-1960s we had entered what Kissick (1970) refers to as the "years of ferment" in the evolution of national health policy. Particular emphasis was placed on community health services.

Community mental health centers. In 1963 President Kennedy signed the Community Mental Health Centers Act. This Act differed from earlier construction assistance acts in that it required centers to provide comprehensive services including outpatient care, consultation, and education. Approximately 400 community mental health centers had been established by 1970, which was significantly behind schedule for the original target of 2,000 by 1975, but the comprehensive approach required and the consequent innovations in delivery systems marked a new departure in organizational arrangements with a community education orientation. Community mental health centers form a network of comprehensive services and continuity of care for patients discharged from state psychiatric facilities, as well as preventive services.

This Act provided specifically for "a State advisory council which shall include representatives of non-government organizations or groups, and of State agencies, concerned with planning, operation, or utilization of community mental health centers or other mental health facilities, *including representatives of consumers* of the services. . . ." This clause was the forerunner of more sweeping provisions for consumer participation in the Economic Opportunity Act and later legislation.

The Community Mental Health Centers Act authorized grants to public or non-profit private agencies to assist "in the establishment and initial operation of community mental health centers providing all or part of a *comprehensive* community mental health program. . . ." A survey in 1967 (Levenson and associates, 1967) revealed that the 250 or so centers existing at that time estimated that approximately 10% of staff time would be spent in consultation, education, and other indirect services. In 1973 nearly 28% of all outpatient mental health episodes were seen at community mental health centers.

MCH, Mental Retardation, and Economic Opportunity Acts of 1963-1964. Also in 1963, the Maternal and Child Health and Mental Retardation Amendments provided for similarly comprehensive, community-based approaches to prenatal and postnatal services for high-risk, low-income groups. Maternity and Infant Care Projects have been funded by grants to many state and local health departments.

The most salient legislation marking the "years of ferment" was the Economic Opportunity Act of 1964. Support for research, demonstration, and training for Neighborhood Health Centers resulted in widespread experimentation with health-care teams, indigenous community workers, or community health aides and—most significantly from an educational perspective—serious attention

to participation of the poor in the planning and evaluation of services. By mid-1969 about fifty projects had been funded, a drop in the bucket in relation to needs and legitimate demands of the poor, but again significant in terms of the concepts demonstrated. Federal support for Neighborhood Health Centers declined in the 1970s.

Regional Medical Programs. The purposes of this 1965 law were (1) to provide federal grants to establish regional cooperative arrangements among medical schools, research institutions, and hospitals for research and training (including continuing education) and for related demonstrations of prevention and patient care in the fields of heart disease, cancer, and stroke; (2) to afford the medical profession the opportunity of making available to patients the latest advances in diagnosis and treatment; and (3) by these means to improve generally the health manpower and facilities available in the nation, ". . . without interfering with the patterns, or the methods of financing, of patient care or professional practice, or with the administration of hospitals, and in cooperation with practicing physicians, medical center officials, hospital administrators, and representatives from appropriate voluntary health agencies."

Note particularly the hesitation in this legislation to offend or challenge the medical establishment. There was no mention of official (state or local) health agencies and no mention of health professionals or paraprofessionals other than those of the hospital "establishment." The Regional Medical Programs were phased out of existence in 1976 with the development of regional Health Systems Agencies, which will be discussed in Chapter 20.

Consumer participation in community health planning. The Community Action Programs (CAP) established under the Economic Opportunity Act of 1964 moved consumer participation from a matter of voluntary action to a matter of public policy. Community action was suddenly defined in legal terms, which carried both opportunities and new obligations for the poor. "Maximum feasible participation" was further legislated in Public Law 89-749 in 1965 (authorizing the establishment of Comprehensive Health Planning Agencies) and in the Model Cities Demonstration Act of 1966. The concept has survived a variety of setbacks and assaults (Green, 1975; Partridge, 1973; Wang and associates, 1975).

For all of the good intentions behind the consumer participation movement, its legislated implementation was misunderstood or mistrusted by many professionals and consumers. The "Maximum feasible misunderstanding" created by the law was summarized by Moynihan (1969, p. 11):

Community action was originally seen as a means of shaping unorganized and even disorganized city dwellers into a coherent and self-conscious group, if necessary by techniques of protest and opposition to established authority. Somehow, however, the higher civil service came to see it as a means for coordinating at the community level the array of conflicting and overlapping departmental programs that proceeded from Washington. . . .

The co-optation of consumer participants in managerial functions undermined the intent of the legislation and left many volunteer participants feeling exploited and suspicious of governmental purposes. If other consumer initiatives in health become similarly enmeshed in governmental relations with health care providers and agencies, they are likely to take a different form, or at least a different flavor for the consumer, than they now take. This caution has special meaning in relation to activities in which voluntary participation of consumers becomes qualitatively a different experience when it is required by law.

The lesson from governmental implementation of maximum feasible participation laws is not necessarily that governmental support should not be offered to voluntary programs but that it should be offered with carefully designed safeguards for the voluntary character of the programs.

VOLUNTARY HEALTH AGENCIES

Nontax-supported, voluntary health agencies are an American creation. The American

way of a free society with opportunities for people to fulfill their needs has led to the formation of organizations to secure for the people what official agencies do not provide. These voluntary health organizations have pioneered in promoting health programs and in demonstrating what can be done. Frequently, when a voluntary health organization demonstrates what can be done the official health agencies then enter the field and supplement what the voluntary health organization does.

Two types of voluntary health agencies— professional health organizations and health foundations—will be discussed in Chapters 20 and 21.

In the late nineteenth and early twentieth centuries, governmental agencies were slow to recognize existing health problems and the need to utilize available means for dealing with these problems and to develop new measures for disease prevention and control. Voluntary agencies were organized in response to the recognized need to take action dealing with the problems of disease, to use all available means for solving problems of disease prevention and control, and to develop new measures. Many such organizations have been formed, several of which will be discussed as representative of the types of voluntary health agencies that have served the public over the past half century or more at both national and community levels.

The National Tuberculosis and Respiratory Disease Association (now the *American Lung Association*) was founded in 1904 and was the first voluntary agency of the educational, promotional type. From the outset, education has been the foundation of the Association's program. This has been based on the premise that, while it is essential to extend knowledge through scientific research, such knowledge is of little value unless it is available to the public, medical practitioners, health personnel, and patients.

With the tuberculosis problem largely under control, the American Lung Association is directing much of its attention and efforts to the problem of emphysema and other disorders of the chest. Some state associations have a subsidiary Thoracic Society composed of physicians who are specialists in thoracic diseases.

From the outset the Association's program has operated primarily on the community level. In part this has been responsible for much of the success of the program. The state association or chapter has supervision over the local units. Financing of the Association's program has been through Christmas seal campaigns, and more people have contributed to this program than to any similar philanthropical enterprise. At no time has the Association paid medical or hospital costs for patients with tuberculosis. The American Lung Association has had an intensive and extensive research program. This research is not limited to tuberculosis but includes research in various diseases of the chest.

The National Foundation was formerly known as the National Foundation for Infantile Paralysis and was founded in 1938. President Franklin D. Roosevelt, stricken by poliomyelitis, gave his personal support to the Foundation and thereby gave great impetus to the organization. From its start the Foundation has been financed through the March of Dimes Program. Several state chapters and more than 3,000 local chapters reach into virtually every county in the nation.

In 1958 the organization shortened its name to the National Foundation and its objectives were expanded to become "an organized force for medical research, patient care and professional education, flexible enough to meet new health problems as they arise." The present program includes investigation into arthritis, birth defects (congenital defects), viral diseases, and other disorders of the central nervous system, as well as poliomyelitis.

Local chapters that are branches of the national organization give direct medical assistance to persons afflicted with infantile paralysis and raise funds to maintain national and local activities. A considerable part of the funds raised locally remains in the community to promote the local program.

Financial assistance from the National Foundation was instrumental in demonstrating the effectiveness of the Salk vaccine in the 1954 Poliomyelitis Vaccine Field Trial. This resulted in the shortest elapsed time between the discovery of a preventive measure and its widespread use.

The American Cancer Society, Inc., was founded in 1913 "to disseminate knowledge concerning the symptoms, diagnosis, treatment, and prevention of cancer; to investigate the conditions under which cancer is found; and to compile statistics in regard thereto." The Society was established largely through the efforts of medical persons, although the work of the organization has been carried on largely by laymen.

The leadoff educational program was designed to acquaint the public with the fact that early cancer can be cured, that early diagnosis is of primary importance, and that prompt, scientific treatment is the acknowledged method of cure. The educational campaign used an impersonal approach in the effort to avoid arousing fear of cancer.

In addition to public health education, the Society encouraged health departments to expand their cancer programs, stimulated medical schools to extend their work in cancer, helped to organize a National Advisory Cancer Council, and influenced the passage of the National Cancer Act and the creation of the National Cancer Institute as a part of the United States Public Health Service.

The state organization is called a division and, as an example, is titled American Cancer Society, Inc., Michigan Division. Operation of the program is basically on the county level and is controlled and supervised by the local medical profession. The women's auxiliary group enlists the active participation of laymen in a program of health education.

Income of the American Cancer Society, Inc., is derived from donations, dues, endowments, and legacies. In many instances citizens losing a family member because of cancer assign life insurance benefits to the society. The official publication of the Society is CA—A Bulletin of Cancer Progress. This is a publication for members of the professions dealing with cancer.

The American Heart Association was originally formed as a scientific and professional organization of physicians interested in heart disease. In 1948 it was reorganized as a voluntary health agency with thousands of nonprofessional members. The objective of the Association is to prevent and control heart disease through research, professional education, public education, and community service.

Each state has a state heart association and county heart councils. A large corps of volunteers composed of physicians and laymen work together to plan and execute the association's programs. The state heart association has a professional staff, which provides consultation services and works with the volunteers in planning and implementing both the education and fundraising aspects of the program.

Through community service the Association provides a work classification service, which determines a patient's work tolerance and makes a vocational recommendation. It provides rheumatic fever control programs to prevent secondary attacks in individuals who have had a first attack. It also provides a nutrition and weight control program, a Speaker's Bureau, a school health program, and a work simplification program, which demonstrates methods to help housekeepers to organize their work in a manner that will prevent unnecessary fatigue. The Association also maintains an information and referral service, which is a directory of cardiac services. Throughout, the Heart Association works through and with physicians by making services available to the physician and to the patient as the physician requests.

Funds are raised by state drives and come from voluntary contributions, endowments, and legacies. At times people losing a family member because of heart disease will turn insurance benefits over to the state heart association. Most of the Heart Association funds go into heart research or an allied activity.

The American National Red Cross techni-cally does not belong in any of the three main categories of voluntary health organizations, although in a sense it is somewhat promotional in nature. It has a quasi-governmental status because it is incorporated under a charter granted by Congress. The President of the United States is president of the American National Red Cross, which is an affiliate of the international organization.

The Red Cross was founded in 1881 in accordance with the Geneva Treaty of 1864, which was ratified by the United States in 1882. The Red Cross provides relief services during wartime and other disasters. In times of peace the American affiliate has established health centers, helped to conduct public health surveys, sponsored health demonstration projects and first aid and water safety programs, and provided public health nursing service for rural areas that were otherwise not served.

It is an established policy of the Red Cross to work closely with private and governmental agencies at all levels—national, state, and community. County chapters are formed but operate under the supervision of the national office, which establishes policies and must approve all local projects.

SCHOOL HEALTH PROGRAM

The school health program properly should be considered as an arm of the public health program and thus be integrated with it. Not only the health of the children but the health of the home and the health of the community should be the concern of the school, because the school can contribute to all three.

Scope of school health program. Six basic policies point up the role of the school health program (Anderson and Creswell, 1976):

1. To provide for healthful school living through standards for safety and sanitation, adequate food service, maintenance of teacher's health, and promotion of mental and emotional health of teachers and pupils
2. To provide health instruction in the entire curriculum, especially in courses

designed for the elementary, junior, and senior high schools, and through school participation in community health education

3. To provide services for health protection and improvement through first aid for emergencies, prevention and control of communicable disease, and health appraisal, guidance, and assistance

4. To emphasize the hygienic aspects of physical education, to seek to adapt programs to individual needs, to secure adequate activity programs, and to develop health safeguards in athletics

5. To designate the education and care of handicapped persons through identification of the need, adjustment of programs, adjustment of individuals, special classes, and properly prepared teachers

6. To denote the needed qualifications of health education personnel

These policies are usually translated into a school health program of health services, health instruction, and healthful living (Eisner and Callan, 1974).

Health services deal with the present health of the school youngster and have three aspects. The first is health *appraisal*, consisting of health examinations, teacher health assessment, vision screening, hearing testing, height and weight determinations, health guidance and supervision, and teacher health. The second is *preventive* aspects, which consist of communicable disease control, safety, emergency care, and first aid. The third is *remedial* aspects, consisting of the follow-up services, correction of remediable defects, practitioner services, and school remedial functions.

Health instruction includes planned instruction, correlated instruction, integrated learning, and incidental instruction. Health education through all possible experiences is the objective of health instruction.

Healthful living is not a static concept but a *dynamic* way of life. It includes a sanitary physical environment but also incorporates the mental health of students and teachers. It is represented in practices that promote the highest level of physical and mental health.

An effective school health program requires elementary school teachers who have preparation in health services, health instruction, and healthful living, certified secondary school health teachers who have specialized in health, and a school health director who has a master's degree in health education. Above all, to have an effective health program a school must have administrators who understand health and provide leadership, counsel, and encouragement for all people involved in the school health program. This properly means everyone in the school.

APPRAISAL OF COMMUNITY HEALTH SERVICES

It is difficult to measure the effectiveness or value of a community health program in terms of lives saved, illnesses prevented, and health improved. There are inferential means of appraising a health program based on the assumption that, if certain activities or services are provided by a health staff, it can be inferred that certain health benefits accrue to the public. This inference is based on independent studies, which have shown that certain services and activities produced certain public health results. This approach to appraisal is simply an accounting of services rendered. A considerable segment of the public health profession prefers to specify the services a health department should provide and contends that appraisal *should* be based on the proficiency with which the health staff performs these services. This approach to evaluation is called quality assurance or quality control.

Full-time county health departments provide a direct health service available to all citizens within the respective county. It provides the various means for reducing the incidence of disease, lowering the death rate, reducing invalidism and dependency, preventing disabilities, correcting remediable defects, decreasing wage losses, reducing hospital and medical costs, and reducing hazards to health and life. Some agencies attempt to get periodic measures of these outcomes to appraise their programs.

In the final analysis the evaluation of community health services is severely compounded by the relationship of health outcomes with aspects of poverty, culture, and the environment over which community health agencies have little control. These relationships are acknowledged in some of the recommendations of the American Health Assembly (1970), which help to cast this chapter in perspective:

It must be recognized that illness produces poverty; and that in turn poverty breeds health problems. Health services will not alone overcome the disadvantages of poverty itself nor be able to correct the disabling impact of inferior nutrition, housing, recreation, and education. As the level of health services rises, a point of diminishing returns from such services may be reached as compared with investment in the quality of the living environment.

Poverty itself involves a variety of handicapping conditions that can result in irreversible health problems. The tragic fact of malnutrition among millions of poor and near poor is a national shame. The economic base of malnutrition should be promptly eliminated by expansion of nutritional support programs.

Because of the vulnerability of infants and young children to the environment of poverty, programs of high quality such as day care and early childhood education should be directed to these age groups.

Special problems of health care delivery exist in poverty areas: urban ghettos and barrios and many rural sections of the country. Until a comprehensive financing system is implemented, we vigorously oppose the curtailment, and instead favor all possible expansion, of existing programs providing health care for the poor or other low-income people.

Consumers have an obviously deep and primary interest in health services. The health professions alone cannot be the sufficient guardians of that interest. Consumers must have effective representation—wherever possible a majority—in the policy-making processes of major health facilities and organizations. This representation must reflect all aspects of the community, including cultural, racial, and linguistic diversities. Special emphasis should be placed on meaningful representation of the poor.

QUESTIONS AND EXERCISES

1. In a republic such as the United States, what individuals or groups are most nearly self-sufficient in dealing with all health matters?
2. About one-third of the counties (and parishes) in the United States are without full-time professional health service. What is the explanation?
3. If you lived in a county or parish without a full-time health department, what measures would you take to obtain full-time public health service?
4. Why do people in the low-income groups benefit most from the county health department program?
5. Is it just or unjust that some people get more service than others from the county health department?
6. Which health department—federal, state, or county—is most likely to give service to the individual citizen? Cite examples to illustrate.
7. What are some nonhealth regulations the state has established through the exercise of the police power?
8. Why not pass laws and regulations identifying as nuisances all conditions and practices that might cause hurt, injury, damage, or inconvenience to people?
9. If a county health department refuses to take court action to stop a condition that citizens regard as a nuisance, what action can the citizens take?
10. A dog in public was thought to have rabies. Rather than risk being bitten, a deputy sheriff shot the dog. What are the possible legal implications?
11. Why not have only medical doctors on the county board of health?
12. Why should decisions by the county board of health be subject to appeal to a court?
13. What justification can you make for the expenditure of $5.00 per person per year for a county health department?
14. What was the national birthrate and death rate for a recent year?
15. Why was mental health promotion not included in the county health department program until recently?
16. Why is it not logical to say that one position on the county health staff is more important to the public than is another?
17. Why should public health education employ a variety of media and methods of communication?
18. If a health council was to be formed in your county, what organizations should be represented?
19. Why should the school be concerned with more than health education?

20. What evidence can you present that people in the United States have better health today than those who lived here at the turn of the century, and what has been the contribution of official and voluntary health agencies?
21. What are some respects in which voluntary health agencies differ from official health agencies?
22. Which voluntary promotional health agency do you regard as being most important? Why?
23. Does the medical profession exercise too great an influence or even control of the voluntary promotional health agencies? What is your line of reasoning?

REFERENCES

American Health Assembly: The health of Americans, New York, 1970, Columbia University Press.

American Public Health Association: Health is a community affair, Cambridge, Mass., 1970, Harvard University Press.

Anderson, C. L., and Creswell, W. H.: School health practice, ed. 6, St. Louis, 1976, The C. V. Mosby Co.

Curran, W. J.: Public health and the law, American Journal of Public Health 60:2208, 1970.

Eisner, V., and Callan, L. B.: Dimensions of school health, Springfield, Ill., 1974, Charles C Thomas, Publisher.

Freeman, R.: Community health nursing, ed. 2, Philadelphia, 1970, W. B. Saunders Co.

Freeman, R.: The expanding role of nursing, some implications, International Nursing Review 19:351, April, 1972.

Fry, H. G., and associates: Educational manpower for community health, Pittsburgh, 1968, University of Pittsburgh Press.

Ginsberg, E.: Urban health services: the case of New York City, New York, 1970, The Columbia University Press.

Grant, J. B.: Health care for the community, Baltimore, 1963, The Johns Hopkins University Press.

Green, L. W.: Constructive consumerism, Health Education 2:3-6, 1975.

Hall, T., and associates: Professional health manpower for community health programs, Chapel Hill, 1973, University of North Carolina School of Public Health.

Hanlon, J. J.: Public health: administration and practice, ed. 6, St. Louis, 1974, The C. V. Mosby Co.

Health resources statistics, 1974, Rockville, Md., 1974, National Center for Health Statistics, DHEW Publication No. (HRA) 75-1509.

Henkle, O. B. M.: Introduction to community health, Boston, 1970, Allyn & Bacon, Inc.

Kissick, W.: Health policy directions for the 1970's, New England Journal of Medicine 282:1343-1354, June 11, 1970.

Kosa, J., and Zola, I. K.: Poverty and health, a sociological analysis, Cambridge, Mass., 1975, Harvard University Press.

Levenson, A. A., and associates: Manpower and training in federally funded mental health centers, Bethesda, Md., 1967, National Institute of Mental Health.

Lilienfeld, A. M., and Gifford, A. J.: Chronic diseases and public health, Baltimore, 1966, The Johns Hopkins University Press.

Maxcy, K. F., and Startwell, P. E.: Preventive medicine and public health, ed. 10, New York, 1976, Appleton-Century-Crofts.

Mayshark, C., Shaw, D. D., and Best, W. H.: Administration of school health programs: its theory and practice, ed. 2, St. Louis, 1976, The C. V. Mosby Co.

Mico, P. R., and Ross, H. S.: Health education and behavioral science, Oakland, 1975, Third-Party Associates.

Moynihan, D. P., editor: Maximum feasible misunderstanding, community action in the War on Poverty, New York, 1969, The Free Press.

National Commission on Community Health Services: Health administration and organization in the decade ahead, Washington, D.C., 1967, Public Affairs Press.

Partridge, K. B.: Community and professional participation in decision making at a health center, Health Services Reports 88:527-534, 1973.

Peters, R. J., and Kinnaird, J.: Health services administration, Baltimore, 1965, The Williams & Wilkins Co.

Richardson, A. H.: Report of the fiscal scheme for the Association of Schools of Public Health (Bureau of Health Manpower Contract NIH 71-4159), Baltimore, 1973, The Johns Hopkins University Press.

Sheps, C. G., chairman: Higher education for public health, a report of the Milbank Memorial Fund Commission, New York, 1976, Prodist.

Smolensky, J., and Haar, F. B.: Community health, ed. 3, Philadelphia, 1972, W. B. Saunders Co.

Taubenhaus, L. J.: A division of community health services, Archives of Environmental Health 20:732, 1970.

Wang, V. L., and associates: An approach to consumer-patient activation in health maintenance, Public Health Reports 90:449-454, 1975.

White, K. L., and Henderson, M. M.: Epidemiology as a fundamental science: its uses in health services planning, administration, and evaluation, New York, 1976, Oxford University Press, Inc.

White, P. E., and associates: A survey of 1956-72 graduates of American schools of public health; Bureau of Health Manpower Contract NIH 71-459, Baltimore, 1974, The Johns Hopkins University Press.

World Health Organization: Postgraduate education and training in public health, Geneva, 1973, Technical Report Series No. 533.

20 ▪ STATE HEALTH SERVICES

States have the recognized authority to include health in their constitutions, and all state constitutions provide for public health services. A state constitution usually provides for a state health agency (SHA) with broad functions. The constitution permits or directs the state legislature to pass supplemental statutory provisions.

State agencies are a backup of the community health department, providing the services of experts when requested or needed for an emergency or for an important health problem. The SHAs also provide local health departments with laboratory services and with equipment and facilities for special surveys and other purposes. Mobile x-ray units and devices for measuring air pollution and other equipment are made available by the state to local authorities for the promotion of community health.

The SHA acts as the link between the federal health agencies and the local health departments. Federal health funds are channeled through the SHA to the local health agency. Through the SHA, community health departments are able to obtain the services of federal health experts to solve unique or difficult health problems or to deal with an emergency when summary action is required.

STATE HEALTH AUTHORITY

Sovereignty, or ultimate authority, in matters of health rests with the people, and this authority is vested in the state government to pass such legislation and take such action as may be necessary to promote the health and general welfare of the people. The state has virtually unlimited authority to do what is necessary to promote the greatest good for the greatest number. There is but one limitation on the state's power to legislate in health matters—a statute may not be contrary to nor violate the provisions of the Federal Constitution. In the exercise of power to act in matters of health the act or performance under the state's police power must be *reasonable* and *constitutional*.

The people of a state approve a state constitution that may merely provide that the state legislature is charged with the responsibility to set up health agencies and make such other provisions as are necessary for the protection and promotion of the health of the public. In some states the constitution delineates in some detail what the state health organization and services shall be. Most public health authorities agree that the constitution should contain broad, general provisions granting to the state legislature authority to establish the necessary health agencies, their responsibilities, and their authority. This provides for changes through legislation as future circumstances develop.

Most legislatures choose to delegate their health authority to a state board of health to pass state health regulations, standards, and requirements, but the health board must restrict itself to health matters. In effect the state board of health acts as a quasi-legislative body. The legislature also charges the health board with the responsibility for the enforcement of these regulations, which have the force of law.

In summary state health authority is exercised through the state constitution, state legislation, and health board regulations. Custom and reasonable action may also enter into matters of state health authority and action so long as it is reasonable and constitutional.

Health agencies in the state

Each state has both official health agencies and voluntary health agencies. Official health agencies and services are those supported by tax funds and recognized as a governmental agency or service. Official health agencies have staffs appointed by some official governmental body, and the staff members are government employees and may be classified as officials.

Voluntary health agencies are those supported entirely by financial contributions from citizens and private organizations. Services of voluntary health agencies are carried on by full-time, salaried, professional personnel. Most of the recognized voluntary health agencies have a national organization with state divisions and local chapters. The effective, principal sphere of operation of voluntary agencies is at the state level. It is at the state level where funds are raised, programs are planned, and services are made available. A small part of the state-raised funds are contributed to the national office, and some of the funds may be channeled to the local chapters, but the main portion of the agency's funds are retained by the state division.

Official health agencies

In every state the state health department is the principal state health agency. Yet each state has many other agencies that are also engaged in health promotion. For most of these agencies health is a secondary service or even an incidental activity. In some instances any health benefits are somewhat in the nature of a by-product of the primary activities of the agency. Yet the composite health contributions of these agencies are significant. In some instances more than one agency may carry on the same health function. At times this duplication is justifiable, but too often the duplication is without merit and is the result of empire building, long-established custom or priority, and political protectionism. On the state level as well as the national level, the institution of politics is not easily changed and agencies multiply and often outgrow their original purpose, so new activities must be created. Too often, tax funds diverted to unnecessary agencies and outmoded services are desperately needed by other essential and worthy services and agencies.

To record all state agencies that are involved in health in some form would mean an almost interminable list. Some of these agencies found in virtually all states will indicate how extensive the spectrum is. In many cases the title of the agency gives some indication of the nature of its health function.

Department of Agriculture
Department of Education
Department of Labor and Industry
Department of Welfare
Department of Conservation
Department of Mines and Minerals
Department of Motor Vehicles
Department of Public Safety
Department of Civil Service and Registration
Department of State Institutions
University
College
Experiment Station
Commissions
   Cancer
   Crippled children's
   Blind
   Mental disease
   Dairy and food
   Hotel
   Workmen's compensation
   Hospital
Boards
   Industrial accident
   Water resources
   Examining and licensing
      Medicine
      Osteopathy
      Dentistry
      Nursing

Medical laboratory
Podiatry
Livestock sanitation
Independent Offices
Toxicologist
Veterinarian

All of the health services given by these agencies are important, but the administrative need for combining agencies and for coordinating services is apparent. Such reorganization could result in a reduction in costs and in an improvement in services but in large states sometimes creates overly complex bureaucracies. A neglected criterion of organization is public familiarity with agency structures and procedures.

State department of health

Every state has an executive agency or department responsible for the activities necessary to protect and promote the health of the state. In four states the state constitution names the department and specifies its functions. In the remaining states the state constitution delegates this authority to the state legislature.

Massachusetts established the first state health board in 1969. Local official health agencies had been in operation for more than a century prior to the creation of the Massachusetts State Board of Health. No two states have precisely the same structure for their health programs, but, generally, state health authority is vested in a board that appoints a full-time health commissioner who administers the health program and agency.

The usual practice is to appoint a board of about nine members. Board members are appointed by the governor—subject to state senate approval—and serve without pay but are reimbursed for personal expenses in connection with their duties, such as attending meetings and participating in special functions. Board members usually are appointed for terms of 6 years, with terms staggered to provide for changes in board membership but with desirable continuity as well. The board is not composed of health specialists but ideally is made up of a cross-section of the population of the state and is represen-

tive of various interests, geographical areas, and backgrounds. The board's role is to reflect the viewpoints, interpretations, desires, and needs of the public. There could be no objection to having one medical doctor on the board, but to have the medical profession dominate would defeat the very purpose for which the board is created. Just as education policies are left to nonexperts in education rather than professional academicians, so too general health policies are decided by lay citizens with the viewpoint and judgment of the general public. Services of experts are provided to the board by the professional staff of the health department.

Powers of the board of health. The state board of health has such powers and functions as have been granted to it by the state constitution and the legislature. There are seven acknowledged powers of any state board of health—code-making, quasi-judicial powers, administration, investigation, supervision and consultation, education, and coordination with other health agencies.

Code-making power of the board is a quasi-legislative function that gives the board the authority to make necessary rules and regulations to carry out the authority and functions granted to it by the legislature. The professional health staff recommends certain health rules and regulations, which are assembled into a state sanitary code. This code has the effect of law when approved by the board of health. Courts have upheld the power of the board to enact binding rules and regulations, providing these rules and regulations do not go outside of health matters.

Quasi-judicial powers are exercised by the board in its authority to summon before it anyone alleged to have violated state health regulations. The board has the further recognized authority to summon witnesses. Hearings may be held by the board before granting or revoking a license. In all cases the citizen concerned has the right to contest any adverse action of the board by filing an appeal in court.

Administrative functions of the state board of health are delegated to the full-time staff of health specialists. In most states the chief administrator is called the health commissioner, although "health officer," "health director," and other titles are used. In some states the board elects the commissioner and in other states the governor appoints the commissioner. State health commissioners are medical doctors usually with preparation and experience in public health. The commissioner has certain recognized responsibilities: (1) general administration, (2) recommendation of health legislation, rules and regulations for consideration by the board, (3) appointment of personnel, (4) preparation of the budget, (5) supervision of divisions or bureaus, (6) enforcement of health rules and regulations, and (7) relationship with official agencies, organizations, and the public.

Department organization. The structure of the health department or organization varies from state to state. At the top of the administrative pyramid is the health commissioner or officer. At the level under the commissioner are the primary administrative units usually called *divisions*, which in turn are divided into bureaus or sections. There may be further subdivisions but this would be necessary only in departments in the heavily populated states. A large state health department may have ten divisions, and a small state health department may have but five administrative divisions. Each division has a director or chief, and each bureau or section has a head as administrator.

In most instances the title of the division or bureau as shown in Fig. 20-1 indicates the function or areas of health service. For present purposes, the distribution of program effort can be illustrated best by reviewing recent expenditures of state health departments in various program areas.

Programs of the state health agencies

The fifty states, the District of Columbia, Guam, Puerto Rico, the Virgin Islands, and the Trust Territory of the Pacific Islands all participated in a 1974 study of the programs and expenditures of state health agencies*

---
*Defined as the agency or department headed by the state or territorial health official.

(SHAs), which was made by the Health Program Reporting System of the Association of State and Territorial Health Officials (1975).

In 1974 the fifty-five SHAs reported expenditures of $5 billion. The range of expenditures was from $3 million in Idaho to $2.5 billion in California. Differences among the SHAs arise primarily from size of population, the wealth of the state, the extent to which local health department expenditures are included, and the wide variance in the responsibility only for traditional public health programs such as maternal and child health, communicable disease control, and specialized chronic disease programs. At the other extreme are states whose health agencies have responsibility for the same traditional areas; for institutional care programs; for environmental health services; for health resources planning, development, and regulation; for Medicaid (Title XIX) programs; and for added social services.

There has been a considerable movement among the states to delegate certain health programs to agencies other than the SHA and to establish "super agencies" or "umbrella agencies" that provide a wide (but not a consistent) variety of services that have been traditionally considered as public health, medical care, environmental health, welfare, and educational services. Therefore, the programs of the SHAs cannot be understood without an awareness of the changing patterns of assignment of function within the larger agency. The expenditures of the SHAs are summarized in three primary groupings:

Program grouping	Number of SHAs reporting	Expenditures	
		Millions of dollars	Percent of total
Public health services	55	2,317.5	47.5
Medicaid single state agencies	10	2,264.5	46.5
Special social services	2	291.0	6.0
Total	55	4,873.0	100.0

It is apparent that the Medicaid and spe-

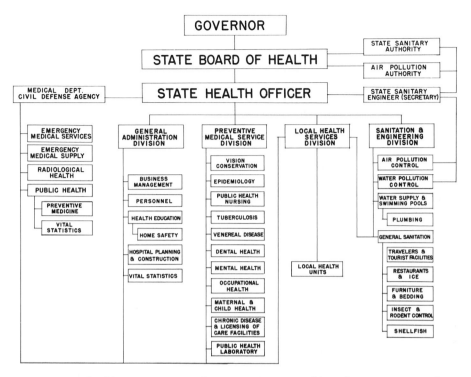

Fig. 20-1. State health organization and services. In states of less than average population, the organization of health services is kept as simple and unified as possible.

cial services programs of ten states account for half of all reported SHA expenditures. Most states do not place these responsibilities in the SHA. Medicaid funding is so different from that of public health programs that it is necessary to identify these state programs separately.

Medicaid single state agencies. In ten states the SHA was the single state agency responsible for the Medicaid program. Together they disbursed $2.3 billion for the purchase of health care for the indigent and medically indigent—almost half of all expenditures of SHAs. Seven of the eight SHAs with expenditures in excess of $100 million are listed on this page.

These Medicaid single state agencies were funded almost 50-50 from federal (Social Security Act Title XIX) and nonfederal sources, primarily state matching funds.

Special social programs. Two of the SHAs —California and Maryland—have responsi-

	Millions of dollars
Alabama	105.5
California	1,685.0
Guam	1.3
Maine	31.4
Maryland	184.3
Puerto Rico	8.5
Tennessee	95.2
Virgin Islands	2.2
Virginia	146.5
Wyoming	4.6
Total	2,264.5

bility for related but unique programs that are really social service rather than health service programs. California reported two such programs—social services and adoption services. The placement of the responsibility for these welfare programs within the Department of Health is unique to California. These programs expended $270 million.

Maryland's Department of Health and Mental Hygiene administers the state's juvenile services programs for delinquent and predelinquent children. Usually considered as correctional or social services programs, the placement of these programs (juvenile court services, institutional care of delinquent juveniles, and community residential care) within the SHA is unique to Maryland. Their reported expenditures were $21 million.

Public health programs. The program areas that comprise the major emphases in almost all SHAs are (1) personal health services, (2) environmental health services, (3) planning, development, and regulation of health resources, and (4) other programs, services, and administration. A fifth category is necessary for funds to local health departments that are not allocated to individual programs.

Public health program area	Number of SHAs reporting	Expenditures Millions of dollars	Percent of total
Personal health services	55	1,734.6	74.8
Environmental health services	51	168.0	7.2
Health resources	54	128.9	5.6
Other programs, services, and administration	55	143.5	6.2
Funds to local health departments not allocated to program areas	20	142.6	6.2
Total	55	2,317.5	100.0

Personal health services programs accounted for $1.7 billion of SHA expenditures in 1974. These included general and supporting services; maternal and child health, family planning, and crippled children's programs; programs for the control of communicable and chronic diseases; and programs for dental services. Over half of the SHAs have some mental health services. Finally, in a number of states these services included the operation of hospitals and other institutions. Expenditures for these several classification groups are in summary:

Personal health services category	Number of SHAs reporting	Expenditures Millions of dollars	Percent of total
General, supporting, and other	55	250.5	14.4
Maternal and child health) $152 million), family planning ($49 million), and crippled children ($109 million)	54	310.1	17.9
Communicable disease control	55	89.2	5.2
Dental services	51	19.2	1.1
Chronic disease	47	36.9	2.1
Mental health (excluding state-operated institutions)	30	317.6	18.3
State-operated institutions	24	711.1	41.0
Total	55	1,734.6	100.0

Programs in the "general, supporting, and other" category were reported primarily for laboratory services for which $55 million was expended. Public health nursing accounted for $49 million. In five states funds to local health departments were allocated to the level of personal health, but not to individual programs—a total of $16 million. Other programs included here are programs of care such as home health services and neighborhood health centers and programs of accident prevention, injury, and poison control. Included in the "other" category were programs for selected population groups such as migrants, medical examiner, and research programs and programs not elsewhere classifiable.

All of the SHAs reported expenditures for *communicable disease* programs with a total of $89 million. This figure does not include expenditures for state-operated institutions (although in some states it does include other patient care).

The SHAs reported another $68 million for operation of tuberculosis or respiratory disease hospitals. As in other areas reported,

Communicable dis- ease program group	Number of SHAs reporting	Millions of dollars
General	41	27.1
Immunization	41	7.8
Tuberculosis and chronic respiratory disease	41	33.3
Venereal disease	47	19.6
Other	10	1.4
Total	55	89.2

the absence of data for a particular program area does not necessarily mean that the state does not have program activities in that area. There is considerable variation among the states in the extent to which program responsibilities are centralized or combined, and this study did not attempt to seek out detail beyond normal budget groupings. In some of the states, programs such as these are carried out as local rather than as state programs.

Most states separately identified *chronic disease* programs. Most of them were general, but the current interest in particular disease problems is reflected in the number of states that reported separate programs concerned with respiratory diseases. The following figures are exclusive of state-operated chronic disease hospitals:

Chronic disease program group	Number of SHAs reporting	Millions of dollars
General chronic disease	23	14.6
Cancer	20	6.4
Cardiovascular disease	20	1.6
Renal disease	15	9.8
Other chronic disease	25	4.6
Total	47	37.0

One-fourth of the reported chronic disease program expenditures are for separately reported renal dialysis programs in fifteen states. Here again the absence of data need not mean the absence of program activity, because services for these and other diseases may be included in reports of institutional services. Virtually every SHA has activities in the cancer and cardiovascular disease prevention areas. However, except

for the twenty states included in the preceding table, funds were reported under other categories such as "general chronic disease." In addition to these expenditures, another $117 million was expended for the operation of state chronic disease hospitals.

In mental health the patterns of state responsibility vary widely. Only eleven SHAs —Maryland, Kentucky, Mississippi, North Dakota, Wyoming, Arizona, California, Hawaii, Puerto Rico, the Virgin Islands, and the Trust Territory—report having the primary responsibility for mental health services. In addition to these jurisdictions, another nineteen SHAs reported discrete fund expenditures in the area of mental health. Among these, programs for alcoholism and drug abuse are the most prominent:

Mental health program group	Number of SHAs reporting	Millions of dollars
Alcoholism and drug abuse	21	83.6
Combined program	6	29.5
Alcoholism	16	25.4
Drug abuse	10	28.7
Mental illness	7	167.5
Mental retardation	19	53.9
General and other	5	12.4
Total	30	317.4

In addition to these expenditures, another $299 million was expended for the operation of mental hospitals and $75 million was expended for institutions for the mentally retarded.

Environmental health programs accounted for $168 million—7% of reported public health expenditures. All but four SHAs reported some environmental health programs —almost always general sanitation, usually potable water (thirty-eight states) and health aspects of water quality (thirty-eight states), less often solid waste management (twenty-nine states), health aspects of occupational safety (twenty states), and air quality (eighteen states).

The largest components were general environmental health services and general sanitation services—$40 million and $34 million,

Environmental health program category	Number of SHAs reporting	Expenditures	
		Millions of dollars	*Percent of total*
General environmental	33	40.0	23.8
General sanitation	30	33.5	19.9
General consumer protection	29	27.3	16.2
Water and water quality	29	20.4	12.1
General	4	3.0	1.8
Potable water	22	6.5	3.9
Water quality	15	10.9	6.5
Laboratory services	24	15.3	9.1
Air quality	18	10.7	6.4
Solid waste management	14	7.1	4.2
Occupational health	25	6.5	3.9
Radiation control	33	5.8	3.5
Other	9	1.3	0.8
Total	51	167.9	100.0

respectively. These represented 24% and 20%, respectively, of the total environmental health program expenditures. General consumer protection followed with $27 million (16%). The above tabulation summarizes the totals.

For fiscal year 1974 SHAs grouped together, under the major program category "Health resources," those programs that dealt with the planning, development, and regulation of health resources, namely, facilities, services, and manpower. To this group were added the health and vital statistics functions of the SHA. All SHAs except the District of Columbia reported health resources programs. This area of responsibility accounted for SHA expenditures of $129 million (6%) of the total. The following tabulation summarizes these expenditures by program category:

Program category	Number of reporting	Millions of dollars
General and other	15	11.3
Planning and development	46	29.7
Facilities and services regulations	48	55.8
Manpower regulation	21	4.7
Vital and health statistics	50	27.4
Total	54	128.9

The previous expenditures reported by the Association of State and Territorial Health Officials (1975) are presented here to provide the student with a sense of the relative magnitude of different state health services and programs. The figures should not be studied literally because their exact meaning is transitory, but they should provide a more realistic picture of the current areas of responsibility and emphasis in state health departments than the organization chart in Fig. 20-1. Organization charts can be deceptive because the boxes are all approximately the same size, giving the illusion that the programs and services are of similar scope. The examination of budgets or expenditure figures casts each program or service into perspective.

One of the noteworthy omissions from the categories used by the Association of State and Territorial Health Officials is health education. As a support service to many programs, it is assumed that health education funds are set aside within the program budgets. This often is not the case, even though the programs require health education services. Hence, certain basic functions such as health education sometimes end up with no budget and their expenditures are from leftover funds. The President's Committee on Health Education (1973) could identify only

0.5% of state health expenditures devoted to health education.

Appraisal of official state health services

No instrument is available to make a precise appraisal of the value and significance of the official state health services. Yet there is ample empirical evidence that, as state health services have expanded and technical know-how has advanced, the health of the public has been advanced, diseases have been prevented, and deaths have been postponed. Many of the state health services do not deal with life and death matters but contribute to the enjoyment and effectiveness of living. While the state health services rarely touch the individual citizen, these services nevertheless serve as a backup for the local health services, medical care, hospital care, and other services related to human well-being. The state health department also serves as the agent of the state in dealings with the federal health agencies and those of other states.

In matters of state public health three cardinal needs exist. The first is the need for more funds to do adequately what is needed in state health promotion. A second need is to relieve the state health department of functions and services that are not strictly the province of the public health department. A third need is to integrate the health functions of all state agencies that provide health services in some form. The state health department, agriculture department, labor department, and other state agencies that have health functions must work closely together and decide what agency has primary responsibility for what health services. Hopefully, this would result in some agencies transferring certain health activities to other agencies where these functions more logically belong. Only when the public demands such coordination and shifting of functions will this actually take place.

HEALTH PLANNING

The Federal Comprehensive Planning Act of 1966 (PL 89-749) and the Partnership for Health Amendments of 1967 (PL 90-174) were enacted to establish comprehensive planning for health services, health manpower, and health facilities essential at every level of government; to strengthen the leadership and capabilities of state health agencies; and to broaden and make more feasible and relevant federal support of health services provided people in their communities. This legislation has been superseded by the National Health Planning and Resource Development Act of 1974.

The new law (PL 93-641) creates a network of health systems agencies responsible for health planning and development throughout the country. In creating such a network, the governors of the states would be asked to designate throughout the country health service areas for planning and development purposes that meet the requirements specified in the legislation. These requirements are as follows:

1. There must be a geographic region appropriate for the effective planning and development of health services, determined on the basis of factors including population and the availability of resources to provide all necessary health services for residents of the area.
2. To the extent practicable, the area must include at least one center for the provision of highly specialized health services, such as a University hospital or major teaching hospital.
3. Each area must have a population of not less than 500,000 or more than three million, except that an area may be less than 500,000 if the area comprises an entire state with a population of less than 500,000 or more than three million if the area includes a standard metropolitan statistical area with a greater population.
4. The area boundaries, to the maximum extent feasible, must be appropriately coordinated with those of Professional Standards Review Organizations, existing regional planning areas, and State planning and administrative areas.
5. The boundaries are also to be established so that, in the planning and development of health services to be offered within the health service area, any economic or geo-

graphic barrier to the receipt of such services in nonmetropolitan areas is taken into account. Determination of boundaries is to reflect the differences in health planning and health services development needs between nonmetropolitan and metropolitan areas.

6. Each standard metropolitan statistical area (SMSA) must be entirely within the boundaries of a single health service area. This requirement may be waived if a governor determines, with the approval of the Secretary,* that in order to meet the above-mentioned requirements, a health service area may contain only part of the SMSA.

The Act also provides that no areas need be designated for states that have no county or municipal public health institution or department and that have maintained a health planning system that complies with the purposes of this title.

In each health service area, the Secretary of the Department of Health, Education and Welfare, after consulting with the governor of the appropriate state, must then designate either a private nonprofit corporation or a public entity as the health systems agency responsible for health planning and development in that area. A health systems agency may not be or operate an educational institution. The legislation specifies minimum criteria for the legal structure, staff, governing body, and functioning of the health systems agencies. They would be generally responsible for preparing and implementing plans designed to improve the health of the residents of their health service area; to increase the accessibility, acceptability, continuity, and quality of health services in the area; to restrain increases in the cost of providing health services; and to prevent unnecessary duplication of health resources. In performing these responsibilities, the health systems agencies are required to:

1. Gather and analyze suitable data
2. Establish health systems plans (goals) and annual implementation plans (objectives and priorities)

3. Provide either technical and/or limited financial assistance to people seeking to implement provisions of the plans
4. Coordinate activities with PSROs* and other appropriate planning and regulatory entities
5. Review and approve or disapprove applications for federal funds for health programs within the area
6. Assist states in the performance of capital expenditures reviews
7. Assist states in making findings as to the need for new institutional health services proposed to be offered in the area
8. Assist states in reviewing existing institutional health services offered with respect to the appropriateness of such services
9. Annually recommend to states projects for the modernization, construction, and conversion of medical facilities in the area

An agency of state government will be chosen by the governor in each state to serve as the state health planning and development agency (state agency). In order to be designated, the state agency must prepare and submit to the Secretary for approval an administrative program for carrying out its functions. The state agency is to be advised by a Statewide Health Coordinating Council whose composition and responsibilities are specified in the legislation, including requirements that the Council:

1. Have 60% of its members appointed by the governor from the state's health systems agencies and have a consumer majority
2. Review annually and coordinate the health systems plans and annual implementation plans of the state's health systems agencies and make comments to the Secretary
3. Prepare a state health plan made up of the health systems plans of the health systems agencies, taking into account the preliminary plan developed by the State Agency
4. Review for the Secretary budgets and applications for assistance of health systems agencies
5. Advise the State Agency on the performance of its functions
6. Review and approve or disapprove state plans and applications for health-type formula grants to the state

---

*Secretary of the U.S. Department of Health, Education and Welfare.

*Professional Standards Review Organizations.

The required functions of the state agency are specified by the Act to include:

1. Conducting the state's health planning activities and implementing the parts of the state health plan and plans of health systems agencies which relate to the government of the state
2. Preparing a preliminary state plan for approval or disapproval by the Council
3. Assisting the Council in the review of the state medical facilities plan and in the performance of its functions
4. Reviewing new institutional health services proposed and making findings as to the need for such services
5. Reviewing existing institutional health services offered with respect to the appropriateness of such services and making public its findings

Any of the functions described above may be performed by another agency of state government on the request of the governor under an agreement with the state agency satisfactory to the Secretary.

The state facilities plan is to include a list of the projects for which assistance will be sought and the priorities for the funding of these projects. For each project an application must be submitted to the Secretary for approval, which must set forth a number of assurances including one that services in assisted facilities will be made available to all persons residing or employed in the areas served by the facilities and that a reasonable volume of services will be available to persons unable to pay.

Allotments to the states will be made on the basis of population, financial need, and the need for medical facilities. Not more than 20% of a state's allotment may be used for projects for construction of new inpatient facilities in areas that have experienced recent rapid population growth, and less than 25% may be used for projects for outpatient facilities that will serve medically underserved populations, half of which must be expended in rural medically underserved areas. The intent to replace expensive inpatient care with less expensive outpatient care is evident here. In the case of a project

to be assisted under an allotment, the federal share may not exceed two-thirds of the costs, except that a project in a rural or urban poverty area may receive 100% federal funding.

The new law also revised the Hill-Burton medical facilities construction program and related their activities more closely than is presently the case to the planning programs created by new Title XV outlined in this chapter. Development funds for each health systems agency will enable the agency to establish and maintain an Area Health Services Development Fund. This fund, together with grants, loans, loan guarantees, and interest subsidies, will support:

1. Modernization of medical facilities
2. Construction of new outpatient medical facilities
3. Construction of new inpatient medical facilities in areas which have experienced recent rapid population growth
4. Conversion of existing medical facilities for the provision of new health services

It is also the purpose to provide grant assistance for construction and modernization projects designed to eliminate or prevent safety hazards or avoid noncompliance with licensure or accreditation standards.

When the health systems agency has determined what health problems are being taken care of adequately and who is dealing with them, the state coordination council's role is to determine whether all concerned agencies are coordinating their efforts to deal efficiently and effectively with these problems. It then follows that areas of health not being adequately provided for is where the planning committees must devote their major attention. This means recruiting the services of all persons and agencies having possible contributions. It means obtaining necessary grants and other funding required for a solution to a particular health problem. A continuing program conceivably could attain the goal of no health problems unrecognized, no problems neglected, and an organized citizenry utilizing its full resources in the protection and promotion of the health of all the people. This is the objective of the health planning legislation.

QUESTIONS AND EXERCISES

1. To what extent are state health agencies the "middleman" of health organization?
2. Is the state's authority over the health of the people too great or not great enough? Why?
3. What check does the public have to prevent health authorities from being too powerful and arrogant?
4. Why should citizens always have the right to appeal to a court when they believe that they have been unjustly dealt with by health officials?
5. What health functions does your state department of agriculture engage in?
6. How do you explain that local health departments were formed long before state health departments were established?
7. How frequently does your state board of health meet?
8. Present the case for and against having the state board of health composed entirely of medical doctors.
9. Obtain a copy of your state sanitary code and report your reactions.
10. Who is your state health commissioner, what has been his professional preparation, what is his experience, and for how many years has he been in his present position?
11. When was the last time you or any member of your family received direct service from personnel of your state health department?
12. What are some health problems in your state on which the state health department should be conducting research?
13. What service now required of or otherwise carried on by your state health department should not be a part of the department's activities?
14. What consolidation of official health services have taken place in your state in the last 10 years?
15. Evaluate comprehensive health planning as it affects the health of your community.
16. Why has Congress enacted laws to regulate health planning in states and regions?

REFERENCES

American Public Health Association: Guidelines for organizing state and area-wide community health planning, New York, 1966, The Association.

Association of State and Territorial Health Officials: Programs and expenditures of state and territorial health agencies, fiscal year 1974, Washington, D. C., 1975, U.S. Government Printing Office.

Carter, R.: The gentle legion: a probing study of the voluntary health organizations, Garden City, N.Y., 1961, Doubleday & Co., Inc.

Ciba Foundation: Health of mankind, Boston, 1967, Little, Brown and Co.

Freeman, R. B., and Holmes, E. M.: Administration of public health services, Philadelphia, 1960, W. B. Saunders Co.

Goerke, L. S., and Stebbins, E. L.: Mustard's introduction to public health, ed. 5, New York, 1968, The Macmillan Co.

Hamilton, J. A., editor: The impact of centralization on the administration of health care services, Minneapolis, 1967, The University of Minnesota Press.

Hanlon, J. J.: Public health: administration and practice, ed. 6, St. Louis, 1974, The C. V. Mosby Co.

Henkle, O. B. M.: Introduction to community health, Boston, 1970, Allyn & Bacon, Inc.

Hilleboe, H. E., and Larimore, G. W.: Preventive medicine, ed. 2, Philadelphia, 1965, W. B. Saunders Co.

Larimore, G.: Health planning, Archives of Environmental Health 20:128, 1970.

Lawrence, C. F.: Public law 89-749: Comprehensive health planning, Journal of American School Health Association 9:261, 1967.

Michael, J.: A basic information system for health planning, Public Health Reports 83:21, 1968.

Mountin, J. W., and Flook, E.: Guide to health organization in the United States, Public Health Service Publication No. 196, Washington, D.C., 1951, U.S. Government Printing Office.

Report of the President's Committee on Health Education, 1973, Rockville, Maryland, Department of Health, Education and Welfare, Health Services and Mental Health Administration.

Sartwell, P. E.: Preventive medicine and public health, ed. 10, New York, 1975, Appleton-Century-Crofts.

Smolensky, J., and Haar, F. B.: Principles of community health, ed. 3, Philadelphia, 1972, W. B. Saunders Co.

21 ▪ NATIONAL AND INTERNATIONAL HEALTH SERVICES

Our true nationality is mankind.

H. G. Wells

The Constitution founding the republic acknowledged that the authority to promote public health rests with the states. Yet the federal government has provided the people with many indispensable health services. The Constitution grants the federal government no direct authority to engage in public health activities, but federal authority to promote health is derived from certain general clauses concerning federal responsibilities.

As a result of these broad, general clauses in the Constitution, the federal government carries on many health functions.

1. Regulation of *interstate commerce* gives Congress the right to pass Pure Food and Drug Acts controlling the interstate shipment of foods and drugs. This power enables Congress to pass legislation governing the movement of people and livestock on interstate carriers. Control of insects, air pollution, stream pollution, and other threats to health become federal functions under the authority to regulate interstate commerce.

2. *Taxing power* is vested in Congress and is used to control narcotics by requiring a tax for a permit to possess and sell narcotics and a tax on each transaction. Oddly, courts have held that these are measures primarily for revenue purposes and not for regulatory reasons.

3. *Postal power* of the national govern-

ment permits the passage of legislation prohibiting the use of the mails in any frauds, including health frauds. Misbranded or fraudulent drugs, patent medicines, and foods cannot be shipped through the mails, nor can any promotional material relating to fraudulent drugs or foods.

4. *Patent authority* enables the national government to require that any newly developed drug or medicine that is to be distributed to the public must be registered or patented.

5. *Treaty-making power* enables the federal government to enter into agreements with other nations on the control of communicable diseases, regulation of sanitation conditions, exchange of health information, and other health matters that are international in nature.

6. *National war power* grants to the national government the authority to protect and maintain the health of all personnel in the armed services.

7. Authority to govern the District of Columbia carries an implied responsibility for the health of residents of the District.

8. Power to appropriate money for the general welfare, together with the right to create agencies, forms the great umbrella under which most federal health activities operate. Appropriating money for health agencies of the national, state, and local governments, for the construction of hospitals under the Hill-Burton Act, for research, for health personnel training, for stream pollution control, and for other health projects has been the major contribution

of the national government in the field of health.

9. Power to create agencies for the general welfare has enabled the federal government to set up agencies to deal with each health problem that arises. Within each of the federal executive departments there exist bureaus, divisions, or branches directly or indirectly concerned with some aspect of health.

OFFICIAL NATIONAL HEALTH AGENCIES

More than fifty federal departments, bureaus, and other agencies are engaged in some sphere of health work. In most cases health is a minor or subordinate function of the agency. No particular overall organizational relationship exists between these agencies. When cooperation does occur it is the result of the judgment and action of the administrators involved or occasionally by legislative requirement for joint action.

Often health functions are assigned to agencies less logically structured for the function than some other agency. This has resulted when a special interest group has succeeded in having a certain health program assigned to a particular agency. Once the program has been lodged with a certain agency, the special interests will guard the agency's prerogative.

Most of the federal agencies with health functions are concerned with special problems or serve special groups. The United States Public Health Service is the only federal agency that truly deals with general health promotion. All others contribute one or more of the health services of the jigsaw puzzle referred to as the federal health program.

EXECUTIVE DEPARTMENTS WITH HEALTH SERVICES

Every executive department of the federal government has one or more branches directly or indirectly involved in health work. In almost every instance, health is a minor concern of the agency. For the purpose of the present discussion, only a limited number of agencies in each executive department will be identified and their health activity indicated. Agencies give direct health services, regulatory services, advisory services, and grants-in-aid, loan personnel, conduct special studies, disseminate information, and conduct research, as well as provide other services related to their primary mission.

Department of Agriculture. Except for the Department of Health, Education and Welfare with its United States Public Health Service, the Department of Agriculture contributes more community health service to the nation than any other executive department. Some of its health services are listed.

Agricultural and industrial chemistry—study of food, feed, and drugs of importance to health

Animal industry—study of the cause, prevention, control, and treatment of diseases affecting man and lower animals

Dairy industry—sanitary methods for handling milk and milk products

Entomology and plant quarantine—control of vectors affecting the health and well-being of man

Extension service—promotion of rural health and environmental sanitation

Human nutrition and home economics—wholesomeness and sanitation of meat or food products

Department of Commerce. Responsibilities in the field of health would appear to be misplaced in the Department of Commerce, but two health functions carried out by this department are of significance and are not too illogically placed.

Bureau of Census—collection and publication of statistics relating to the population, which is of value in planning health programs

Maritime Administration—medical and dental services for members of the Merchant Marine Cadet Corps and operation of the health program at merchant marine training stations

Department of Defense. As the title indicates, the health responsibilities of this department would be that of providing health and medical care programs for military

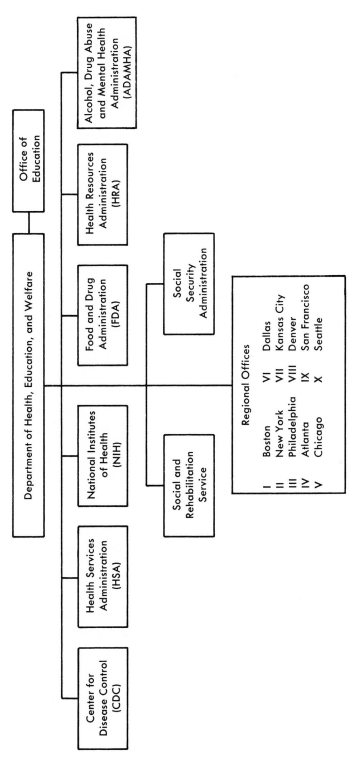

Fig. 21-1. Organizational plan of Department of Health, Education and Welfare. The six units on the second row make up the Public Health Service.

personnel and their dependents. This includes the provision of healthful environmental conditions and the training of personnel for duties in the field of health. The department cooperates with other federal agencies on health and medical problems.

Department of Health, Education and Welfare (DHEW). This department is continually restructuring its operating divisions, all of which are involved in matters of health in one form or another.

The six units of the Public Health Service contain numerous offices, bureaus, centers, institutes, and divisions that change their names, locations, and functions to some degree with every major health bill passed by Congress. They grow, shrink, split, or disappear with each year's appropriations. Of the sixty-two units of DHEW listed in this space in the last edition of this book (1973), only a few still exist under the same administrative division and with the same name in 1977, and it is expected that President Carter will make major bureaucratic changes as promised in his campaign. Rather than list them here again by their bureaucratic names, which are sure to change, Fig. 21-2 presents the major program or service areas of the six units of the Public Health Service. Most of the budgeted areas shown are identified organizationally with a bureau, center, office, institute, or division containing the name (for example, the $819 million budgeted for cancer is the entire 1978 budget of the National Cancer Institute).

For administration closer to the grass roots, the Department of Health, Education and Welfare has ten regional offices. See list on this page.

All divisions of the Department of Health, Education and Welfare will have offices and personnel complements in these regional headquarters. This is especially true as it relates to the Public Health Service. The organization and functions of this unit and the National Institutes of Health will be presented in more detail following a brief account of some of the health activities of

Region	Area	Office location
I	Connecticut, Maine, Massachusetts, New Hampshire, Rhode Island, Vermont	Boston, Mass.
II	New Jersey, New York	New York, N.Y.
III	Delaware, Maryland, Pennsylvania, Virginia, West Virginia	Philadelphia, Pa.
IV	Alabama, Florida, Georgia, Kentucky, Mississippi, North Carolina, South Carolina, Tennessee	Atlanta, Ga.
V	Illinois, Indiana, Michigan, Minnesota, Ohio, Wisconsin	Chicago, Ill.
VI	Arkansas, Louisiana, New Mexico, Oklahoma, Texas	Dallas, Tex.
VII	Iowa, Kansas, Missouri, Nebraska	Kansas City, Mo.
VIII	Colorado, Montana, North Dakota, South Dakota, Utah, Wyoming	Denver, Colo.
IX	Arizona, California, Hawaii, Nevada	San Francisco, Calif.
X	Alaska, Idaho, Oregon, Washington	Seattle, Wash.

other departments of the executive branch of the federal government.

Department of the Interior. Many highly significant health problems are the responsibility of the Department of the Interior. These responsibilities are adjuncts of the primary purpose of the department and are an essential service.

Bureau of Mines—inspection of mines, investigation of mine accidents, and training personnel in mine rescue work

Fish and Wildlife Service—research on sanitary processing of fishery products, elimination of hazards of stream pollution, and the destruction of wildlife that jeopardize the health and life of man

National Park Service—provision of environmental sanitation measures in national parks

Department of Justice. At first glance one would be inclined to disbelieve that the

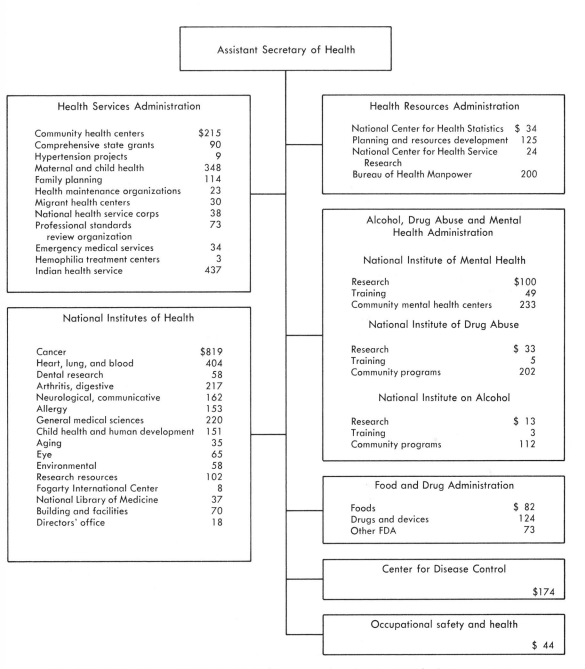

Fig. 21-2. United States Public Health Service programs, showing 1978 budget requests in millions.

Department of Justice could have any health responsibilities. Yet the duties of the Justice Department encompass certain social responsibilities that logically incorporate health.

Bureau of Prisons—With the assistance of the Public Health Service, provision of medical and dental services to inmates in federal correctional institutions and prisons

Immigration and Naturalization Service—With assistance from the Public Health Service, provision of medical examinations and medical care of immigrants

Department of Labor. Responsibility for the welfare of the worker includes responsibility for health and health conditions. Indeed, health of workers is a primary consideration of the department.

Bureau of Employment Security—health and medical services for migrant farm workers en route from one contractor to another and at reception centers

Bureau of Labor Standards—promotion of health in industry of all descriptions and magnitude

Bureau of Labor Statistics—collection, analysis, and application of data relating to significant health conditions in industry

Women's Bureau—studies on health and working conditions of women in industry and the promotion of the health and welfare of working women

Other agencies. A considerable number of somewhat independent federal agencies provide health services to a significant degree. From a long list, a few of these agencies are identified as examples.

Atomic Energy Commission—production and distribution of radioactive materials for research and medical purposes and training of personnel in radiology

Federal Trade Commission—control of deceptive advertising of foods, drugs, cosmetics, and devices shipped in interstate commerce

Interstate Commerce Commission—enforcement and promotion of health standards in the operation of interstate carriers

National Science Foundation—development of fundamental research in biological, physical, medical, and health sciences

Veterans Administration—providing health and medical services, including hospitalization and

rehabilitation to armed forces veterans; training of personnel in health work

It is thus apparent that scores of federal agencies are engaged in health work. In each case the service is significant and in some essential. Yet, the principal health organization in the federal government, the one that carries on virtually all health functions to an extended degree, is the United States Public Health Service. In terms of classic public health, this is perhaps the largest, most formidable, and most effective health organization in the world.

UNITED STATES PUBLIC HEALTH SERVICE

What began in 1798 as the Marine Hospital Service in the Treasury Department evolved into the Public Health and Marine Hospital Service in 1902. In 1912 the name was changed to the United States Public Health Service. The responsibilities of the agency continued to be increased. In 1917 the Health Service was charged with responsibility for the physical and mental examinations of all aliens entering the country. In the same year a national leprosarium was opened in Carville, Louisiana, and the Health Service was designated as the operating agency. In 1929 the medical care of federal prisoners and narcotic addicts became a responsibility of the United States Public Health Service. In the same year a program in mental hygiene was launched. The Social Security Act of 1935 extended the responsibilities of the Public Health Service. All grants-in-aid to states to strengthen local and state health departments were administered by the Public Health Service.

In subsequent years a series of Congressional Acts increased the functions of the Service. In 1937 The National Cancer Act was passed, followed by the Venereal Disease Control Act a year later. In 1939 the United States Public Health Service was moved from the Treasury Department to the Federal Security Agencies. Health agencies of other departments were also affected by this action.

The Public Health Law enacted in 1944

was a landmark in the development of the Public Health Service, because this Act provided for an expansion, reorganization, and consolidation of the Service and a revision of laws relating to public health. When the Department of Health, Education and Welfare was established in 1953, the United States Public Health Service became a part of the new department.

In the reorganization of the Department of Health, Education and Welfare in 1968, Health Services and Mental Health Administration became the designation of what had largely been the United States Public Health Service. In the same reorganization the National Institutes of Health became independent of the Health Services and Mental Health Administration as a division of the Department of Health, Education and Welfare. Food and Drug Administration became the third major division along with the Health Services and Health Institutes. Today, the Assistant Secretary for Health is the administrative head of the six divisions of the Public Health Service shown in Figs. 21-1 and 21-2.

The Environmental Health Service is no longer operational. Its pollution control programs—National Pollution Control Administration, Bureau of Solid Wastes Managements, Bureau of Water Hygiene, and elements of the Bureau of Radiological Health—were transferred out of the service to the Environmental Protection Agency. In 1971 Community Environmental Management and the Bureau of Occupational Safety and Health became the National Institute of Occupational Safety and Health.

The Communicable Disease Center, although located in Atlanta, Georgia, is the responsibility of the Public Health Service. This center supports and promotes tuberculosis control programs, combats epidemics, trains personnel for international health work, assists in malaria control programs in affected nations, promotes programs to eliminate smallpox and measles in the world, sponsors immunization and health education programs, and develops insecticides to control vector-borne diseases.

National Institutes of Health. In 1887 the Marine Hospital Service founded a research laboratory at the Marine Hospital, Staten Island, New York. In 1891 the name was changed to Hygienic Laboratory, and the unit was moved to Washington, D.C. In 1930 the Hygienic Laboratory became the National Institutes of Health and moved to Bethesda, Maryland, on land donated by Mr. and Mrs. Luke I. Wilson of Bethesda. The use of the plural, Institutes, was but a natural transition as the agency expanded its operations.

The mission of the National Institutes of Health is the discovery of knowledge for the prevention and control of disease and the extension of life. A broad, complex program is designed to meet the needs in biomedical science. Scientists in the laboratories and Clinical Center of the Institutes carry on part of the program of research. Most of the research is done outside of the Institutes through grants administered by the National Institutes of Health. About 85% of the Institute's appropriation of more than 2 billion dollars yearly goes to the extramural program of grants to scientists and research institutions throughout the nation.

The grants program is planned to provide a continuous supply of competent scientists in biomedical disciplines. In addition to the training grants, fellowships, and traineeships, the program also provides facilities, equipment, and other resources, including such things as computers and primate centers. Basic research now cuts across several of the traditional areas. Special attention is given to national trends and to neglected research areas.

The National Institutes of Health has an international research program, which seeks to make use of the abilities of qualified scientists the world over. Grants have been made to scientists in various health disciplines in many countries. The NIH has also provided opportunities for promising young American scientists to work abroad as members of the established research groups. No foreign grants are made unless they are of a high value and are related to

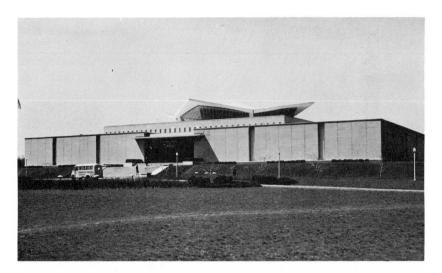

Fig. 21-3. National Library of Medicine in the National Institutes of Health campus in Bethesda, Maryland. A central national repository of the accumulated medical knowledge available in many forms and through various media. (Courtesy National Library of Medicine)

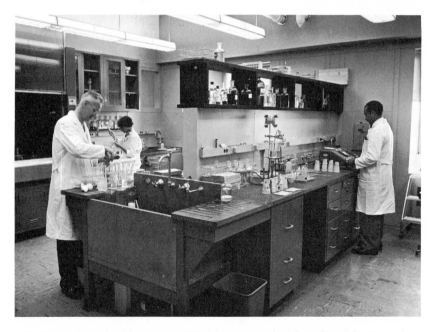

Fig. 21-4. Research in health. Over 1,000 laboratories for clinical and basic studies are a part of the 500-bed Clinical Center at the National Institutes of Health. Scientists working in a variety of disciplines are able to consult with each other in solving the problems of human health. (Courtesy National Institutes of Health)

health objectives of value to the United States. Nobel Prize awards in medicine and physiology have been made to foreign investigators who were working under grants from the National Institutes of Health.

The NIH makes contracts with foreign institutions to conduct research and provides fellowships to American scientists to study at foreign centers of excellence. NIH also promotes a visiting program that brings distinguished scientists to this country to work in the NIH laboratories or the Fogarty International Center.

Appraisal of the United States Public Health Service

No one can say precisely how many lives have been saved or how many people have had the quality of their health improved by the work of the United States Public Health Service. Yet, through mere observation, one can infer that the general health of the nation has been affected favorably and death has been postponed for millions of citizens. All of the professional personnel of the United States Public Health Service should be regarded as dedicated public servants who guard the nation's health and strive constantly to improve the quality of health and extend life expectancy.

Vision and perseverance have characterized the history of the Health Service. Frequently, the Health Service has anticipated health problems and crises before they developed. At other times the Health Service has thrown its full resources into a critical disease situation. Service to states and communities has been invaluable. The people of the United States get good value from a tax dollar spent by the Public Health Service.

PROFESSIONAL HEALTH ORGANIZATIONS

Professional societies or associations are formed by people who have completed a prescribed curriculum and training and have met standards of certification. These people of common purpose organize to uphold professional standards and to serve society

better through their organized efforts. While the primary purpose of a professional society is to promote the interests of the profession and its members, its image and prestige depend on its service to mankind, and members of these professional societies are fully aware of this fact. What best serves the public should be in the best interests of the professional organization.

American Medical Association. The American Medical Association was founded in 1847. Its constitution states that "the object of the Association is to promote the art of medicine and the betterment of public health." Primarily, the Association serves the interests of private medical practitioners, but its activities are planned to protect and serve the interests of the public and particularly to provide the best possible medical service.

The American Medical Association is a federation of state societies, and these in turn are made up of county societies, which means that the national organization is an association of state societies rather than of individual practitioners. The Association strives to improve the quality of medical service by informing members of advancements in medicine and related fields. It has three different agencies investigating possible quackery in drugs, nostrums, foods, cosmetics, and other possible health frauds that might jeopardize the health of the public. The Association participates in the accreditation of hospital standards.

The *Journal of the American Medical Association* is a weekly publication and is generally regarded as a leading journal in its field. For the general lay public, the Association publishes *Today's Health*, the health education publication. This publication deals with topics of personal and community health. The Association also publishes much pamphlet material for distribution.

American Dental Association. The American Dental Association was formed in 1860 to advance the dental profession by raising the quality of dental education and dental practice. The Association is the profession's agency for keeping practitioners informed of new developments in equipment, procedures, and techniques.

In its early years the American Dental Association was an organization of individual dental practitioners; later it became an association of state societies, which in turn are composed of representatives from county societies. The American Dental Association publishes the *Journal of the American Dental Association* and a yearly index of periodical dental literature. The Association also publishes pamphlets for distribution.

American Public Health Association. The American Public Health Association was established in September, 1872, and rapidly expanded from a limited interest in sanitation to a broad public health program to encompass all factors affecting the health of the people.

The American Public Health Association carries on a wide variety of activities through 22 sections including laboratory, health administration, statistics, environment, radiological health, food and nutrition, injury control, maternal and child health, public health education, veterinary public health, social work, population, public health nursing, epidemiology, school health, dental health, mental health, occupational health, and medical care. The Association has developed standards that have been widely accepted and adopted. These include methods for the examination of water, milk, and sewage, the operation of swimming pools, diagnostic reagents and procedures, the appraisal of local health work, a model health code for cities, the accreditation of public health training, and many other standards, procedures, and guides. The Association conducts surveys and other studies, which it initiates and carries out at the request of organizations or of individuals. Its publication, *American Journal of Public Health*, is issued each month. In addition the Association publishes *The Nation's Health*, a monthly newsletter, pamphlets, special reports, and other material.

National League for Nursing. The National League for Nursing was formed in 1952 when three national nursing organizations and four national committees combined their resources and programs—the National League of Nursing Education (founded in 1893), the National Organization for Public Health Nursing (1912), the Association of Collegiate Schools of Nursing (1933), the Joint Committee on Practical Nurses and Auxiliary workers in Nursing Services (1945), the Joint Committee on Careers in Nursing (1948), the National Committee for the Improvement of Nursing Services (1949), and the National Nursing Accrediting Service (1949).

The principal purpose of the National League for Nursing is simply stated, "That the nursing needs of the people may be met." The Department of Public Health Nursing continues the practices and objectives of the previous National Organization for Public Health Nursing. The following are the objectives of the Department of Public Health Nursing:

1. To stimulate responsibility for the health of the community by establishing and extending public health nursing
2. To bring about cooperation among nurses, physicians, and all others interested in public health
3. To develop standards of public health nursing
4. To maintain a central bureau of information and assistance in such services
5. To publish periodicals and bulletins

The league has both professional and nonprofessional members including both public health nurses and friends of public health nurses. The official periodical of the National League for Nursing is *Nursing Outlook*. The league is also the sponsor of *Nursing Research*.

Society for Public Health Education. The Society for Public Health Education was formed in 1958 as the Society of Public Health Educators. Its change in name reflects its commitment to promotion of health education of the public more than the interests of its professional members. With a membership of less than 1500, the Society has been remarkably effective in influencing national policy related to health education, including the Health Information and Promotion Act of 1976 (PL 94-317). The Society publishes *Health Education Monographs* and meets annually in conjunction with American Public Health Association.

American Alliance for Health, Physical Education, and Recreation. The American Alliance for Health, Physical Education, and Recreation began in 1885 as the American Association for the Advancement of Physical Education and became a department of the National Education Association in 1937. Several areas of Alliance activity are related to health, such as school nursing, school medical service, health teaching, nutrition education, dental health, mental health, and recreation. The Alliance recommends program standards for communities. The Alliance publishes the monthly *Journal of the American Association for Health, Physical Education and Recreation,* the bimonthly *Health Education,* and the *Research Quarterly.*

HEALTH FOUNDATIONS

The United States is blessed with a considerable number of philanthropical foundations, many of which are engaged in public health programs. Some foundations have broad programs and operate in a variety of fields. Others are more specific in their activities and tend to concentrate on relatively few projects. Four foundations will be described as examples of the different types that engage in health projects.

Rockefeller Foundation. The Rockefeller Foundation was chartered in 1913 under the laws of the state of New York for the purpose of "promoting the well-being of mankind throughout the world." In part, the charter states:

It shall be within the purposes of said corporation to use as means to that end research, publications, the establishment and maintenance of charitable, benevolent, religious, missionary, and public

education activities, agencies, and institutions already established and any other means and agencies which from time to time shall seem expedient to its members or trustees.

In its organization the Foundation consists of five divisions: (1) International Health, (2) Medical Sciences, (3) Natural Sciences, (4) Social Sciences, and (5) Humanities.

Only the International Health Division is an operating agency with its own laboratories and staff of scientists. Three phases of work have been pursued: (1) control of specific diseases such as yellow fever, tuberculosis, and influenza, (2) aid to health departments, (3) health demonstrations, aid to selected schools, public health education, and grants of postgraduate fellowships in public health. Out of the research laboratories of the foundation have come many significant contributions in the treatment of yellow fever, typhus, influenza, and malaria.

The four nonoperating divisions support university, laboratory, and other research groups. Fellowships for postdoctoral work are also granted. These divisions support a wide range of activities through various grants and appropriations.

Milbank Memorial Fund. The Milbank Memorial Fund was established in 1905 with the objective "to improve the physical, mental, and moral condition of humanity and generally to advance charitable and benevolent objects." Its activities for the most part have been in preventive medicine. Objectives of the organization have been attained through grants and fellowships. Contributions of the fund have been to the fields of public health, medicine, social welfare, research, and education. The fund has sponsored population studies, demonstrations, projects, and the measurement of various aspects of public health services. The organization has extended its activities to mental hygiene, school lunches, food research, defective vision, dental studies, prenatal and postnatal instruction, and public health demonstrations.

Commonwealth Fund. The Commonwealth Fund was founded in 1918 with a simple but meaningful objective: "To do something for the welfare of mankind." Activities have included health, medical education and research, education, and mental hygiene. The fund has been instrumental in advancing public health practices and procedures through research, improved teaching in medical schools, extension of public health services to rural communities, provision and improvement of hospital facilities, and strengthening mental health services in the United States and in Great Britain.

W. K. Kellogg Foundation. The W. K. Kellogg Foundation was established in 1930 for "the promotion of health, education, and the welfare of mankind, but principally of children and youth, directly or indirectly, without regard to sex, race, creed, or nationality." The nineteen points listed in the Children's Charter of the White House Conference on Child Health and Protection in 1930 have been accepted as goals. A functional problem-solving approach has been used rather than one of research or relief.

The foundation's program begins in the home by teaching people to help themselves. Grants have been made to various counties to establish county health departments. Health education programs have been sponsored to link the school and community in public health promotion.

Cooperation and coordination. Voluntary health agencies have made a significant contribution to the health of the nation and the world. Each agency is free to choose its own course of action and is sufficiently flexible to adjust to changing conditions and needs. These agencies tend to specialize and demonstrate what can be done in a specific field of health. In theory, when this has been accomplished, the task or field is taken over by an official health agency and the need for the voluntary agency no longer exists. In practice, few voluntary agencies are ever dissolved.

Overlapping of programs exists to some degree. In addition the need for cooperation and coordination has long existed, and in

1921 the National Health Council was organized with about fifty voluntary national groups represented. The United States Public Health Service served as an advisory member. At the outset the council was well financed and well staffed. Within 5 years after its inception, the council had become ineffective and had abandoned many of its projects. Some revitalization has occurred in recent years through the organization of National Health Forums, the inauguration of Community Health Week, the creation of working committees, and various publications. The Council recently assisted in the establishment of a National Center for Health Education based in San Francisco.

Voluntary health agencies perform a unique and important role in the promotion of health in every state and in most nations. No health program is complete in the sense that it serves every individual who could benefit from the program. Thus these agencies have a need to expand and intensify their services. Further, there are areas of health needs that receive little attention and less service. Perhaps the National Foundation for Infantile Paralysis charted the course that all existing voluntary as well as official agencies might consider. When the agency's original goal is virtually achieved, the agency directs its attention and energies to other health problems in need of solution rather than returning to the public with requests for funds to do more of the same.

OFFICIAL INTERNATIONAL HEALTH ORGANIZATIONS

For more than a century, health scientists of the world have worked cooperatively and harmoniously in promoting the health of all people. National interests have given way to world interests. Exchange of health knowledge, loan of the services of experts, and united efforts in preventing the spread of disease have characterized the international activities of public health personnel the world over. In the early years of international health activities, virtually all attention was directed to the control of communicable diseases, but programs have expanded to encompass the entire spectrum of health promotion.

International congresses on hygiene and epidemiology have been held at irregular intervals since 1852, when the first congress met in Brussels. After a series of such meetings, the International Office of Public Health was created on December 9, 1907, by agreement among forty nations. Until the formation of the Health Section in the Secretariat of the League of Nations, the International Office of Public Health served as the medium for the international exchange of health knowledge and for cooperation on health matters. In 1950 the International Office of Public Health was absorbed by the World Health Organization.

Pan American Health Organization. Creation of the Pan American Sanitary Bureau was authorized by the Second International Conference of the American States, which met in Mexico City in 1901. It was formally organized as the International Sanitary Office at the First Inter-American Sanitary Conference, held in Washington, D.C. in 1902. The Fifth Conference, which met in Santiago, Chile, in 1911, changed the name to Pan American Sanitary Bureau.

From its inception the Pan American Sanitary Bureau has devoted its attention primarily to the control of communicable diseases. This has been done through cooperation between the participating nations by exchanging vital statistics reports, exchanging health information on travellers, reporting new advances in disease control, exchanging knowledge on advances in sanitation procedures, training health personnel, and making technical experts available to other nations on a consulting basis. The Pan American Sanitary Bureau is now known as the Pan American Health Organization and is an independent health organization, but at present is essentially an agency integrated with the World Health Organization as one of its regional offices.

League of Nations Health Section. In September, 1923, under Article 23 of the covenant of the League of Nations, participating nations established a Health Section in the Secretariat of the League of Nations. The Health Section developed a moderately effective program. In cooperation with the International Office of Public Health, the Health Section took steps to control epidemics, improved the worldwide epidemiological reporting system, initiated research in the control of communicable diseases, established standards for biological products, began studies on the underlying foundations of health, and assisted governments in improving their public health services.

With the formation of the United Nations and the creation of the World Health Organization, the Health Section of the League of Nations was duly dissolved. The World Health Organization took over all functions of the Health Section of the League of Nations and of the International Office of Public Health.

WORLD HEALTH ORGANIZATION

The International Health Conference that convened in New York City on June 19, 1946, ushered in a new era in health cooperation. The Conference was attended by representatives from all of the member states of the United Nations and by observers from thirteen countries that were not members. At the closing session on June 22, the final instruments were approved and signed by the Conference. This included a protocol providing for the absorption by the World Health Organization of the International Office of Health and the Health Section of the League of Nations. The Constitution provided for the eventual integration of the Pan American Sanitary Bureau with the World Health Organization. By April 7, 1948, the required twenty-six countries that were members of the United Nations had confirmed their approval of the Constitution and their membership in the World Health Organization.

The founding principles of the World Health Organization and a widely quoted definition of health are set forth in the preamble of its Constitution:

Health is a state of complete physical, mental, and social wellbeing and not merely the the absence of disease or infirmity.

The enjoyment of the highest attainable standard of health is one of the fundamental rights of every human being without distinction of race, religion, political belief, or economic or social conditions.

The health of all peoples is fundamental to the attainment of peace and security and is dependent upon the fullest cooperation of individuals and states.

The achievement of any state in the promotion and protection of health is of value to all.

Unequal development in different countries in the promotion of health and control of disease, especially communicable disease, is a common danger.

Healthy development of the child is of basic importance; the ability to live harmoniously in a changing total environment is essential to such development.

The extension to all peoples of the benefits of medical, psychologic, and related knowledge is essential to the fullest attainment of health.

Informed opinion and active cooperation on the part of the public are of the utmost importance in the improvement of the health of the people.

Governments have a responsibility for the health of their peoples that can be fulfilled only by the provision of adequate health and social measures.

Financing. The WHO budget is raised by assessments of Member States according to a formula, with a limitation that no nation shall pay more than 33⅓% of the total assessment. In addition, the organization receives funds from various other sources— Pan American Health Organization and voluntary contributions from governments, institutions, and individuals.

Organization. The democratic nature of WHO is reflected in its organization, where legislation, administration, and services are under the direction of the Member States. A great deal of the services of participants are contributed without any cost to the organization.

World Health Assembly is the legislative branch of WHO. Delegates of the Member States and Associate Members meet annually in Geneva, Switzerland. The Assembly establishes policy and decides on the program and budget for the next year.

Executive Board is the board of directors of the organization. The Board is composed of twenty-four persons qualified in health matters. It meets at least twice a year to advise and act for the Assembly. Each year the Assembly elects eight governments to designate members to serve for 3 years and to replace eight retiring members.

Secretariat designates the professional management of the World Health Organization at Headquarters in Geneva and in 140 countries of the world. The Director-General is the chief executive, and in organization the Secretariat is composed of three departments—advisory services, central technical services, and administration and finance. Each department is composed of divisions that, in turn, are made up of sections.

Regions are used for effectiveness in organization and operation. For WHO purposes, the world is divided into six regions, each with its own organization consisting of a regional committee composed of delegates from governments in the region, and a regional office that administers WHO-aided projects and supervises the staff in the various projects. Regional offices of WHO are logically distributed.

Region	Regional office
Southeast Asia	New Delhi
Eastern Mediterranean	Alexandria
The Americas (Pan American Health Organization)	Washington, D.C.
Western Pacific	Manila
Africa	Brazzaville
Europe	Copenhagen

Each regional office has its own staff and method of operation.

Advisory panels consist of more than 12,000 scientists, health administrators, and educators from many nations. These forty-four panels provide expert advice in their re-

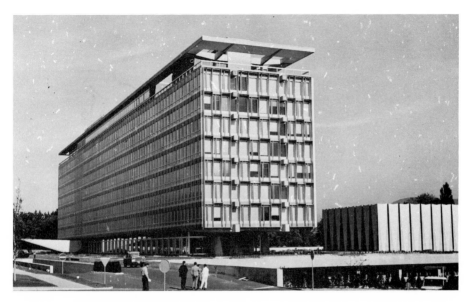

Fig. 21-5. World Health Organization Headquarters in Geneva is a monument to man's concern for his fellow man and a symbol of cooperation in a world of conflict. (Courtesy World Health Organization)

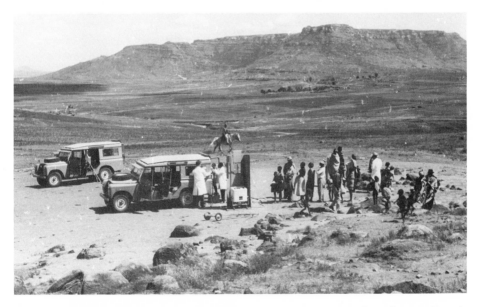

Fig. 21-6. Mobile WHO-assisted x-ray unit in a remote area. Tuberculosis still ranks among the world's greatest scourges. WHO is helping to develop large-scale programs in diagnosis and control. (Courtesy World Health Organization)

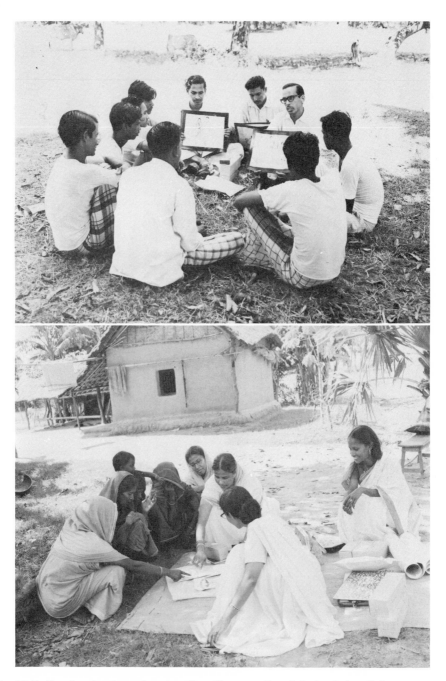

Fig. 21-7. Family planning education for villages in Bangladesh. Cultural factors require local adaptations of media and channels of communication in traditional societies. (Courtesy Public Health Education Research Project, University of California, Berkeley)

spective fields. Committees of experts are chosen from these panels to provide the necessary expertise to deal with particular health problems.

Functions of WHO. To meet the objectives of its charter, the World Health Organization recognizes specific functions that are its responsibilities.

1. International health—to act as the directing and coordinating authority on world health
2. International conventions—to propose conventions, agreements, and regulations and make recommendations concerning international health matters
3. International standards—to develop, establish, and promote international standards for food, biologic, pharmaceutical, and similar products
4. Nongovernmental organizations—to promote cooperation among scientific and professional groups that contribute to the advancement of science
5. Research—to promote and conduct research in health
6. Public health—to study and report on public health and medical care from preventive and curative points of view, including hospital services and social security
7. Health services—to assist governments, upon request, in strengthening health services
8. Maternal and child health—to promote

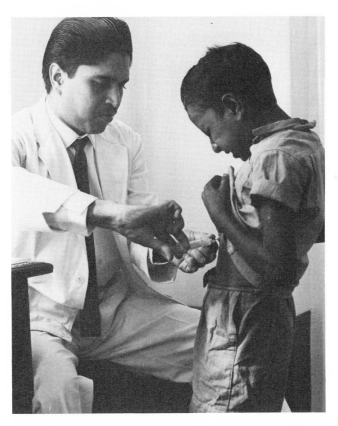

Fig. 21-8. Rabies immunization, WHO International Reference Centre, Coonoor, India. The long incubation period provides the victim the chance to be immunized before the virus reaches the brain. Rabies must be eliminated in lower animals if rabies is to be eradicated in man. (Courtesy World Health Organization)

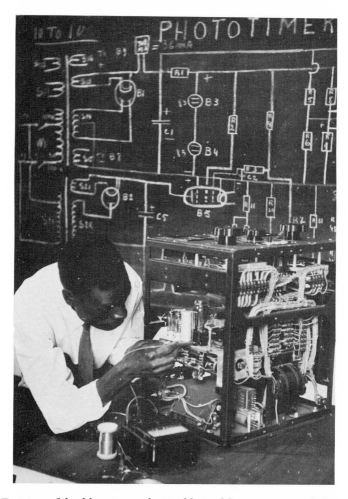

Fig. 21-9. Training of health personnel. World Health Organization helps to build up national and regional teaching and training institutions. At the Tuberculosis Chemotherapy Laboratory in Nairobi, Kenya, trainees learn to repair x-ray equipment. (Courtesy World Health Organization)

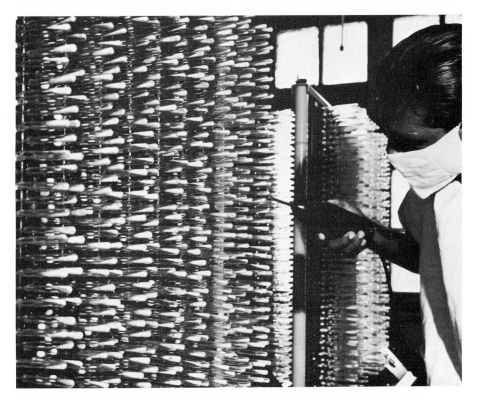

Fig. 21-10. Smallpox eradication. Modern freeze-dried and tropical stable vaccine production in India. In a massive 10-year assault (1967-1977), WHO has worked together with all the countries of the world to defeat one of the greatest killers of all times. In 1977 smallpox became a fear of the past. (Courtesy World Health Organization)

maternal and child health and welfare and to foster the ability to live harmoniously in a changing environment

9. Diseases—to stimulate and advance work to eradicate epidemic, endemic, and other disease
10. Diagnosis—to standardize diagnostic procedures as necessary
11. Living conditions—to promote the improvement of nutrition, housing, sanitation, recreation, economic, or working conditions, and other aspects of environmental hygiene
12. Accidents—to promote the prevention of accidental injuries
13. Mental health—to foster activities in mental health, especially those affecting human relations
14. Education—to promote improved standards of teaching and training in health, medical, and related professions

The World Health Organization is helping many nations to solve many health problems. In helping a nation, it is always the objective of WHO to build up the nation's potential and train its personnel so that eventually outside help will not be needed. In some instances the services of WHO are merely advisory, but in many instances WHO personnel are on the scene to do the job that is necessary. WHO also takes part in the United Nations Expanded Programme of Technical Assistance for economic development of underdeveloped countries. WHO operates closely with the United Nations Children's Fund, the United Nations Specialized Agencies, especially the Food and Agriculture Organization, and the United Nations Educational, Scientific and Cultural Organization, the Technical As-

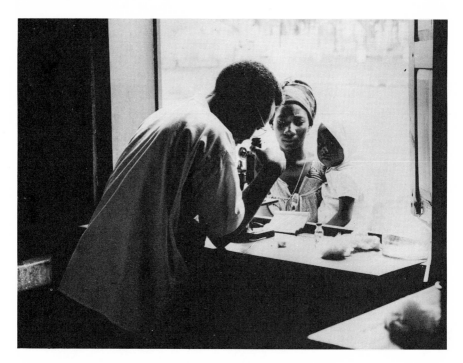

Fig. 21-11. Rural health services. Well-organized rural health services are essential to improve health conditions of the areas concerned and to help in the consolidation and integration phases of eradication campaigns against communicable diseases. (Courtesy World Health Organization)

sistance Board, and the International Labor Organization.

It is significant that public health people from all over the world can work together harmoniously and cooperatively. This is possible in a profession guided by the idea of service to humanity. Professional public health people are motivated to improve the health and general well-being and to extend the life expectancy of all people.

QUESTIONS AND EXERCISES

1. In your judgment, which of the eight broad general clauses of the Constitution provides the federal government with the best means for the promotion of health, and what is your reasoning?
2. Give some examples of how the federal government has used the taxing power in matters of health.
3. Evaluate this statement: "One price paid for democracy is inefficiency and illogical organization."
4. Recall any time that you or any member of your family received a direct health service from a federal agency. Why is such service rare for a student?
5. Identify one health service in a federal agency, other than the United States Public Health Service, which should be assigned to the Public Health Service, and explain your reasons.
6. What reasons can you give for and against lodging the function of stream pollution prevention and control in the Department of the Interior?
7. What are your reasons for or against establishing the United States Public Health Services as an independent agency?
8. What is your reaction to the United States Public Health Service having a semimilitary character?
9. What is the significance of the fact that 95% of the professional public health people in the United States are nonmedical people?
10. Evaluate this statement: "Appropriations for the United States Public Health Service represent investments rather than expenditures."
11. Justify the grants for Public Health Traineeships. Present a case for extending these grants to other traineeship programs.
12. What justification is there for the National Institutes of Health subsidizing the research of scientists in other countries?
13. Why should the federal government concern itself with research in the health sciences?
14. In your judgment, what specific health problem is most in need of more extensive and intensive research?

15. What voice does a local medical practitioner have in the policies of the American Medical Association?

16. Which of the professional health organizations do you regard as most public spirited and least self-interested? Why?

17. The United States gives far more to the World Health Organization than it receives. What is your comment?

18. Why does the World Health Organization place so much emphasis on communicable disease control in view of all the recent technologic advances in this field?

19. Why is it so very important that the World Health Organization place primary emphasis on helping nations to help themselves?

20. What do you regard as the number one health problem in the world today and why?

REFERENCES

Bryant, J.: Health and the developing world, Ithaca, N.Y., 1969, Cornell University Press.

Elliott, K. M.: The world health service, Postgraduate Medical Journal 43:447, 1967.

Epstein S., and Epstein, B.: First book of the World Health Organization, New York, 1964, Franklin Watts, Inc.

Goerke, L. S., and Stebbins, E. L.: Mustard's introduction to public health, ed. 5, New York, 1968, The Macmillan Co.

Hanlon, J. J.: Public health: administration and practice, ed. 6, St. Louis, 1974, The C. V. Mosby Co.

Health and development: an annotated, indexed bibliography, Baltimore, 1972, The Johns Hopkins University Press.

Hilleboe, H. E., and Larimore, G. W.: Preventive medicine, ed. 2, Philadelphia, 1965, W. B. Saunders Co.

King, M., editor: Medical care in developing countries, London, 1966, Oxford University Press, Inc.

National Nutrition Policy Study—1974: hearings before the Select Committee on Nutrition and Human Needs, United States Senate, 93rd Congress, Part I: Famine and the world situation, Washington, D.C., 1974, U.S. Government Printing Office.

Pflanz, M., and Schach, E., editors: Cross-national sociomedical research: concepts, methods, practice, Stuttgart, 1976, Georg Thieme Publishers.

Sivin, I.: Contraception and fertility change in the international postpartum program, New York, 1974, The Population Council.

Smoking and health programs around the world, Bethesda, 1973, DHEW Publication No. 74-8707, National Clearinghouse for Smoking and Health, Center for Smoking and Health, Center for Disease Control.

Smolensky, J., and Harr, F. B.: Principles of community health, ed. 3, Philadelphia, 1972, W. B. Saunders Co.

UNESCO: World of promise, Dobbs Ferry, N.Y., 1965, Oceana Publications, Inc.

World Health Organization, what it is, what it does, how it works, Irvington-on-Hudson, N.Y., 1965, Columbia University Press.

PUBLICATIONS

The following publications of the World Health Organization may be obtained from Q Corporation, 49 Sheridan Avenue, Albany, New York 12210 (variably priced):

Technical report series

No. 548—Planning and organization of geriatric services. Report of a WHO expert Committee, 1974, 46 pages.

No. 553—Ecology and control of rodents of public health importance. Report of a WHO Scientific Group, 1974, 42 pages.

No. 554—Health aspects of environmental pollution control: planning and implementation of national programmes. Report of a WHO Expert Committee, 1974, 57 pages.

No. 558—Community health nursing. Report of a WHO Expert Committee, 1974, 28 pages.

No. 559—New approaches in health statistics. Report of the Second International Conference of National Committees on Vital and Health Statistics, 1974, 40 pages.

No. 562—Services for cardiovascular emergencies. Report of a WHO Expert Committee, 1975, 129 pages.

No. 564—Organization of mental health services in developing countries. Sixteenth Report of the WHO Expert Committee on Mental Health, 1975, 41 pages.

No. 569—Evaluation of family planning in health services. Report of a WHO Expert Committee, 1975, 67 pages.

No. 571—Early detection of health impairment in occupational exposure to health hazards. Report of a WHO Study Group, 1975, 80 pages.

No. 573—Veterinary contribution to public health practice. Report of a joint FAO/WHO Committee, 1975, 79 pages.

No. 584—Food and nutrition strategies in national development. Ninth report of the Joint FAO/WHO Expert Committee on Nutrition, 1976, 64 pages.

No. 586—Health hazards from new environment pollutants. Report of a WHO Study Group, 1976, 96 pages.

No. 589—Planning and evaluation of public dental health services. Report of a WHO Expert Committee, 1976, 35 pages.

Public health papers

No. 57—The teaching of human sexuality in schools for health professionals, 1974, 47 pages.

No. 58—Suicide and attempted suicide, 1974, 127 pages.

No. 59—Administration of environmental health programs. A systems view, 1974, 242 pages.

No. 61—Educational strategies for the health professions, 1974, 106 pages.

INDEX